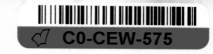

EXERCISE PHYSIOLOGY

CONTRIBUTORS

THOMAS ADAMS

K. LANGE ANDERSEN

ERLING ASMUSSEN

BRUNO BALKE

E. W. BANISTER

ALBERT R. BEHNKE

GEOFFREY H. BOURNE

S. R. BROWN

PAOLO CERRETELLI

JOHN A. FAULKNER

RICHARD V. GANSLEN

P. F. IAMPIETRO

A. H. ISMAIL

RODOLFO MARGARIA

P. J. RASCH

ALLAN J. RYAN

JAMES S. SKINNER

I. DODD WILSON

FRED WILT

EXERCISE PHYSIOLOGY

Edited by HAROLD B. FALLS

DIRECTOR
KINETOENERGETICS LABORATORY
DEPARTMENT OF PHYSICAL EDUCATION
SOUTHWEST MISSOURI STATE COLLEGE
SPRINGFIELD, MISSOURI

ACADEMIC PRESS   New York and London   1968

ACADEMIC PRESS, INC.
111 Fifth Avenue, New York, New York 10003

United Kingdom Edition published by
ACADEMIC PRESS, INC. (LONDON) LTD.
Berkeley Square House, London W.1

LIBRARY OF CONGRESS CATALOG CARD NUMBER: 68-14665

PRINTED IN THE UNITED STATES OF AMERICA

LIST OF CONTRIBUTORS

Numbers in parentheses indicate the pages on which authors' contributions begin.

Thomas Adams,* *Physiology Laboratory, Civil Aeromedical Institute, Federal Aviation Administration, Oklahoma City, Oklahoma* (173)

K. Lange Andersen,† *Institute of Physiology, University of Bergen, Bergen, Norway* (79)

Erling Asmussen, *Laboratory for the Theory of Gymnastics, University of Copenhagen, Copenhagen, Denmark* (3)

Bruno Balke, *Departments of Physiology and Physical Education, University of Wisconsin, Madison, Wisconsin* (239)

E. W. Banister,‡ *Human Performance Laboratory, University of British Columbia, Vancouver, British Columbia, Canada* (267)

Albert R. Behnke, *University of California Medical Center, San Francisco, California* (359)

Geoffrey H. Bourne, *Yerkes Regional Primate Research Center, Emory University, Atlanta, Georgia* (155)

S. R. Brown, *Human Performance Laboratory, University of British Columbia, Vancouver, British Columbia, Canada* (267)

Paolo Cerretelli, *Department of Physiology, University of Milan, Milan, Italy* (43)

John A. Faulkner, *Departments of Physiology and Physical Education, University of Michigan, Ann Arbor, Michigan* (415)

* Present address: Department of Physiology, Michigan State University, East Lansing, Michigan.
† Present address: School of Physiotherapy, Oslo, Trondheimsvein, Oslo, Norway.
‡ Present address: Human Performance Laboratory, Physical Development Centre, Simon Fraser University, Burnaby, British Columbia, Canada.

Richard V. Ganslen,* *Aerospace Medicine, McDonnell Aircraft Corporation, St. Louis, Missouri* (197)

P. F. Iampietro, *Physiology Laboratory, Civil Aeromedical Institute, Federal Aviation Administration, Oklahoma City, Oklahoma* (173)

A. H. Ismail, *Department of Physical Education for Men, Purdue University, Lafayette, Indiana* (387)

Rodolfo Margaria, *Department of Physiology, University of Milan, Milan, Italy* (43)

P. J. Rasch, *Physiology Division, U.S. Naval Medical Field Research Laboratory, Camp Lejeune, North Carolina* (129)

Allan J. Ryan, *Department of Physical Education and Athletic Teams Physician, University of Wisconsin, Madison, Wisconsin* (323)

James S. Skinner,† *Division of Cardiology, University of Washington School of Medicine, Seattle, Washington* (219)

I. Dodd Wilson, *Department of Medicine, University of Minnesota Medical School, Minneapolis, Minnesota* (129)

Fred Wilt, *Editor, Track Technique, Lafayette, Indiana* (395)

  * Present address: College of Health, Physical Education and Recreation, Texas Woman's University, Denton, Texas.
  † Present address: Laboratory for Human Performance Research, Institute for Science and Engineering, The Pennsylvania State University, University Park, Pennsylvania.

PREFACE

The physiology of exercise has become an increasingly important topic for research and discussion over the past few years. There are several important reasons for this increased emphasis. Among them are space flight and the tremendous physiological stresses associated with it; the increased quality of athletic records making necessary more intensive training and more sophisticated training methods; the emphasis placed on physical fitness by the executive branch of the federal government which has created a need for better understanding of the multiple phenomena involved in optimum physiological functioning; and the wider participation and interest in athletics by all persons making necessary new knowledge aimed at protecting the participant and enhancing his enjoyment.

Due to the above emphasis the physiology of exercise has participated in the knowledge explosion along with many other areas of scientific study. Not many years ago, it was possible for a physical educator, athletic coach, trainer, or physiologist to be quite knowledgeable in most areas related to exercise participation. This is no longer true. Today, it is no more possible for one exercise scientist to keep abreast of all the facets of exercise than it is for the general practitioner of medicine to keep abreast of the various medical specialities. There are specialists in exercise physiology just as there are specialists in other scientific fields.

These trends have brought about the need for a book on the physiology of exercise written by experts on the various topics. This work is directed toward meeting that need. The topics have been selected because it was felt that they represented important and pressing problems in exercise physiology today. The authors were selected because of their research competencies and/or knowledge in the various topics toward which their efforts were directed.

The book should be viewed as three related sections. Chapters 1 through 4 deal with the general effects of exercise on specific body systems and organs. Chapters 5 through 13 are directed at what are considered important problems in exercise physiology today. Chapters 14 and 15 are intended as a synthesis. The purpose of these two chapters is to apply the material of the foregoing chapters to specific sports. The sports chosen were competitive running and swimming and diving. The authors are both competent exercise scientists as well as outstanding coaches of their specialities.

It is hoped that this work will serve two major purposes: find use as a textbook for college and university courses dealing with the physiology of exercise and provide a source of reference for physicians, physical educators, physiologists, psychologists, coaches, trainers, and other exercise scientists throughout the world.

Special appreciation is extended to the international group of distinguished persons who so willingly collaborated on this volume. Without their cooperation and the cooperation and special help of Academic Press this work would not have been possible.

March, 1968   H.B. FALLS

CONTENTS

Part I: **Basic Physiology**

Chapter 1

The Neuromuscular System and Exercise

ERLING ASMUSSEN

Chapter 2

The Respiratory System and Exercise

RODOLFO MARGARIA AND PAOLO CERRETELLI

Chapter 3

The Cardiovascular System in Exercise

K. LANGE ANDERSEN

Chapter 4
Other Body Systems and Exercise
P. J. Rasch and I. Dodd Wilson

Part II: **Special Problems**

Chapter 5
Nutrition and Exercise
Geoffrey H. Bourne

Chapter 6
Temperature Regulation

Thomas Adams and P. F. Iampietro

P. F. Iampietro and Thomas Adams

Chapter 7
Doping and Athletic Performance
Richard V. Ganslen

Chapter 8

Longevity, General Health, and Exercise

JAMES S. SKINNER

Chapter 9

Variation in Altitude and Its Effects on Exercise Performance

BRUNO BALKE

Chapter 10

The Relative Energy Requirements of Physical Activity

E. W. BANISTER AND S. R. BROWN

Chapter 11

The Physician and Exercise Physiology

ALLAN J. RYAN

Chapter 12

Physique and Exercise

ALBERT R. BEHNKE

Chapter 13

Body Composition and Relationships to Physical Activity

A. H. ISMAIL

Part III: **Running and Water Sports**

Chapter 14

Training for Competitive Running

FRED WILT

Chapter 15

Physiology of Swimming and Diving

JOHN A. FAULKNER

PART I: **BASIC PHYSIOLOGY**

I

THE NEUROMUSCULAR SYSTEM AND EXERCISE

Erling Asmussen

I. The Skeletal Muscle

Man, like most other animals, is endowed with the ability to move in relation to his environment and to move the different parts of his body in relation to each other, thus taking up and maintaining different postures or stances and counterbalancing the impact of outer forces such as gravitation and wind movement. He is further able to transfer mechanical energy to the outer world, i.e., doing work on it. Likewise he is able to absorb mechanical work being done on his body, e.g., by gravitation and by other beings. These abilities are lodged in the skeletal muscles and are due to their gift of transforming chemical energy into mechanical energy during their so-called contractions.

From a functional point of view the total mass of skeletal muscles in the organism may be looked upon as one large organ, the organ of movement and posture, constituting about 40% of the weight of the human body. This is so because most activities, especially those connected with the more vigorous

3

activities of sport and labor, are the result of the integrated activity of nearly all the muscles in the body. However, the instantaneous distribution of activity in this large organ is changing continuously as the individual muscles are called into play or released at the proper moment, directed by the central nervous system according to the plan or intent of the activity. Individual, anatomically defined muscles seldom act as a functional unit—in most cases they are members of muscle groups that may be "flexors," "extensors," "supinators," etc. But also the composition of such groups may vary, both with respect to which muscles are called upon to become members in a given situation, and with respect to the relative importance of the single members of the group. In most cases it is possible to point out one or a few prime movers in a given situation. These are assisted by synergists, and the movements may be controlled by or stopped by antagonists that are placed on the other side of the instantaneous axis of movement. A permanent functional or physiological subdivision of the musculature is consequently not possible. Anatomically, however, it is possible to define a muscle, and by tradition and practice the usual number of named single muscles have been established.

HISTOLOGICAL BUILDUP

1. Connective Tissue, Tendons

The typical skeletal muscle is separated from its surroundings by a membranous layer of connective tissue, the perimysium (Fig. 1). Connective tissue

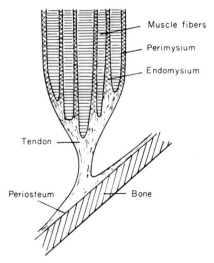

Fig. 1. Schematic drawing of a muscle and its connective tissue.

also extends into the interior, the belly, of the muscle as septa of decreasing order of coarseness, the endomysium, subdividing the muscle into smaller and smaller compartments. The smallest of these form fasciculi, containing various numbers of muscle fibers bound together and to the endomysium by looser connective tissue. At both ends of the muscle this "skeleton" of connective tissue converges to form the tendons, tough and almost unyielding bands or membranes of tightly packed fibers of collagenous substance, that mediate the connection with the bones. The collagenous membrane that covers the outside of the bones, the periosteum, is in intimate connection with the collagenous part of the bone substance itself, and into this mass of fibers the tendinous fibers are woven so as to form a very resistant and continuous connection between muscle and bone. The connective tissue of the muscle thus serves as the transmitter of mechanical tension from the collagenous outer layer of each individual muscle fiber to the bony skeleton. There are no other connections from the contractile substance in the muscle fibers to the tendons than the intramuscular network of connective tissue.

The intramuscular connective tissue is not an altogether passive part of the muscle. There is good evidence to show that it develops with training, becoming tougher and thicker. This growth is preceded by a period with increased formation of mucopolysaccharides, probably induced by high mechanical tensions in the muscles. The possible connection between these phenomena and the edema and soreness that follow strenuous exercise with untrained muscles still has to be studied in detail.

2. Vascularization

Inside the muscle the connective tissue also envelops the larger vessels and the nerves that supply the muscle. The vessels are numerous and widely

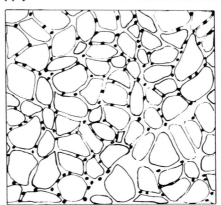

Fig. 2. Capillaries between muscle fibers in a horse's muscle. (Redrawn after Spalteholz, 1888.)

branching, generally orientated in parallel with the muscle fibers. Especially numerous are the capillaries that run in the interspace between the single muscle fibers. Their number is so great that each individual muscle fiber may have contact with 5 to 6 capillaries (Fig. 2). These capillaries—or the pre-capillary arterioles—can be constricted and dilated, possibly under both nervous (sympathetic) and humoral control so that the blood flow through the muscles can be regulated within very wide limits in relation to the demand for oxygen during rest and exercise. According to Krogh (1922) the number of open capillaries in the muscles of guinea pigs varied between $30/mm^2$ transectional area in rest and $2500/mm^2$ in heavy exercise. A hormone from the posterior lobe of the hypophysis (vasopressin) acts in a constrictive way if the oxygen tension around the capillaries is sufficiently high, whereas oxygen lack and certain metabolites—CO_2, lactic acid, H^+—induce dilatation. By this self-regulating device the blood flow through the muscles can be shown to vary from rest to maximum exercise with a factor of about 100.

3. Sense Organs

The nerves entering a muscle are mixed nerves, containing both motor and sensory axons. The former originate in the motor neurons of the spinal cord and in the corresponding parts of the brain stem. Some are thick, $8–12\,\mu$, and supply the normal muscle fibers; others are thin, $3–5\,\mu$, and supply the so-called intrafusal muscle fibers of the muscle spindles (see below). The sensory nerves, which have their trophic centers in the spinal ganglia, supply the sense organs in the muscles, and are usually of the thick variety.

There is a whole series of different sense organs in the muscles and tendons: mechanoreceptors, thermoreceptors, pain receptors, and others of more hypothetical character, e.g., "metaboloreceptors" and "ergoreceptors." Of these, only certain mechanoreceptors have been identified and thoroughly studied. These are the muscle spindles, situated in the belly of the muscles, and the Golgi tendon organs within the tendons.

The muscle spindles are small (a few millimeters long) and cigar-shaped, and are suspended in the intramuscular network of connective tissue in parallel with the muscle fibers. Each spindle contains, within a capsule of connective tissue, a small number of thin, modified muscle fibers, the intra-fusal muscle fibers (from fusum = spindle). Each intrafusal fiber consists of two polar portions, built and striated in the same way as normal (extrafusal) muscle fibers (see Section II), and a midportion, the nuclear bag, in which the striation is missing (Fig. 3). The two striated polar portions are contractile and are supplied with a branch from a thin motor nerve, a so-called γ-fiber. The nuclear bag is surrounded with the annulospiral endings of a sensory nerve, and the transitional parts between the striated parts and the nuclear bag may also have sensory nerve endings of a different kind ("flower-spray endings" according to the old terminology of Ruffini, 1897).

Sensory impulses are generated in the nuclear bag and transmitted to the nerves when this portion of the intrafusal fiber undergoes lengthening. This can happen in two ways: (1) if the whole muscle, containing the muscle spindle, is passively stretched, and (2) if the striated polar portions of the intrafusal fibers contract under the influence of the γ-fibers. These portions are anchored in the connective tissue of the whole muscle, and their shortening will consequently result in a stretching of the nuclear bag. A contraction (shortening) of the whole muscle, on the other hand, will unload the muscle spindle and thus stop the generation of impulses from the nuclear bag.

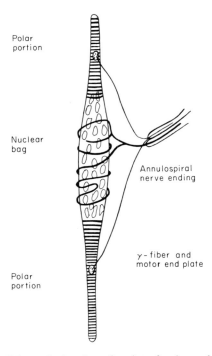

Polar portion

Nuclear bag

Annulospiral nerve ending

γ-fiber and motor end plate

Polar portion

Fig. 3. Schematic drawing of an intrafusal muscle fiber.

The Golgi tendon organs are less well circumscribed. Their nerve endings are located at the insertion of the tendons into the muscles, but may also be found elsewhere in the connective tissue of the muscles. They record tension in the tendons, independent of whether this is caused by stretching of the whole muscle or by contraction of its muscle fibers.

Both muscle spindles and Golgi tendon organs are receptors in important reflexes, the myotatic reflex and the antimyotatic reflex, respectively. These will be described in Section III, B.

II. The Striated Muscle Fiber

The all-dominant space within the skeletal muscle is taken up by the contractile cells, the muscle fibers (Fig. 4). They are long (from a few mm up to

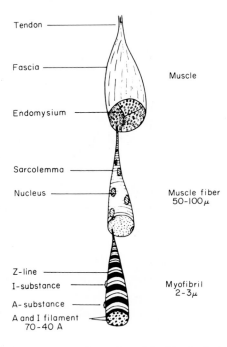

Fig. 4. Schematic drawing of muscle and its histological subdivisions.

about 30 cm in the sartorius of man), thin (50–100 μ), cylindrical threads, running from end to end in the muscles. In most cases they insert at an angle to the main direction of the tendons, thus making the muscles in longitudinal section look semipennate, pennate, or multipennate. In other cases tendons and muscle fibers are parallel. Within a given space, pennate muscles can contain more, although shorter, muscle fibers than parallel fibered muscles. The former can consequently produce higher tensions, but with less shortening than the latter.

A. Microscopical Description

Viewed through a light microscope a muscle fiber appears to be regularly striated, light and dark parts alternating at regular intervals (Fig. 5). The dark parts are referred to as the A-substance and the light parts as the I-substance (from anisotropic and isotropic, describing their effect on polarized light). In

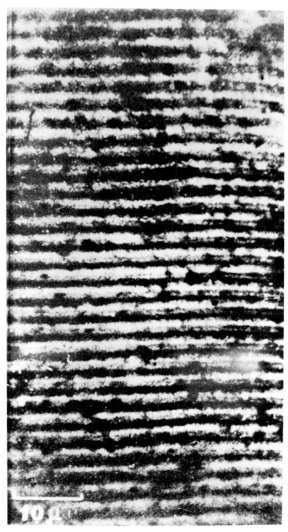

Fig. 5. Microphotogram of living striated muscle fiber in the frog. (Data from Carlsen and Knappeis, Institute of Neurophysiology, University of Copenhagen.)

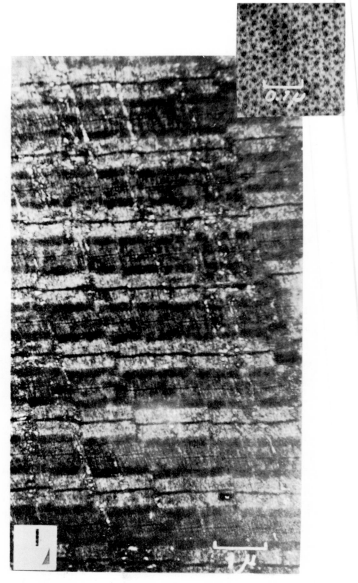

Fig. 6. An electron micrograph of part of a myofibril showing thin Z-lines in light I-zones and dark A-zones. Upper corner: transectional cut showing thick A-filaments, surrounded by thin I-filaments. (Data from Carlsen and Knappeis, Institute of Neurophysiology, University of Copenhagen.)

the middle of the I-substance a dark line, the Z-line (from German zwischen, i.e., between), marks the borders of what has been termed the sarcomeres, which are 1 to 2 μ long. Each muscle fiber is surrounded by a seemingly homogeneous membrane, the sarcolemma, which in its outer layers contains collagenous fibrils that connect it to the intramuscular connective tissue. Its innermost layer is the cell membrane proper, built of a few molecular layers of lipid and protein, which plays an important role in the production and conduction of excitation along the fiber. The interior of the tubelike sarcolemma is filled with sarcoplasma, a usually red, viscous fluid containing numerous nuclei and mitochondria, and 500–600 threadlike, 2 to 3 μ thick myofibrils (Fig. 4), continuous from end to end in the muscle fiber. While the sarcoplasma mainly subserves the metabolic processes of the muscle fiber, the myofibrils constitute the contractile part of it. Fat, glycogen, creatine phosphate, and adenosine triphosphate (ATP) are found as energy stores in the sarcoplasma, and likewise varying amounts of myoglobin, which besides giving the muscles their red color, by its combination with oxygen to form the easily dissociable oxymyoglobin, acts as a carrier of oxygen (cf., the related hemoglobin in the red cells of the blood).

A close study of the myofibrils reveals that these consist of alternating light and dark parts and that it is the precise arrangement of all the light and dark portions of the numerous fibrils side by side that gives the muscle fiber its striated appearance. The Z-line, which presumably is a special structure, seems to play an important part in this sidewise alignment. Further examination by means of the electron microscope (Fig. 6) has shown that the myofibrils are built of even finer threads, filaments, of which two kinds have been described: Thin filaments (about 40 Å), and thicker filaments (about 100 Å). The arrangement of these filaments seems to be characteristic for muscles and offers an explanation of the contraction process.

In longitudinal section of resting myofibrils electron micrographs show that the thin filaments apparently are fixed to the substance of the Z-line and extend through the I-substance and a short way into the A-substance. The thicker filaments, on the other hand, are found in the A-substance in spaces between the ends of the thin filaments. In the gap between the thin filaments (I-filaments) from one Z-line and those from the next Z-line some even thinner filaments have been described; they may serve to keep the two

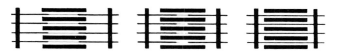

Fig. 7. Schematic representation of the filaments in a sarcomere. Left, stretched; middle, resting; right, contracted.

sets of I-filaments aligned. When a myofibril is passively stretched, micro-photos show that the I-filaments are drawn to both sides, out from the A-substance, so that the overlap zone between the I-filaments and the thicker A-filaments diminishes or—at extreme lengthening—disappears. In con-tracted myofibrils, on the other hand, the I-filaments appear to be drawn further in between the A-filaments, increasing the overlap zone and mak-ing the gap between the two opposite sets of I-filaments diminish or vanish (Fig. 7).

B. CONTRACTION

On the basis of these observations a "sliding filament" hypothesis (Huxley and Hanson, 1954) of muscle contraction has been offered. According to this, contraction appears as the result of a chemical reaction between the I-filaments and the A-filaments, which causes the I-filaments to be drawn in between the A-filaments in a sliding movement. This hypothesis is strength-ened by the fact that the I-filaments have been found to consist of a protein, actin, the A-filaments of another protein, myosin, and that these two proteins will combine to form actomyosin under the influence of ATP. Artificially produced fibers of these proteins will shorten when ATP is added; muscle fibers, from which all other substances except myosin and actin have been extracted by glycerol, will shorten when ATP is added, showing sliding of the filaments.

1. Excitation

In the living muscle fiber the processes leading to a contraction are in-itiated by an excitation, a sudden change in the muscle fiber that in an un-known way leads to the activation of the enzymatic system ATP-myosin-actin.

The excitation and its spreading along and into the muscle fiber is bound up with the membrane that surrounds the muscle fiber. This membrane has the ability of actively transporting Na^+ from the interior of the muscle fiber to the surrounding extracellular fluid. The so-called "Na^+-pump" is driven by energy derived from cell metabolism. As a result of the extrusion of Na^+, a surplus of K^+ will passively build up inside the muscle fiber. Of the anions, Cl^- diffuses freely through the membrane, whereas other anions inside the cell are unable to pass out. The net result will be a high Na^+ and Cl^- con-centration on the outside of the membrane, and a high K^+ and a low Cl^- concentration on the inside. These concentration differences result in an electric polarization of the membrane which becomes positively charged on the outside and negatively charged on the inside (Fig. 8). A microelectrode placed inside the muscle fiber will register a potential difference of 50 to 100 mV between the two sides.

The membrane potential can be disturbed in different ways, e.g., by an electric current, that may "depolarize" a part of the membrane. If, as a result of the depolarization the membrane potential falls below a critical value of 30–40 mV, a change takes place in the membrane. It suddenly becomes freely permeable to Na$^+$, which consequently will rush into the cell from the outside, thereby causing a further, rapid fall in the membrane potential, even

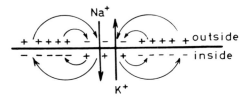

Fig. 8. Schematic representation of muscle fiber membrane with local depolarization. The arrows indicate movements of ions and electric currents.

with a reversal of signs. The inside becomes momentarily positive as compared to the outside, which becomes negative ("overshoot"). The rapidly following diffusion of K$^+$ from the inside to the outside will, however, soon restore the potential and bring the membrane back to its resting state again. These changes in polarity last only some few milliseconds and are called action potentials when recorded as ":spikes" (Fig. 9) in an electromyogram.

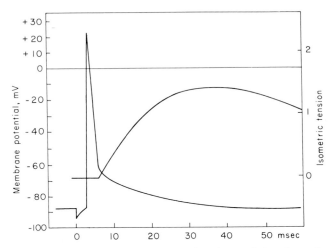

Fig. 9. Action potential recorded by means of an intracellular electrode near site of stimulation and mechanical tension in single muscle fiber. (Data from Buchthal and Steen-Knudsen, Institute of Neurophysiology, University of Copenhagen.)

During the short interval in which the membrane was depolarized, or the polarization was reversed, currents of electric charges will flow from the adjacent parts of the membrane to the depolarized part, both inside and outside the membrane, causing a depolarization of these more remote parts (Fig. 8). As soon as the membrane potential here has fallen to the critical value of 30–40 mV, a new action potential will be triggered. This again will cause new currents to flow—and in this way the state of excitation spreads along the muscle fiber with a velocity of about 5 m/sec at body temperature. It is believed that "pockets" from the external membrane extend into the interior of the fiber, thus somehow providing for an approximately simultaneous arrival of the excitation to all myofibrils in a sarcomere. In a long muscle fiber, however, it is evident that the excitation cannot reach all parts simultaneously. The relatively slow development of the mechanical tension in a muscle fiber may be partly due to this fact.

2. The Motor End Plate

Under natural conditions the initial depolarization of the muscle membrane is initiated by the arrival to the muscle fiber of a nervous impulse. While nervous impulses travel along the axons in much the same way as the excitation spreads along the muscle fiber, the transfer from nerve to muscle takes place by means of a chemical transmitter, acetylcholine (ACh). This substance is produced in the nerve cells and transported by fluid currents inside the hollow nerve fiber to its fine terminal branches. These end in a special organelle, the motor end plate, situated at about the middle of the muscle fiber and, in mammals, reptiles, and birds, consisting of a slight thickening of the sarcoplasma and the muscle membrane. The membrane has "troughs" or "synaptic gutters" in which the terminal nerve branches lie (Fig. 10). When

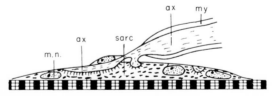

Fig. 10. Schematic drawing of a motor end plate; *m.n.*, muscle nucleus; *sarc*, sarcoplasm; *my*, myelin sheath; *ax*, nerve axon.

a nervous impulse reaches the terminal branches, a small amount of ACh is set free into the "gap" that separates nerve and muscle. By diffusion it reaches the muscle membrane and acts upon it in such a way that it suddenly becomes freely permeable to both Na^+ and K^+. The membrane thereby loses its potential, and electric currents from adjacent parts of the membrane will flow into this "hole," thus depolarizing the membrane outside the end plate eventually giving rise to an action potential and a spreading of excitation. The chemical transmitter is immediately broken down by an enzyme, cholinesterase, that is found in the end plates and in the extracellular fluid around it.

The transmission from nerve to muscle can be blocked, e.g., by curarine that "occupies" the sites on the membrane where ACh should act, or by anticholinesterases ("nerve gas," some insecticides) that inhibit the breakdown of ACh.

3. Active State, Mechanical Reaction

Immediately after the passing of the wave of excitation over the muscle fiber the contraction begins. The short interval between the two processes is the latent period, lasting 3 to 4 msec in frog's muscle at room temperature. During this period a slight relaxation, the latency relaxation, is observed, presumably indicating a loosening of the bonds between the actin-myosin filaments before the actual development of tension begins. Experiments with suddenly applied stretches to the muscle during contraction have revealed that the muscle after the latent period immediately passes into a so-called "active state" (Hill, 1949), which is maintained for a short time and then gradually disappears (Fig. 11). The development of mechanical tension begins

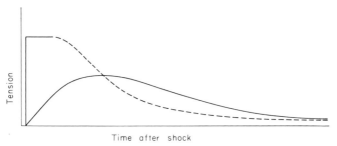

Fig. 11. Schematic drawing of the relation between "active state" and mechanical tension in a twitch.

at the same time, but due to the passive elastic elements present in series with the contractile elements, tension development is relatively slow. Peak tension or shortening is reached only some time after the "active state" has begun to wane, and then relaxation sets in. The duration of such a twitch contraction varies with the kind of muscle fiber and with temperature. In mammalian muscles at body temperature it lasts about 30 msec, but there is a wide range of speeds from rapid fibers to slow fibers.

The "active state" can be prolonged by repetitive stimulation of the fibers, thus allowing the elastic elements in the fibers to be fully stretched before relaxation sets in. The tension developed, or the shortening performed, will thus reach considerably higher values than in a twitch (Fig. 12). Outwardly the

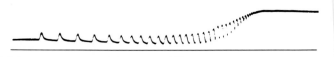

Fig. 12. Contractions of a single muscle fiber (frog) at increasing stimulation frequency. The twitches gradually fuse into a tetanus. (Data from Buchthal (1942), Institute of Neurophysiology, University of Copenhagen.)

muscle fiber will appear to be in a permanent state of contraction, a tetanus, but recording of the action potential reveals the rhythmic character of the process (Fig. 13).

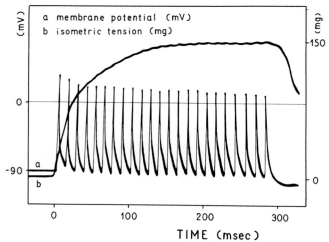

Fig. 13. Intracellularly recorded action potentials and mechanical tension during tetanization of a single muscle fiber. (Data from Guld and Steen-Knudsen, Institute of Neurophysiology, University of Copenhagen.)

4. Isometric and Isotonic Recording

The external appearance of the mechanical events that take place in a muscle during contraction depends on the conditions: If the muscle fiber is fixed between two immovable points, the increased attachment between the actin and myosin filaments will lead to no visible movement, and the contraction will manifest itself as development of tension in the fiber (isometric contraction). If, however, a movement is possible the actin filaments will

motor neuron, through its axon with branches, thus serves a number of muscle fibers. A nervous impulse, traveling down along an axon in a motor nerve, will consequently branch out to a number of muscle fibers and cause depolarization under their motor end plates. Assuming the condition of the different muscle fibers to be about equal, all of them will either (1) not respond or (2) respond with a conducted action potential, followed by contraction of all the fibers. A group of muscle fibers united in this way through their connection with the same motor neuron is called a motor unit. Their response to a nervous stimulus is said to obey the "all-or-none law."

2. Gradation of Contraction

Voluntary and reflex contractions of whole muscles are the result of the concerted activity of a smaller or larger number of such motor units. How these contractions are graduated in strength can be deduced from (a) the known behavior of single muscle fibers and (b) a study of the electromyograms of contracting muscles *in situ*.

(a) It must be recalled that, mechanically, a muscle fiber responds to a single effective stimulus by a twitch lasting about 30 msec at body temperature and of a constant height. Repeated stimuli at frequencies above ca. 60 per second, will produce a tetanus, with considerably higher tension than the twitch.

(b) Electromyograms (EMG's) are recorded action potentials picked up by skin electrodes placed over the contracting muscle or, better, by needle electrodes thrust into the muscle or by fine wires sewn into it. They record the electrical activity, the action potentials, of the motor units in the neighborhood, and by careful placement they may register the activity of individual motor units as distinct "spikes." EMG's from muscles during sustained voluntary contractions of increasing strength show that the frequency of stimulation may vary between about 5 per second in weak contractions and 60 to 70 per second in strong contractions. Hence it may be deduced that the

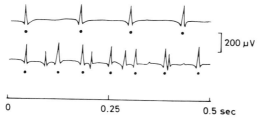

0   0.25   0.5 sec

Fig. 19. EMG's from human muscle. Upper trace: weak isometric contraction. Lower trace: stronger contraction. The dots mark spikes from the same motor unit. Note increased frequency and recruitment of new motor units at stronger contraction. (Data from Rosenfalck and Rosenfalck, Institute of Neurophysiology, University of Copenhagen.)

individual muscle fibers in cases perform twitches, with relatively long inactive periods, but that these pauses may be shortened and disappear completely as the frequency reaches such values that twitches are fused into a
tetanus. EMG's further show that as the voluntary contraction increases in
strength an increasing number of motor units is called into action. The active
units contract rhythmically, but out of phase with one another, asynchronously.
As even weak contractions of whole muscles demand the cooperation of
many motor units, the contraction will appear smooth, the pauses between the
individual twitches being filled out by the contraction of other motor units.
This gives the appearance of a tetanus even to weak contractions with low
frequencies.

An increase in strength of a whole muscle's contraction can thus be effected: (1) by increasing the frequency of stimulation of the active motor units,
and (2) by mobilizing an increasing number of motor units (Fig. 19).

Movements of a body segment are controlled in the same way, i.e., by
varying the number of active motor units and the frequency of their stimulation. The lifting or lowering of a load, although it outwardly resembles and
also is often called an isotonic contraction, is in reality the integrated result
of numerous twitches or tetani of a varying number of motor units. In weak
slow movements these twitches must come very close to being isometric contractions. Another difference between true isotonic contractions of isolated
muscles, and for instance, the lifting of a burden with the elbow flexors, is that
in the latter case the muscles are not initially weighted and stretched by the
burden which is carried by the passive ligaments and joint capsule of the
elbow. In lifting, the muscles are contracting at first isometrically, until their
torque surpasses that of the burden, which then is lifted by a seemingly isotonic contraction. The changing lengths of lever arms of both burden and
muscles during the movement, however, necessitate a steadily changing total
tension of the muscles involved, and this is effected by variations in stimulus
frequency and recruitment or dismissal of motor units. The seemingly simple
"isotonic" contraction thus in reality is a rather complex cooperative action
of the many motor units involved.

3. Direct and Indirect Motor Pathways

The motor neurons that directly control the activity of the muscle fibers
usually command a rather large number of fibers; the size of a motor unit
varies between about 50 and 1700 individual fibers. Muscles which perform
finely graduated movements, e.g., those of the eye, have small motor units,
whereas those that partake in coarser movements of larger masses, e.g., the
trunk, and the legs have larger motor units. The motor neurons are activated
by nervous impulses, either through descending motor nerves from the brain,

or reflexly through sensory nerves from receptors in the skin (e.g., touch receptors, pain receptors), or in the muscles (e.g., muscle spindles).

The descending pathways from the cortex of the brain [corticospinal (pyramidal) and extrapyramidal tracts] permit quick and direct innervation of the muscles for the performance of volitional movements. The corticospinal tract (Fig. 20A) runs uninterruptedly from motor centers in the cortex

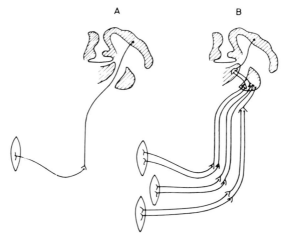

A   B

Fig. 20. Schematic representation of a direct corticospinal (pyramidal) tract (A) and some extrapyramidal tracts (B).

to the lower motor neurons and is especially well developed in humans. It initiates discrete contractions in all the different muscles but is singularly well developed with respect to the muscles connected with speech and with finger movements. The extrapyramidal tracts (Fig. 20B) originate also in other subcortical centers and in the brain stem. Their nerves are interrupted by synapses on their passage through the brain, and the movements that are initiated through them are larger, more complex movements involving several muscles and joints. In life's daily movements the two systems act in close cooperation; the extrapyramidal system initiating the larger more diffuse muscle contractions, upon the background of which the more detailed localized contractions governed by the corticospinal system are superimposed.

B. REFLEXES

The peripheral motor neurons may also be activated through sensory nerves as in reflexes. Such reflexes involving the skeletal muscles are numerous, serving a wide variety of purposes: the acquisition of food, protection and

withdrawal from dangers and painful stimuli, mating, resistance to external
forces such as gravity, etc. Many of these reflexes are very "old," i.e., we find
them in primitive forms of vertebrates. Others are of more recent origin, restricted to the higher forms of mammals. Some are highly complicated involving a large part of the neuromuscular system. Others are simple and
restricted to but a few motor neurons.

1. Myotatic and Antimyotatic Reflexes

As a typical example of the simple reflex the myotatic reflex must be
mentioned. Its receptors are in the muscle spindles, presumably in the nuclear
bag with its annulospiral nerve endings. When this part of the muscle spindle
is stretched, nervous impulses will travel to the spinal cord where motor
neurons will be stimulated and start "firing," with the result that a number of
motor units in the same muscle that contains the stretched muscle spindle will
contract. Another motor reflex, initiated from the Golgi tendon organ, is the
antimyotatic reflex. It is elicited by powerful tensions applied to the tendons,
passively or by the contraction of the muscle. The tendon receptors have a
considerably higher threshold to stretching than the muscle spindles, and the
response to the stimulus is not a muscle contraction but a reflex relaxation.
This is probably caused by an inhibition of the γ-neurons, which in their turn
will reduce their tonic stimulation of the intrafusal muscle fibers of the muscle
spindles and thus cause a decrease in the reflex (myotatic) tension of the
muscle (Granit, 1956). It must be assumed that the tendon organs—besides
simply recording the tensions in the tendons—play an important part in the
controlling of movements by preventing overstretching of muscles (Sherrington, 1913; Granit, 1956).

As mentioned earlier (Section I), a stretching of the nuclear bag can happen
in two different ways: because the whole muscle and spindle is stretched by
some external force, or because the contractile polar ends of the intrafusal
fibers contract and stretch the nuclear bag. An example of the first way of
eliciting the myotatic reflex is the tendon reflex, in which a tap on the tendon
of a muscle results in a short, jerklike contraction of the muscle.

Of more general interest is the role played by the myotatic reflex in the
postural reflexes. In man, for instance, the line of gravity for the body above
the ankle joints in the erect position will pass in front of the axis of movements
in these joints (Fig. 21). Gravity will consequently tend to pull the body forward in a fall, thereby causing a dorsal flexion of the ankle joints and a
stretching of the plantar flexors of these joints. The muscle spindles in the
flexors—mainly the soleus muscle—will be stimulated, and the resulting contraction of the extrafusal muscle fibers in the soleus will pull the body back,
thereby relieving the stretch on the muscle spindles. A corresponding play
between gravity and muscle force will take place in other joints of the body,

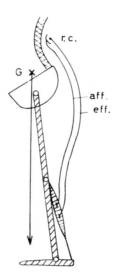

Fig. 21. Schematic drawing to explain the myotatic reflex as part of the postural reflexes. *G*, center of gravity of body; *r.c.*, reflex center in spinal cord; *aff.*, sensory nerve; *eff.*, motor nerve.

and the erect posture can thus be maintained reflexly as a dynamic, ever-changing state of equilibrium between gravity and muscle force.

2. The γ-System

The other situation, in which no external force but the contraction of the intrafusal fibers themselves elicits a reflex contraction in the muscle, is probably found in a number of postural and probably also locomotor muscle contractions that are initiated in the higher motor centers of the brain, but which are not elicited through the direct pathways of the pyramidal and extrapyramidal tracts. The sequence of events may be described as follows (see Fig. 22). From that part of the central nervous system in which movements are initiated a stream of impulses flows to the reticular formation. Here the nerve cells that control the small motor neurons in the spinal cord (the γ-neurons), innervating the intrafusal muscle fibers, are stimulated, causing the contractile end portions of the intrafusal fibers to shorten. The ensuing stretching of the nuclear bag portion will then elicit a myotatic reflex, and a number of extrafusal fibers in the muscle will contract. The result—a postural or a locomotor muscle contraction—has thus been produced without the involvement of the direct descending pathways to the motor neurons by means of what is now generally termed "the γ-loop" (Granit, 1956). There seems, therefore, to be two independent ways of causing contraction in the skeletal muscles: via the direct pathway and via the γ-loop. The first one probably is of greatest importance for sudden, skilled movements; the latter for postural control and maybe for such automatized movements as walking and running.

The supraspinal control of the muscle spindles through the γ-system affords an explanation of how spinal reflexes such as the myotatic reflex may be influenced by the alertness or "state of wakefulness" of the subject. It is known that the reticular formation is the anatomical substrate for the "state of wakefulness." This is regulated by means of the numerous nervous impulses

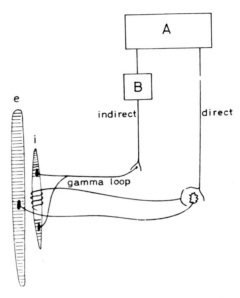

Fig. 22. Schemes of indirect motor pathway via γ-loop, and direct pathway. *A*, higher motor centers; *B*, centers in reticular formation; *i*, intrafusal; *e*, extrafusal muscle fibers.

from all parts of the central nervous system and from the sense organs that impinge upon its cells. Some of these cells keep the γ-system in a tonic state of excitation that can wax and wane in parallel to the general state of wakefulness. In an alerted condition the polar portions of the intrafusal fibers of the muscle spindles consequently will be more contracted and the nuclear bag pulled more taut. A slight further stretching will immediately "fire" the sensory organ, resulting in a very brisk reflex. As the psychological condition of the subject will influence the level of activity in the reticular formation, we have perhaps here the explanation of how a man's state of mind may influence his posture, his gait, and his other movements.

C. Voluntary Movements

Voluntary movements are the result of an act of volition. The precise site in the brain of the will is not known. It has been assumed that the motor cortex from which the descending motor pathways of the pyramidal tract and some of the extrapyramidal pathways originate is the center for voluntary skilled movements. However, finely localized electrical stimulation of the motor cortex results in contraction of single muscles or parts of muscles, never in coordinated movements. The well-known notion that "the brain does not know muscles, only movements" (Taylor, 1932) thus does not hold for the motor cortex. It is now believed that some subcortical centers are the place of origin for the complex patterns of nervous activity that will result in a movement, and that the cortical motor centers are the "keyboard" upon which the subcortical centers can play different "kinetic melodies." The precise execution of a skilled movement demands a control system, and this is afforded partly by means of an "input controlled feedback system," which controls the "orders" that leave the motor centers—partly by means of an "output-controlled feedback system" controlling the movement by way of incoming sensory impulses from many different sense organs. The "comparator" for both feedback systems is the cerebellum, which thus becomes the coordinating center for all skilled movements.

The complex interplay of muscles—agonists, synergists, and antagonists—is the result of the "integrative action of the nervous system" (Sherrington, 1947) on all levels, from brain to spinal cord. The activity of the individual muscles in this interplay can be studied by means of electromyography. In many cases it is enough to use skin electrodes for this purpose. They will

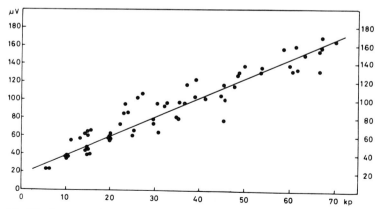

Fig. 23. The "mean peak voltage" in relation to the isometric pull of the back muscles. Skin electrodes on lumbar portion of m.m. erectores spinae. Pull exerted on strap at shoulder height. One subject studied at 7 different days within a month.

pick up the action potentials from an indeterminable number of motor units in the environment of the electrode, and the recorded interference EMG's will show if and when the underlying muscles are active, e.g., in a movement or in maintaining a posture. In certain cases a quantitation of the muscle activity may be obtained by "integration" of the EMG's. This can be done electronically by rectifying all the spikes in the EMG and measuring the "mean peak voltage." With the electrodes on the same site, experiments have shown that the "mean peak voltage" is nearly rectilinearly related to the mechanical isometric tension in the muscles. Mechanical tension may, therefore, in some cases be estimated from the EMG's by means of a calibration curve (see Fig. 23).

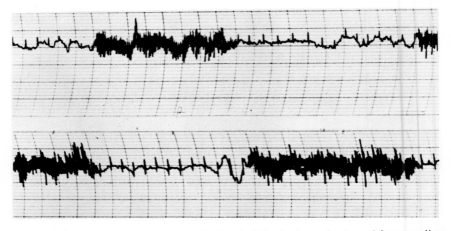

Fig. 24. EMG's from back muscles (top) and abdominal muscles (lower) in a standing subject. By leaning slightly forward and backward in the ankle joints, the pull of gravity shifts and is opposed alternately by the muscles of the back and of the abdominal wall. Note: no overlapping of activity.

Electromyographic recordings of muscles during movements or in different postures disclose the ways in which muscular force is applied. For maintaining a given position of limbs or body against the pull of gravity only those muscles that oppose gravity will be active so that a balance is struck between the two forces, gravitation and muscle force (Fig. 24). If gravity plays no role, the antagonistic muscles on the two sides of the fixated joint will alternate in making small corrective movements around the established position. For small body parts such as fingers, the passive resistance of the tissues around the joints may act as one of the pair of forces that keep the position. Only in voluntarily stiff positions, or in certain pathological conditions, will muscles on both sides of a joint be active at the same time.

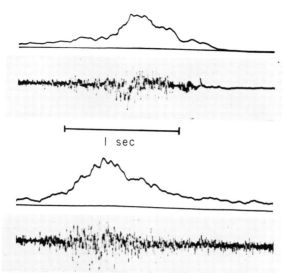

Fig. 25. EMG's and "mean peak voltage" recorded from the rectus femoris muscle during standing knee bending (top) and extension.

In slow movements the prime movers and synergists will be active throughout the movement although the relative importance of the individual muscles may be altered during various phases: If the movement consists of lifting the whole or a part of the body against gravity, the same muscles will be active during a slow return to the initial position, but at a lower level of activity (Fig. 25). If gravity is not antagonistic to the movement, the muscles on the other side of the joint will take over and bring the body part back to the starting position. In quicker movements, the muscles may stop being active before the movement has reached its end point. A limb may then "sail" through a smaller or larger part of its path by the momentum given it during the first part of the movement ("ballistic" or "thrown" movements). The movement may then be stopped either by some external force, by stretching of the passive tissues, or by the activation of the antagonistic muscles. In very fast repeated movements the shift between agonists and antagonists occurs before the movements have reached their end point, and there may be periods in the middle of the movements when no muscles are active.

IV. Muscular Strength

A. MEASUREMENT OF STRENGTH

In sports, physical education, rehabilitation work, and also for scientific purposes it often is of advantage to be able to measure muscle strength, e.g., the maximum tension that a muscle can produce. This of course can be done in isolated muscles outside the organism, but with the muscles *in situ* it is much more difficult. The reason for this is twofold. First, in the organism no muscle contracts individually. It is always a member of a group, and it is difficult to determine the relative part taken by the different members of the group in developing the total tension. Second, in the organism the muscles act on the skeletal lever arms, and so do ordinarily also the dynamometers, loads, or other measuring equipment that are used. The force that is measured cannot, therefore, be referred directly to the muscle or its tendon without rather elaborate measurements of lever arms and their changes during movement. For these reasons most measurements of strength are expressed as the maximal tension or work that a synergistic group of muscles can produce in a standard position or during a standard movement.

Strength measurements can be undertaken in several ways. In the main they may be divided according to the conditions under which the muscles are activated during the test. A maximally innervated (or stimulated) muscle may contract in three different ways, depending on the external conditions.

1. They may contract against an outer resistance which is immovable. There will be no external movements, only minor internal stretchings of the weaker parts of the muscles, of tendons, connective tissue, etc. The muscles contract isometrically and this activity takes the form of tension. The maximum tension is a measure of the isometric strength of the muscle group.

2. The muscles may contract against an outer resistance which they can overcome and move, e.g., against the force of gravity on a load. The muscles will be shortening during the contraction and will do work to an amount equalling the product fd, in which f is the resistance they overcome (e.g., the weight they lift) and d is the distance of movement (e.g., the height to which f is lifted). If d is prescribed—for instance, as the full movement of the joint which the muscles can move—the maximum resistance which can be overcome through the whole movement is a measure of muscular strength. (More precisely, it is a measure of maximum work under the given conditions.) Muscular strength measured in this way is often referred to as "dynamic strength."

3. Finally, the muscles may contract against an outer force which lengthens them by moving the skeletal segments to which the muscles are attached. The activity of the muscles takes the form of resistance to the outer force, and the maximum resistance exerted during a forced movement over a prescribed course can also be used as an expression of the muscles' strength.

All three forms of strength measurement—the isometric or static and the two forms of dynamic—are used and have been elaborated into routine methods. In most cases, however, isometric strength measurements have certain advantages over the two others.

For one thing, isometric strength measuring is less time-consuming and less fatiguing to the subject. As opposed to the dynamic, weight-lifting method, the maximum strength can in principle be determined by one single maximum contraction, whereas several trials with changing loads are necessary to determine the maximum load that can be lifted. Further, both weight lifting and resistance measurements are dependent on the velocity with which the movements take place. This adds a new uncertainty to the methods unless speed is carefully controlled. No such problems exist in isometric measurements. Technically, dynamometers for isometric tension measurements are simple in construction and can be made for practically all purposes with the same basic equipment, whereas dynamic strength measurements, although apparently simple, demand a wide variety of weights, pulleys, etc.

One apparent advantage of the weight-lifting method is that it measures the whole range of movement in which the muscles under investigation participate. This, however, is only an apparent advantage. In reality, since the lifting power of a muscle changes with the position of the joints, the maximum weight that can be moved through the whole range is the maximum only for the position where the lifting ability is the least.

This last-mentioned fact is of course also of great importance for isometric muscle strength measurements. It necessitates strict observance of standard positions in which the measurements are to be made. The reasons for the great importance of standardized positions are threefold. First, the maximum isometric tension that any muscle fiber can develop depends on the relative length of the muscle fiber at the time of stimulation (cf. length-tension diagram in Section II, B). Second, the lever arms in the body through which the muscle tensions are transformed into pulls, pushes, etc., alter with changing positions of the movable joints. Finally, as no natural muscle contraction in

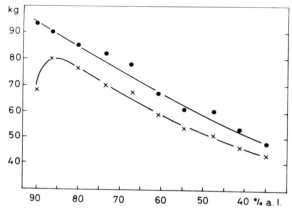

Fig. 26. Isometric (upper curve) and dynamic (lower curve) maximum tensions in the arm-shoulder muscles during horizontal pull on a handle. Abscissa: position of handle in percentage of arm length (100% = extended arm).

the body is restricted to one single muscle but rather is the combined effect of several anatomically different muscles, the content of the muscle group that acts in synergism may change with the position of the body parts.

The combined effect of these three factors is quite considerable, as seen for instance in the maximum horizontal pull that can be exerted on a handle by the muscles of the arm and shoulder (Fig. 26). Isometric strength measurements should, therefore, be performed in well-defined, easily reproducible positions of the joints. They will then give fairly constant results, even if repeated with intervals of several days.

Interindividually there are large differences between the isometric strength of identical muscles. This is due to several factors. In isolated muscles the isometric strength is proportional to the transectional area of the muscle. If this also holds for muscles *in situ*, and if geometrical similarity is assumed to exist between small and large persons, muscle strength should vary in proportion to a factor, h^2, where h is some linear dimension, e.g., body height. According to this, a person A who is 20% taller than another B should be 44% stronger than B. This of course gives tall persons an advantage over small persons when it comes to handling loads, weights, sport implements, etc. In moving his own body, however, A does not necessarily have any advantage,

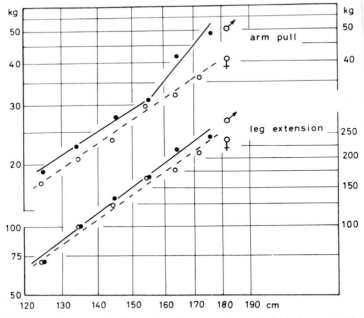

Fig. 27. Isometric strength of arm-shoulder muscles and of hip-knee muscles in relation to height. Logarithmic ordinates.

because his body weight will increase nearly as h^3. In exercises such as chinning the bar, push-ups, etc., he will have a handicap relative to B of the size $1.0/1.2$, because his stronger muscles ($\simeq 1.2^2$) are opposed by his heavier body ($\simeq 1.2^3$). In running, etc., these differences, however, cancel out, because his longer legs will make up for the slower movements of his heavier body.

Isometric strength, besides being related to size, also varies with sex and age. The sex difference is less pronounced before puberty, but after that boys become increasingly stronger especially in the upper extremity in relation to size, whereas girls tend to level off (Fig. 27). This difference may account for

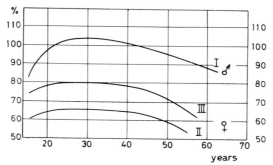

Fig. 28. Isometric strength in relation to age. Average of 25 different muscle groups. I, men; II, women; III, women corrected for size under the assumption that strength is proportional to (height)^2. The strength of 22-year-old men is used as standard.

the failing interest in athletics and other strength-demanding activities so often noticed in adolescent girls. Adult women have about 65% of the strength of adult men (Fig. 28). Part of this is due to the difference in average height, but even with this factor eliminated, women have only about 80% of the strength of men.

In adults maximum isometric strength is attained at about 30 years of age. From this point, maximum strength seems to decrease with age in most

TABLE I

CORRELATION COEFFICIENTS FOR STRENGTH IN DIFFERENT MUSCLE GROUPS IN 96 YOUNG MEN

	Left handgrip	Left arm pull	Trunk extension	Trunk flexion	Left leg extension
Right handgrip	0.78	0.51	0.30	0.25	0.40
Right arm pull		0.82	0.36	0.34	0.44
Trunk extension				0.57	0.39
Trunk flexion					0.47
Right leg extension					0.81

people (Fig. 28). It decreases faster in the big muscles of the leg and trunk than in the smaller muscles, e.g., hand muscles.

A person who is strong in his arms is usually also strong in his trunk or legs, but the correlation is not particularly high. Table I shows the correlation coefficients between isometric strength measurements in different muscle groups for 96 young Danish draftees. It will be noticed that the correlation is high between left and right side muscles, but not between different muscle groups.

Average values of isometric strength in some muscle groups are presented in Table II. The subjects were about 600 Danish adults (average height: 171 cm for the men, 167 cm for the women).

TABLE II

AVERAGE VALUES FOR ISOMETRIC STRENGTH IN SOME MUSCLE GROUPS

	Age (years)				
	20	25	35	45	55
Handgrip in kp $\pm 16\%$ SD[a]					
Men	55.9	59.9	58.5	55.6	51.6
Women	37.5	38.5	38.0	35.6	32.7
Arm pull downward in kp $\pm 14\%$ SD[a]					
Men	56.8	57.4	56.5	55.6	54.5
Women	35.3	36.0	36.0	36.0	32.4
Trunk extension in kp $\pm 16\%$ SD[a]					
Men	81.6	87.4	90.7	89.8	85.7
Women	56.6	58.3	59.2	57.7	49.1
Trunk flexion in kp $\pm 17\%$ SD[a]					
Men	60.6	64.2	66.7	66.0	63.0
Women	40.9	42.2	42.4	41.5	33.6
Leg extension, sitting in kp $\pm 18.5\%$ SD[a]					
Men	295	310	312	296	263
Women	214	225	212	197	162

[a] Standard deviation.

The dynamic strength—i.e., the maximum tension that a muscle can produce during a movement—differs from the isometric strength (cf. Section II, 5). If the muscle shortens during contraction it falls short of the corresponding isometric values. If it is being lengthened during contraction it resists with a force that is higher than the corresponding isometric tensions. These differences will increase with the velocity of movement, as seen in an example of the arm-shoulder muscles in Fig. 29. These facts are similar to

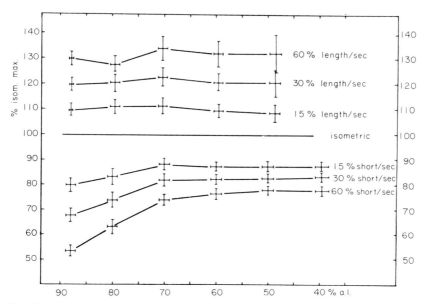

Fig. 29. Maximum tensions in the arm-shoulder muscles in contractions during shortening (lower curves) and during lengthening (upper curves). Tensions are expressed as percentages of isometric strength in the same position. Abscissa: position of handle with arm length as measure. Velocities are given as percentage arm length per second.

those expressed in the force-velocity curve of the single muscle fiber and may be due to the same underlying phenomena. But it must be remembered that the function of a whole muscle is an interplay of numerous individual muscle fibers going in and out of activity according to the frequency of stimulation.

The decreasing tension at the higher velocities may result in decreased tension during very rapid movements. In sprint running, for instance, this may be a limiting factor for the speed of limb movements as pointed out by Fenn *et al.* (1931).

B. Training of Muscular Strength

1. Methods and Results

As a general principle for an effective training of muscular strength it must be emphasized that only repeated maximal or near maximal contractions will produce measurable results. The widely publicized postulation (Hettinger, 1961) that one daily, submaximal isometric contraction should have the same training effect as several maximal contractions has been disputed (Müller and

Rohmert, 1963), and it is now generally accepted that both the number of daily contractions and their magnitude must be large in order to obtain measurable increases in muscular strength. The actual training program can consist either of series of isometric exercises or of series of dynamic exercises. The former kind have attained a certain popularity mainly because they can be performed without any apparatus. All that is needed is a firm resistance against which the muscles can push or pull. Even one's own muscles can be used—one group pulling or pushing against the other. There is no doubt that isometric muscle training, performed daily, and with greatest possible intensity and frequency, will result in an increase in isometric muscle strength. The question is only: For what use? If the object of the training is "body building," i.e., the acquisition of large bulging muscles that can produce great tension during isometric contractions, the method is adequate. But if the muscle strength is intended for something useful—for performing certain tasks in labor or sport—isometric training probably is rather worthless. This is because the obtained isometric strength apparently can not be transferred directly to other forms of activity where the muscles are to be used under other conditions. Further, it must be remembered that even strong and long-lasting isometric contractions put only very light demands on the cardio-respiratory and vascular systems and, therefore, are a very poor training form for endurance.

In dynamic muscle training (e.g., weight lifting, step tests, gymnastic exercises) the load on the muscles is seldom maximal, but here also the rule applies that the heavier the load and the more often it is applied the better the result. Dynamic muscle training will increase the isometric strength of the muscles undergoing training in proportion to the loads they have been opposing, and at the same time it will increase the capacity for performing the training exercises and the endurance in performing them.

A few examples will illustrate the effect of muscle training: About half the number (ca. 500) of boys and girls in a Danish school spent 5 min three times each day, 3 days a week for 2 months, practicing "chinning the bar." The other half of the children served as controls. After 2 months the isometric strength of the arm-shoulder muscles in the training group had not increased measurably compared to the control group, but the ability to perform chin-ups had increased about 100% in the training group, none in the controls. Under stricter laboratory conditions the following experiments were performed (Petersen *et al.*, 1961; Hansen, 1961): Two groups of female student nurses trained 5 days a week for 6 weeks. One group trained by lifting a weight corresponding to 60% of their maximum capacity with their elbow flexors 150 times per session. Another group produced the same tension isometrically, maintained it for 5 sec, rested for 2 sec, and repeated this procedure 150 times per session. Before and after, the following tests were made: isometric strength; dynamic strength, i.e., maximum weight that could be lifted once by the elbow flexors; dynamic endurance, measured as the maximum number of lifts performed with the training load; isometric endurance, i.e., maximum number of isometric contractions with the training load. The combined results are tabulated in Table III.

TABLE III

INCREASE IN STRENGTH AND ENDURANCE DUE TO ISOMETRIC AND DYNAMIC TRAINING (PERCENTAGE OF PRETRAINING VALUE)[a]

Training	Isometric strength	Dynamic strength	Dynamic endurance	Static endurance
Dynamic	5	29	5040	Not measured[b]
Isometric	4	6	41	1058

[a] Data from Petersen et al. (1961) and Hansen (1961).
[b] Later experiments (Hansen, 1967) showed no increase.

The striking results are the tremendous increases in performance in the kind of exercise that was used in the training program and the modest increases in the other tests. These specific effects of the methods used for muscle training make the indiscriminate use of any strength training method seem of dubious value. Strength should not be developed as an isolated function but in connection with the task for which it is desired.

The increase in isometric strength, even with optimal loads and frequencies, has been found by several authors to be a rather slow process. It is found to be 2 to 3% per week in the first few weeks of a training period, but then it gradually slows down.

2. What Happens to the Muscle?

Intensive muscle training resulting in an increase in isometric strength is usually accompanied by an increase in circumference of the muscle. The often much larger increase in dynamic strength and endurance need not manifest itself in an increase in bulk.

Whether a muscle grows by increasing the number of muscle fibers, or whether the growth is due only to an increase in thickness of the existing fibers has been discussed. The latter view is at present prevalent. However, in young rats in which the small m. plantaris was transplanted so as to take the place of the much larger m. gastrocnemius, Van Linge (1962) found indications of a splitting up of muscle fibers and thus a growth involving formation of new muscle fibers. The fibers had also increased in thickness, contained more sarcoplasma but no more myofibrils than the controls, and the intramuscular connective tissue had increased very much.

The slow and rather modest increases in isometric strength thus are explained as the result of a growth in thickness of the individual muscle fibers and the connective tissue, which becomes more tough and presumably less yielding in the well-trained muscle. The increase in dynamic strength is probably due to the same factors, plus possibly a better neuromuscular coordination. This latter factor may also play an important role in the very large increases in endurance, but here a third factor is added—an increase in number of capillaries that will enhance the transport of oxygen and nutrients to the muscle and of metabolites like lactate and CO_2 from the muscle. In animal experiments, Petrén *et al.* (1937) found that the number of visible capillaries in the gastrocnemius of trained guinea pigs had increased by 45%.

It is natural to assume that training also leads to beneficial changes in the chemical composition of the muscles, such as increases in content of myoglobin, glycogen, creatine phosphate, ATP, and diverse enzymes. Such changes have been found by various authors in animals, but precise information from experiments with humans are still lacking.

V. Muscular Fatigue

When muscles have been called upon to function over a certain time, they may become fatigued. In isolated muscles this is seen as a decreasing shortening, or tension production, in spite of constant stimulation. *In situ*, the same is seen if the muscle contractions are maximal. In the classic experiments of Mosso (1892) with his ergograph, the contractions became gradually smaller.

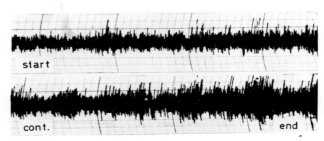

Fig. 30. EMG's from finger flexors during continued contraction at 50% maximal strength.

In submaximal contractions a constant work level may be maintained for some time, depending on the load, because it is possible to draw upon the reserves of motor units that are not engaged in submaximal contractions. As the first active fibers become fatigued their output per twitch decreases, but new units are then mobilized to make up for the loss in contractile power. After a while, even in originally submaximal contractions, all mobilizable motor units may be engaged, and from then on fatigue will show as a decrease in contraction. Electromyograms of the muscles show increasing electrical activity as fatigue sets in (Fig. 30).

A fatigued muscle will recuperate after a period of rest if blood is allowed to flow through it. The blood will carry oxygen and nutrients to the muscle and will remove metabolites that inhibit the processes in the muscle. Rest alone will not do it, as seen when the blood flow through a fatigued muscle group is blocked by pressure cuffs. It is obvious that local muscle fatigue has to do with the chemical reactions that deliver energy to the contractile mechanism in the muscle fibers. This energy can be delivered through aerobic or anaerobic processes.

1. Aerobic Muscle Metabolism

By oxidation of foodstuffs brought to the muscles by the blood, energy is set free and used directly for the resynthesis of ATP. Both glucose (and lactic acid) and free fatty acids can be utilized by the muscles in this way. The waste products are CO_2 and H_2O, and the intensity of the aerobic processes will therefore be limited by the perfusion of the muscles. Blood flow through a contracting muscle is hindered by the high intramuscular pressure that accompanies contraction, and in strong contractions blood flow is completely blocked. If the muscular activity, however, is rhythmic, a much increased blood flow will pass through the muscle capillaries in the periods of relaxation, and within limits a steady state can be reached in which oxygen and nutrients are brought to the muscles as fast as they are needed. Above a certain level, different for different muscles and depending on the fitness of the subject, the delivery of oxygen cannot keep up with the energy demands, and energy must then be produced anaerobically. The muscles do, however, contain a small reserve of stored oxygen, bound to myoglobin as oxymyoglobin. In short bursts of maximal activity this oxygen is probably used to keep the metabolism going aerobically, e.g., during the very first seconds of any strenuous exercise before the blood flow has been stepped up. It has been suggested by Christensen et al. (1960) that the ability to run at top speed in short intervals of 5 to 10 sec with pauses in between for a considerable time without signs of accumulating fatigue, may at least partly be explained by this store of oxygen. The actual amount of myoglobin in muscles of well-trained athletes is, however, not known, but in animals it is found to be higher in trained rats and rabbits than in untrained animals (Lawrie, 1953).

2. Anaerobic Muscle Metabolism

In all situations where the blood flow through the muscles is unable to deliver oxygen fast enough for the energy demand, energy for the resynthesis of ATP is liberated by the breakdown of creatine phosphate, of which the muscle contains a small store, or of glycogen, which is present in considerably larger amounts. As both ATP and creatine phosphate can be rebuilt by energy from the breakdown of glycogen to lactic acid, it is this last process that usually leads to fatigue of the muscle. This can happen in two ways: If the blood flow through the muscle is too slow to remove lactate as fast as it is formed, it will accumulate in the muscles and inhibit further muscle contractions. This is what happens in sustained isometric (static) contractions, and in rhythmic contractions with high loads and/or frequencies. In isometric (static) contractions the time a certain tension can be maintained decreases with increasing tension (Fig. 31). In rhythmic contractions, the

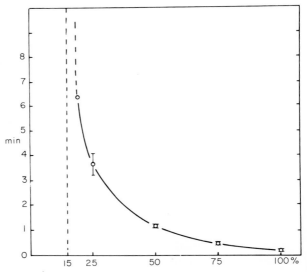

Fig. 31. Relation between isometric tension (in percentage of maximal isometric tension) and time it can be maintained. (After Rohmert, 1960.)

time one can continue will depend both on the load or tension, and on the frequency. High loads at high frequencies resemble static exercise and will soon cause fatigue. Lower loads, at a slower tempo, may allow the lactic acid to be removed from the muscles as fast as it is formed so that work can go on "indefinitely."

The other way in which the anaerobic processes may cause muscular fatigue is by exhaustion of the stores of glycogen in the muscles. With fairly high loads, although not so high as to cause a steadily increasing concentration of lactic acid in the muscles, the glycogen may be used up. This will cause fatigue. While the fatigue caused by lactic acid accumulation may be alleviated within the hour, the wearing down of the glycogen stores may take several days to repair, as shown by experiments with muscle biopsies performed on athletes during and after hard exercise (Hultman and Bergström, 1967).

The above-mentioned forms of muscular fatigue could be explained as results of an impairment of the contractile mechanism itself. Other forms of general fatigue caused by muscular exercise may be traced back to hypoglycemia, hyperthermia, dehydration, and, perhaps, to sensory impulses from muscles and joints, signaling disturbances of the homeostasis. The subjective feeling of fatigue is a complex phenomenon and has not yet been fully explained.

Acknowledgments

Figures 5, 6, 9, 12, 13, 16, 17, 18, 19 are originals or are redrawn from data of the Institute of Neurophysiology, University of Copenhagen. I thank my colleagues Drs. F. Buchthal, I. Carlsen, C. Guld, G. Knappeis, A. L. Rosenfalck, and Steen-Knudsen for kind permission to use their material.

Figures 15, 23, 24, 25, 26, 27, 28, 29, 30 are based on material from the Laboratory for Theory of Gymnastics, University of Copenhagen, and the Polio-institute, Hellerup, Denmark. I am grateful to my co-workers O. Hansen, K. Jørgensen, K. Klausen, O. Lammert, S. Molbech, H. Nielsen, E. Poulsen, and B. Rasmussen for their kind cooperation.

REFERENCES

Buchthal, F. (1942). *Danish Biol. Med.* **17**.
Buchthal, F., and Kaiser, E. (1951). *Danish Biol. Med.* **21**.
Christensen, E. H., Hedman, R., and Saltin, B. (1960). *Acta Physiol. Scand.* **50**, 269.
Fenn, W. O., Brody, H., and Petrilli, A. (1931). *Am. J. Physiol.* **97**, 1.
Granit, R. (1956). "Receptors and Sensory Perception." Yale Univ. Press, New Haven, Connecticut.
Hansen, J. W. (1961). *Intern. Z. Angew. Physiol.* **18**, 474.
Hansen, J. W. (1967). *Intern. Z. Angew. Physiol.* **23**, 367.
Hettinger, T. (1961). "Physiology of Strength." Thomas, Springfield, Illinois.
Hill, A. V. (1949). *Proc. Roy. Soc.* **B136**, 399.
Hultman, E., and Bergström, J. (1967). *Acta Med. Scand.* (in press).
Huxley, H. E., and Hanson, J. (1954). *Nature* **173**, 973.
Krogh, A. (1922). "The Anatomy and Physiology of Capillaries." Yale Univ. Press, New Haven, Connecticut.
Lawrie, R. A. (1953). *Nature* **171**, 1069.
Mosso, U. (1892). "Die Ermüdung." Hirzel, Leipzig.
Müller, E. A., and Rohmert, W. (1963). *Intern. Z. Angew. Physiol.* **19**, 403.
Petersen, F. B., Graudal, H., Hansen, J. W., and Hvid, N. (1961). *Intern. Z. Angew. Physiol.* **18**, 468.
Petrén, T., Sjöstrand, T., and Silvén, B. (1937). *Intern. Z. Angew. Physiol.* **9**, 376.
Reichel, H. (1960). "Muskelphysiologie." Springer, Berlin.
Rohmert, W. (1960). *Intern. Z. Angew. Physiol.* **18**, 123.
Ruffini, A. (1897). *Brain* **20**, 368.
Sherrington, C. (1913). *Quart. J. Exptl. Physiol.* **6**, 251.

Sherrington, C. (1947). "The Integrative Action of the Nervous System." Cambridge
    Univ. Press, London and New York.
Spalteholz, W. (1888). *Abhandl. Saechs. Ges. Akad. Wiss.* **14**, 509.
Taylor, J. (1932). "Selected Writings of John Hughling Jackson." Hodder & Stoughton,
    London.
Van Linge, B. (1962). *J. Bone Joint Surg.* **44B**, 711.

2

THE RESPIRATORY SYSTEM AND EXERCISE

Rodolfo Margaria and Paolo Cerretelli

I. Mechanics of Breathing during Exercise

A. Lung Volumes and Ventilation at Exercise

Pulmonary ventilation ($\dot{V}_E$), which is at rest 5–6 liters/min, may exceed in a short spell of exercise 150 liters/min, i.e., more than 25 times the resting value. Such an increase is brought about by a fourfold increase of the breathing rate (f) (up to 50 breaths/min) coupled with an increase by a factor of six of the tidal volume (V_T), which from a rest value of about 0.5 liters may reach a value of 3 liters (about 60% of the vital capacity, V.C.). These changes involve a very high increase of the work of breathing ($\dot{W}b$), which may exceed one hundred times the rest value.

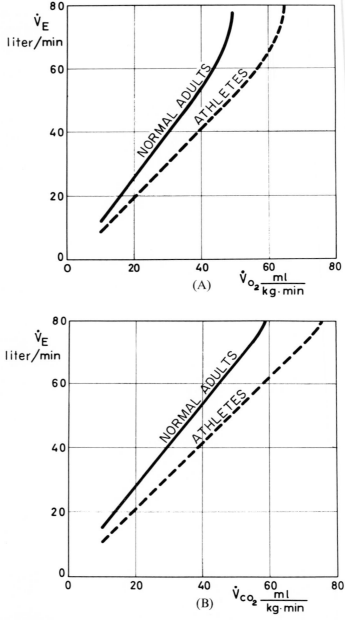

Fig. 1. Pulmonary ventilation (V_E) as a function of oxygen uptake (V_{O_2}) (A) or (B) of carbon dioxide output ($\dot{V}_{CO_2}$).

Pulmonary ventilation has been found to increase in muscular exercise in strict relation to the increased metabolic demand. In an exercise of long duration, such that a steady state can be attained, the maximal ventilation value is of the order of magnitude of 80–100 liters/min.

In Fig. 1, $\dot{V}_E$ is plotted against $\dot{V}_{O_2}$ (A) and $\dot{V}_{CO_2}$ (B). Both functions are straight lines within a certain range: the slope of the lines, dV_E/dV_{O_2} or dV_E/dV_{CO_2} is the reciprocal of the efficiency of the ventilation in terms of liters of air that are to be carried to the lungs per liter of O_2 consumed or CO_2 produced. It appears to have a lower value for athletes, thus indicating a more efficient ventilation in these subjects. The efficiency of ventilation is perhaps better given by d kcal/dV_E, or kcal per liter ventilated, this value being about 0.22–0.24 (Margaria, 1937).

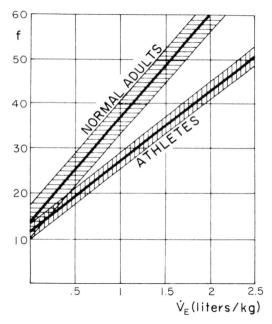

Fig. 2. Respiration rate (f) as a function of ventilation $\dot{V}_E$ in liters/kg of body weight. (From Brambilla *et al.*, 1958.)

From Fig. 1 it appears that when the work load is very high and the aerobic energy supply becomes insufficient, i.e., when glycolysis enters into the picture and lactic acid is produced, dV_E/dV_{O_2} increases. This is an evidence that an additional stimulus is given to the respiratory center, this being possibly the H^+ ion concentration increase in the blood, or the CO_2 released, as a consequence of the lactic acid produced. This interpretation is supported also by the fact that the $\dot{V}_{CO_2}$ line does not seem to deflect until much higher metabolic rates than the $\dot{V}_{O_2}$ line are reached, thus indicating that pulmonary ventilation seems to be more directly related to the needs of eliminating CO_2 than of absorbing O_2.

The deflection from the straight line both for the $\dot{V}_{O_2}$ and for the $\dot{V}_{CO_2}$ curve of Fig. 1 takes place at a much higher metabolic rate in athletic subjects. This is in agreement with the observation that lactic acid production also sets in at higher work loads (for details, see Margaria, 1967, and Margaria *et al.*, 1963b).

As $\dot{V}_E = f \cdot V_T$, where f is the breathing rate and V_T the tidal volume, the contribution of each factor f and V_T to an increase of ventilation must be known. In Fig. 2 the relationship between $\dot{V}_E$ and f is given for both ordinary

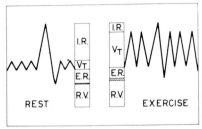

Fig. 3. Lung volumes at rest and exercise. The hatched areas indicate the changes of the intrathoracic blood volume.

men (N) and athletes. The function is approximately linear for both groups of subjects. The line for athletes, however, is less inclined, thus showing a greater contribution of the tidal volume to the increased ventilation. This is possibly related to (1) a greater compliance of the chest and the lungs or (2) a lower resistance to the air flow in the athletes.

The total lung volume (T.L.V.) decreases very slightly during exercise. This is due to an increased central blood volume, i.e., a more complete filling of the vessels of the lungs to cope with the increased circulation.

The tidal volume increases at the expense of the inspiratory reserve (I.R.), which is correspondingly reduced. The expiratory reserve volume (E.R.) does not seem to change appreciably even at the highest levels of ventilation (Petit *et al.*, 1959) provided no postural changes of the subject are taking place in relation to the type of exercise.

The vital capacity (V.C.) decreases about 300–400 ml, i.e., more than can be accounted for by the increased central blood volume. Consequently the residual volume (R.V.) must be slightly increased at exercise.

An increased residual volume might play an important physiological role at exercise, as it involves an increased functional residual capacity (F.R.C. =

R.V. + E.R.). The volume oscillations of the air in the lungs due to the respiratory movements are obviously much larger at exercise (see Fig. 5). With a greater value of F.R.C. the pressure damping would be more pronounced, and the fluctuations of the $P_{A_{CO_2}}$ reduced. A tendency to a more constant $P_{A_{CO_2}}$ value all throughout the respiratory cycle is thus obtained.

A schematic description of the lung volumes at rest and at exercise is given in Fig. 3.

B. The Forces Involved

In pumping air in and out the chest, work is done not only to overcome the resistance (viscosity) of the fluid displaced from one compartment to another or to the outside, but also part of the structures undergo internal frictions, and changes of position, size, and shape (rib cage, abdomen, and lung) take place. Several components are therefore at work.

The overall driving forces can be schematically classified into static and dynamic. Static forces are
1. Elasticity of the chest wall and lung
2. Surface tension of the alveoli
3. Gravitational effect of the different structures
Dynamic forces are
1. Viscous resistance of the tissues
2. Resistance to the laminar and turbulent flow of the gas through the airways

Condition	At low ventilation rate	At 50 liters/min and above[a]
Inspiratory	Diaphragm Intercostal (external and intercartilagineous) Scaleni (only in some subjects)	Diaphragm Intercostal (external and intercartilagineous) Scaleni (only in some subjects) Sternocleidomastoids Extensors of the vertebral column
Condition	Above 30–40 liters/min	
Expiratory	Muscles of the abdominal wall Internal intercostal	

[a] From Campbell, 1958.

In absence of a sizable inertial component even at relatively high ventilation rates, the main opposing forces involved in hyperventilation are the flow-resistive ones. Most of the increased work of breathing observed during exercise is spent to overcome these forces. The forces employed to overcome the elastic resistance to expansion during inspiration are in fact temporarily stored and utilized completely in the following expiratory phase to drive the air out of the lungs, so that the overall balance of the elastic forces throughout a complete respiratory cycle is practically even for $\dot{V}_E$ values greater than 30 liters/min.

The forces applied to the system (driving forces) are provided by the activity of the muscles shown in the table on p. 47 (Agostoni, 1963).

C. Work of Breathing

In Fig. 4 the pressure–volume diagrams of the respiratory apparatus (1) with the inspiratory muscles maximally contracted (left), (2) with the expiratory muscles maximally contracted (right), and (3) at relaxation (middle) are shown. The maximum potential work of breathing in static conditions is given by the area included by the curves indicating the maximum inspiratory and expiratory pressures. It can be approximated as the product of the vital capacity by the sum of the maximal inspiratory and expiratory pressures measured at midexpiration. This has been proved to be a significant index of the mechanical possibilities of the respiratory function that can be utilized as

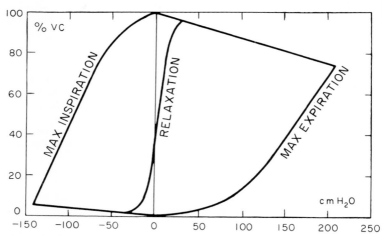

Fig. 4. Lung volume in percent of the vital capacity (V.C.), as a function of the endopulmonary pressure in cm H_2O at relaxation and during maximum inspiratory and expiratory efforts. (Modified after Rahn et al., 1946.)

a clinical test in sport medicine or in population survey analysis (Margaria and Marro, 1955).

The horizontal distance between the relaxation curve and the maximum inspiratory or the maximum expiratory curves indicates the pressure exerted by the inspiratory and expiratory muscles, respectively.

This "net" pressure is plotted in Fig. 5 against the volume expressed as percentage of the vital capacity. In the same graph the dotted loops indicate the $P-V$ path during a single breath at different ventilation levels (Fenn, 1951). As it appears from the graph, the work of breathing done even at

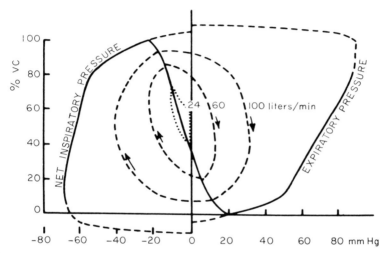

Fig. 5. Net maximum voluntary inspiratory and expiratory pressures (full lines on the sides). The full line crossing the ordinate describes the pressure exerted by the respiratory muscles to balance the elastic forces of the respiratory system. Dotted loops indicate the pressure–volume path during a single breath at ventilation levels of 24, 60, and 100 liters/min. (Modified after Fenn, 1951.)

maximum exercise is a small fraction only of the maximum potential work.

In spite of the relatively large increase of the work of breathing during exercise as compared to rest, the overall energy required by the exercise hyperventilation is still very low, as compared with the total energy expenditure. In fact, at a ventilation level of 130 liters/min it amounts to only 450–650 cal/min, about 5% of the maximum aerobic power that the subject is able to develop.

The elastic work done by the inspiratory muscles to introduce a given amount of air into the lungs, say 1 liter, starting from the end of a normal expiration, and neglecting the frictional component, is that indicated in Fig. 6

by the hatched triangle. Increasing V_T from 1 to 2 liters, the work required is 4 times higher (pointed and hatched area). For a constant ventilation, of say 10 liters/min, taking into account that the frequency of the breaths drops to one-half, the cost of inspiration per minute will increase by a factor of two. The higher cost of inspiration is in part counterbalanced by the increased efficiency of the ventilation. In fact, assuming that the respiratory dead space does not change and the alveolar ventilation keeps constant, $\dot{V}_E$ should increase only 1.8 times instead of two. The lower efficiency of inspiration at high-tidal-volume values, due to the increased elastic work, does not involve a parallel lower efficiency of the whole respiratory cycle. As it has been mentioned

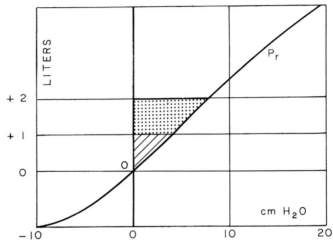

Fig. 6. Elastic component of the work of breathing during a single inspiration of 1 liter (hatched area) and 2 liters (dotted plus hatched area), respectively. P_r indicates the relaxation curve of the chest and lung. 0 is the volume at the end of a normal expiration.

earlier, this is because the elastic work done at inspiration (when $\dot{V}_E < 30$ liters/min) is utilized to support the work of expiration that can then take place without the expiratory muscles taking any, or any sizable, part.

During a quiet breathing cycle the muscle contribution to respiration is indicated schematically in Fig. 7A. The double hatched area is the work done by the inspiratory muscles. Part of this area, i.e., that included between the ordinate and the relaxation curve, P_r, corresponds to the static work, while the part between the ordinate and the endopulmonary pressure curve, P_{mus}, corresponds to dynamic work. The distance between P_{mus} and P_r of the figure indicates the total pressure exerted by the inspiratory muscles.

While the static component of the inspiratory work is stored as potential energy, and is more than sufficient to support a quiet passive expiration, the

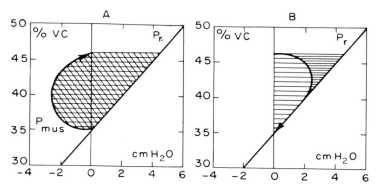

Fig. 7. Schematic diagram showing the pressure applied to the respiratory system during a quiet breathing cycle: A, inspiration; B, expiration. The P_{mus} curve indicates the dynamic pressure, the P_r line the relaxation pressure–volume curve. The horizontal distance between P_{mus} and P_r indicates the pressure exerted by the inspiratory muscles. The double hatched area of A is the work of inspiration. The spaced hatched area of B is the energy spent for expiration that corresponds to a fraction of the elastic energy stored during inspiration (area between the ordinate and the P_r line). The thick hatched area between P_{mus} and P_r of B indicates the elastic energy spent to overcome the persistent activity of the inspiratory muscles in the early phase of expiration. (Redrawn from Agostoni, 1963.)

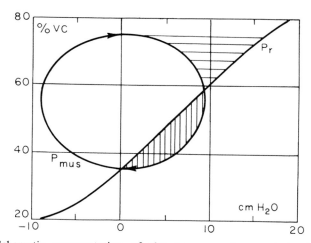

Fig. 8. Schematic representation of the pressure–volume relationship within a breathing cycle when ventilation is at 50 liters/min. The area circumscribed by the inspiratory section of curve P_{mus} (left of the ordinate) and P_r corresponds to the work of inspiration (dynamic + static). The horizontal hatched area at the left of curve P_r represents work done by the inspiratory muscles during the early expiration phase to oppose the overwhelming static forces; the vertical hatched area to the right of curve P_r is the work performed by the expiratory muscles. (Redrawn from Agostoni, 1963.)

dynamic component is lost as heat. During expiration (Fig. 7B) the excess pressure exerted by the elasticity of the chest must be counterbalanced by the persistent contraction of the inspiratory muscles to control the expiratory flow and make of it a continuous smooth process. This is indicated in diagram B by the distance between the P_r curve and the endopulmonary expiratory pressure curve. The thick hatched area included between these curves is the work done by the inspiratory muscles to support this activity (Campbell, 1958; Agostoni *et al.*, 1960; Petit *et al.*, 1960).

Figure 8 is a schematic representation of the pressure–volume relationship within a breathing cycle when the ventilation is 50 liters/min. Again, the area circumscribed by the part at the left of the ordinate of the curve P_{mus} and the curve P_r corresponds to the inspiratory work, both dynamic and static. During expiration, part of the static work stored as potential energy by the

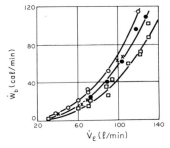

Fig. 9. Work of breathing [cal/min] at different ventilatory rates ($\dot{V}_E$) in three subjects. (Redrawn from Margaria *et al.*, 1960.)

system (area included between the segment of ordinate limited by the curve P_{mus} and the curve P_r) is used to overcome the frictional resistance of the system for that given flow. The hatched area at the left of the curve P_r represents again the work done by the inspiratory muscles to oppose the exceeding elastic force at the beginning of expiration, while the hatched area to the right of curve P_r is the actual work performed by the expiratory muscles, the elastic energy of the chest at the end of expiration being insufficient to drive the air out.

The work of breathing at rest as well as during exercise is measured practically by recording simultaneously esophageal pressure, indicative of the intrathoracic pressure, and the tidal volume (Margaria *et al.*, 1960), and by plotting them on a Cartesian diagram. A loop is thus obtained of the type shown in Fig. 8 by the curve P_{mus}, the area of which is dimensionally work. This method of measuring the work of breathing tends to underestimate the total work, as the energy required for overcoming the viscous resistance of the rib cage and abdomen is not taken into account.

The relationship between the work of breathing so obtained and the pulmonary ventilation is given for 3 subjects in Fig. 9. Even during severe exercise at steady state, the work of breathing does not reach its maximal value in the normal individual. Evidently the limiting factor to the maximal exercise is set by other factors, presumably by the cardiac activity.

The analysis of the pressure–volume relationship of the lung and of the chest components of the respiratory system, as given in Fig. 8, however, is incomplete, because it has been constructed on the assumption that the respiratory system is made only by the lungs and by the rib cage. In reality the base of the thoracic cavity has a completely different structure from its sides; here the structures that separate the thoracic cavity from the external air are the diaphragm and the abdomen. To measure the contribution of this system also in respiration, Agostoni (1961) has recorded the abdominal pressure simultaneously with the intrathoracic pressure and the tidal volume. The transdiaphragmatic (abdominal minus intrathoracic) pressure and the transabdominal (abdominal minus atmospheric) pressure could thus be calculated, the first being an index of the diaphragm activity, the second of the elastic, gravitational, and muscular forces of the abdominal system. The data so collected are presented in Fig. 10 for rest, and working conditions, respectively.

In this diagram the horizontal distance between the P_i (intrathoracic pressure) and P_{ab} curves is the pressure given by the activity of the diaphragm. On the assumption that the volume of air introduced in the chest is due only to the activity of the diaphragm, the area limited by these two curves is a

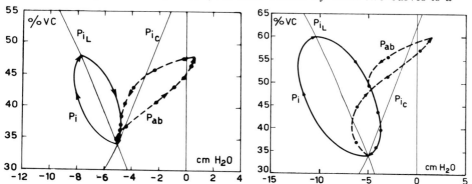

Fig. 10. Pulmonary volume, in percentage of vital capacity, as a function of the intrathoracic pressure P_i and of the intra-abdominal (immediately below the diaphragm) pressure P_{ab} during a respiratory cycle at rest (left) and, on the same subject, at a ventilation level of 35 liters/min, the breathing rate being 30/min (right). The lines P_{i_L} and P_{i_c} indicate the static intrathoracic pressures due to the elastic force of the lung and chest, respectively. The transdiaphragmatic pressure is given by the horizontal distance between P_{ab} and P_i. (From Agostoni, 1961.)

measure of the work of the diaphragm. However, as the diaphragm contribution to the tidal volume is only 70% of the total, the work performed by the diaphragm is correspondingly 70% of this area. The remaining 30% of the tidal volume has to be supported by a change of volume of the chest. The corresponding work will then be given in Fig. 10 by the corresponding fraction of the area circumscribed by the line P_i, representative of the work contribution by the chest wall.

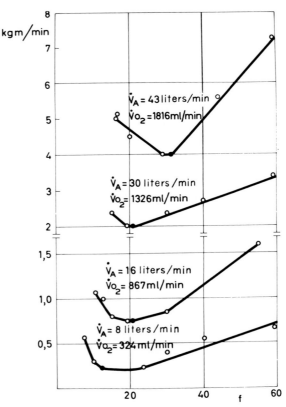

Fig. 11. Work of breathing (kgm/min) as a function of the respiratory rate (f) for different $\dot{V}_A$ and $\dot{V}_{O_2}$ values (indicated in the graphs). ●, Spontaneous breathing rate; ○, data obtained at imposed breathing rates. (Redrawn from Milic-Emili and Petit, 1959.)

When the respiratory work is measured as the area circumscribed by the intrathoracic pressure loop (P_i) only, as indicated in Fig. 8, without considering the diaphragm–abdominal component, an error is made, which will be larger the greater the average distance of the loop line P_{ab} from the line P_{i_c}.

For a given alveolar ventilation the mechanical work of breathing is affected by the respiratory rate. It is high at very low and at very high frequency of respiration and it attains a minimal value at an intermediate optimal value. It has been observed that the body tends spontaneously to regulate the ventilation to this optimal breathing frequency (Fig. 11).

Of the two fractions of the dynamic resistances (resistance to flow in the airways and viscous resistance offered by the chest), that due to the gas flow prevails at exercise, due particularly to the increased resistance to flow occurring at high ventilation rates as the laminar flow shifts to turbulent.

The resistance of the air flow through the nose during breathing is higher than through the mouth. At rest, with a flow of about 0.5 liters/sec the resistance in "nose" breathing is about 30–40% higher than in "mouth" breathing (Mead, 1960). With increasing flow, this difference tends to increase to much higher values. At exercise the nose resistance reaches soon such a high value that the respiration is switched from nose to mouth, in order to allow the attainment of the required minute volume. This takes place at a critical ventilation value, constant for each individual, at about 40 liters/min (Saibene *et al.*, 1965).

II. Gas Exchange and Gas Transport at Exercise

A. Processes Affecting Gas Intake, Transport, Transfer, and Output

The respiratory function, i.e., the O_2 transport to and the CO_2 removal from the tissues, is secured by two active processes, the pulmonary ventilation and the circulation. The diffusion of the respiratory gases through the alveolar and capillary membranes in the lung, and across the capillary walls and the cell membranes in the tissues, is a passive process, carried out by the gas pressure gradient between blood in the capillaries and the active tissues (or alveoli) and depending on the physical characteristics of the tissue or other layers between the two systems.

The blood, the function of which is to carry O_2 from the lungs to the tissues and CO_2 from the active tissues to the lungs, has the peculiarity of having a high capacity for these 2 gases. The high capacity for O_2 is due to the hemoglobin content in the erythrocytes and the capacity for CO_2 is due to the high buffer capacity, particularly by the high bicarbonate and proteinate content of both plasma and blood cells.

Oxidation being the final step of all energy giving processes in the muscle, the goal of the respiratory function is that of securing an adequate supply of O_2 to the tissues, so as to maintain a sufficiently high partial pressure of this gas at the cellular enzymatic system level, even when the oxygen consumption is increased 10 to 12 times, as during strenuous exercise.

The respiratory and circulatory functions must, therefore, undergo a definite change during exercise.

In Fig. 12 the average normal values for P_{O_2} at different levels along the path from external air to active muscle cells are given. Such values do not change appreciably as an effect of exercise within the lung and the arteries, whereas remarkable changes occur in the working tissues and consequently in the venous blood. At the level of the alveoli, the mixed venous blood (O_2 and CO_2 contents are at rest 15 and 54 vol %, respectively) undergoes arterialization, thus increasing the O_2 content to about 20 vol % and decreasing the CO_2 content to about 50 vol %. During heavy exercise, the mixed venous

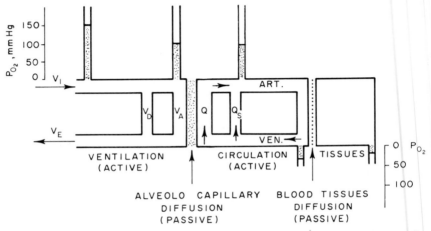

Fig. 12. Schematic representation of the respiratory and circulatory system. P_{O_2} values at different levels along the path from external air to active muscle cells are also given, part in the upper, part in the lower section of the drawing.

blood oxygen content may drop to 5 vol % and the CO_2 rise to about 65 vol %.

The pulmonary ventilation, together with gas diffusion through the lungs, keeps the O_2 and the CO_2 pressures in the arterial blood constant at 100–110 and 40 mm Hg respectively, independent of the work load. The P_{CO_2} value of the arterial blood together with the amount of alkali present in the blood sets the pH value, which is 7.4 for a man at rest under ordinary conditions. Therefore, the pH of the arterial blood is also unaffected by exercise as long as the P_{CO_2} value does not change. Only during very heavy exercise carried out in anaerobic conditions and involving production of lactic acid does the arterial H^+ ion concentration increase, in some cases up to 60% or more (Fig. 13).

The increased acidity of the blood due to lactic acid affects both O_2 and the CO_2 carrying power of the blood. Because of the Bohr effect, the dissociation curve of the blood for oxygen is displaced to the right, thus facilitating the delivery of O_2 from the blood to the tissues. The uptake of O_2 by the blood at the lung level, on the contrary, is not appreciably affected because of the flattening of the dissociation curve at high P_{O_2} values.

The lactic acid entering the blood brings about a corresponding decrease of the alkali reserve and a flattening of the CO_2 dissociation curve of the blood. This involves a higher difference of P_{CO_2} necessary to change the total CO_2 content of the blood of a given amount. In other words, the buffer power of the blood is decreased.

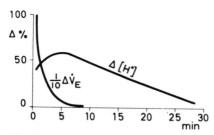

Fig. 13. Changes of blood H^+ ion concentration and pulmonary ventilation during recovery following a maximal exercise (standing running) of 30-sec duration in percentage of the rest value (from Margaria and Talenti, 1933). Note that the scale for $\dot{V}_E$ is one-tenth that for H^+ indicated on the ordinate.

Consequently, lactic acid favors the oxygen uptake by the tissues while it hampers the CO_2 uptake by the blood flowing through the active muscles.

The effect of the lactic acid on the respiratory center in increasing the pulmonary ventilation through an increased H^+ ion concentration is very meager. It is evident from the experiments of Fig. 13, in which the subject performed an exhausting exercise for 30 sec, that in the first few minutes of recovery, the H^+ ion concentration in the blood kept increasing, while the pulmonary ventilation decreased very rapidly toward the rest values. The maximal H^+ ion concentration in the blood was not reached until after about 5 min of recovery. By then the pulmonary ventilation had subsided nearly to normal rest levels.

A decrease of the blood hemoglobin concentration such as in anemic subjects causes a reduction of the blood O_2 carrying capacity and, as a consequence, a reduction of the maximum aerobic power of the subjects (see Figs. 15 and 16). Conversely, a moderate increase of blood hemoglobin should lead to a higher aerobic power. The effect of a decrease or an increase of the erythrocytes in blood should be counterbalanced by a corresponding decrease or increase of the blood viscosity, and, therefore, of the resistance to circulation.

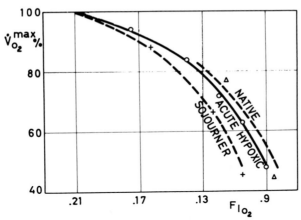

Fig. 14. Maximum O_2 uptake as percentage of the value at sea level as a function of $F_{I_{O_2}}$ for acute hypoxic subjects and sojourners at altitude. (Data on natives from Elsner *et al.*, 1964, are also added for reference.)

Small changes in erythrocyte concentration, however, do not seem to appreciably affect the dynamic flow resistance. Only a very substantial increase of the blood cells such as is met in plethora or high altitude dwellers affects the circulation of the blood negatively more than the increased capacity for oxygen may improve the respiratory conditions (Cerretelli and Margaria, 1961).

A reduction of the inspired oxygen pressure, such as takes place at altitude, is necessarily followed by a decreased O_2 partial pressure at the alveolar level,

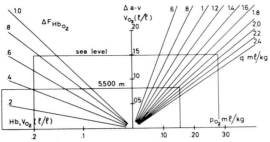

Fig. 15. Arteriovenous O_2 difference in liters per liter of blood as a function of the O_2 pulse in milliliters per kilogram of body weight (right) and of the O_2 capacity of the blood (Hb) in liters per liter of blood (left). The lines irradiating from the origin give the stroke volume, q, in milliliters per kilogram, and the arteriovenous difference in saturation fraction ($\Delta F_{Hb_{O_2}}$). Data for a subject at maximal exercise at sea level are given, together with the data on the same subject after a sojourn at about 5500 m altitude, as calculated from direct observation of Hb and P_{O_2} and on the assumption that the stroke volume at exercise is the same as at sea level. (Modified after Margaria, 1966.)

by a decreased arterial blood oxygen saturation, and consequently, through a reduction of the arteriovenous O_2 difference (see Figs. 15 and 16) by a reduced maximum $\dot{V}_{O_2}$.

In Fig. 14 the maximum O_2 uptake versus $F_{I_{O_2}}$ is plotted for acute hypoxic subjects, sojourners at altitude for more than 4 weeks, and natives of the

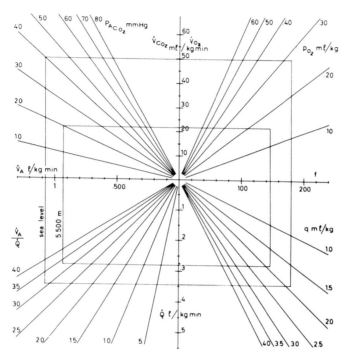

Fig. 16. Maximal O_2 consumption ($\dot{V}_{O_2}$) or CO_2 production ($\dot{V}_{CO_2}$) in milliliters per kilogram of body weight and minute volume of the heart ($\dot{Q}$) in liters per kilogram, as a function of the heart rate f (right) and of the alveolar ventilation ($\dot{V}_A$) in liters per minute per kilogram of body weight. The lines radiating from the origin give the O_2 pulse, p_{O_2}, in milliliters per kilogram of body weight, the stroke volume, q, in milliliters per kilogram of body weight, the alveolar P_{CO_2} in mm Hg and the $\dot{V}_A/\dot{Q}$ ratio. The lines refer to the condition of maximal exercise for a young fit subject at sea level, and after a sojourn at 5500 m altitude (see also Fig. 14). (From Margaria, 1966.)

Andes. The lower maximal $\dot{V}_{O_2}$ found in chronic hypoxic subjects is probably due to the higher erythrocyte content of the blood in this condition as compared to the high altitude natives.

Some of the most significant changes that take place in exercise are represented in Figs. 15 and 16. In the first, the arteriovenous oxygen difference is plotted as a function of the oxygen capacity of the blood (Hb) in liters per liter of blood, and of the oxygen pulse, p_{O_2}. The oxygen capacity of the blood is easily measured. The oxygen pulse can be calculated when the maximum oxygen consumption in exercise and the maximal heart rate are known. The lines irradiating from the origin give the stroke volume, q, at the right, and the difference in oxygen saturation between arterial and venous blood at the left. Assuming that the arterial oxygen saturation is 0.95 even in strenuous exercise, and that the lowest mixed venous blood saturation is 0.2, the arteriovenous difference in saturation with oxygen is 0.75. If this assumption is correct, then also the other two variables $(a\text{-}v)$ and q are defined.

Data on the changes of hemoglobin, maximum heart rate, and maximum oxygen consumption after a sojourn of 2 months at about 5000 m have been collected by Cerretelli and Margaria (1961). From them, and assuming that the stroke volume does not change as an effect of altitude, the data for all the variables indicated at maximum exercise at altitude are shown by the smaller (shifted to the left) parallelogram. The rest values for both sea level and altitude conditions have not been indicated for simplicity.

In Fig. 16 four functions are represented. The upper right diagram gives the heart rate as a function of the oxygen consumption. As is well known, this is a linear function, and when the heart rates at two submaximal work levels are known, the maximal oxygen consumption is easily obtained by extrapolating the line at the value of maximal heart rate, which is ordinarily 180. Then, also the oxygen pulse, p_{O_2}, is obtained.

In the upper left diagram the CO_2 output per minute, $\dot{V}_{CO_2}$, is plotted against $\dot{V}_A$. The two lower diagrams give the minute volume of the heart, $\dot{Q}$, as a function of the heart rate (right) and of $\dot{V}_A$ (left).

The lines irradiating from the origin in the upper left diagram give the partial pressure of CO_2 in the alveoli. This seems to be constant at about 40 mm Hg independent of the work load. On this assumption (or measurement) then also the alveolar ventilation is defined.

If the stroke volume, q (lower right diagram) is quantitated as described above, discussing Fig. 15, the minute volume of the heart, $\dot{Q}$, and the ventilation perfusion coefficient, $\dot{V}_A/\dot{Q}$ (lower left diagram), are defined. This last value increases from a rest value of about 0.8 to a value of over 3.0 in maximal exercise, showing that, in this condition, the alveolar ventilation is in excess relative to the blood circulation through the alveoli. A limit to the maximum O_2 consumption (aerobic power) may, therefore, be set by a limitation of the blood minute volume, rather than by the capacity of the respiratory pump.

The changes between the sea level and the altitude conditions taking place at maximal exercise are given by the two parallelograms. Rest conditions have been omitted from the diagram.

In an acute hypoxic subject the Hb would remain at approximately the normal level but the arteriovenous difference in O_2 saturation decreases appreciably probably of the same order of magnitude as shown for chronic hypoxia. Then $(a\text{-}\bar{v})_{O_2}$ necessarily decreases, and assuming that the stroke volume, q, does not change, the oxygen pulse, p_{O_2}, correspondingly decreases. This involves a decrease of the maximum O_2 consumption. However, this decrease is not so pronounced as in chronic hypoxia (Fig. 14), in spite of the increased Hb content of the blood in the latter case. Evidently the decreased P_{O_2} in acute hypoxia is probably compensated by a higher heart rate than in chronic hypoxia. The increased resistance to circulation due to the increased erythrocyte concentration in the blood is possibly a limiting factor to the heart rate. A lower heart rate may be the only mechanism by which the minute volume of the heart can be decreased to meet the working possibilities of the anoxic heart.

Alternatively, the slightly lesser maximal O_2 consumption of chronic hypoxia could be related to a reduced stroke volume. This hypothesis however does not seem to be very plausible, and more data need to be collected to clarify this problem.

B. FACTORS LIMITING THE MAXIMUM AEROBIC POWER

The possible limiting factors to O_2 utilization by the tissues are
Lung factors:
  1. Alveolar ventilation ($\dot{V}_A$)
  2. Alveolocapillary diffusion of the respiratory gases through the lung (D_L)
Blood factors:
  3. O_2 and CO_2 uptake by the blood
Cardiovascular factors:
  4. Cardiac output ($\dot{Q}$)
  5. Perfusion of the active muscles ($\dot{Q}_{musc}$)
Tissue factors:
  6. Diffusion of the oxygen from the capillary to the cells ($D_{t_{O_2}}$)
  7. Ability of the cell itself to utilize oxygen

The pulmonary function does not seem to be a limiting factor to the maximum performance both in man (Asmussen and Nielsen, 1960) and in the dog (Cuttica et al., 1965). This is clearly demonstrated by the fact that $P_{a_{O_2}}$ and $P_{a_{CO_2}}$ seem to be unchanged even at the highest work load thus showing that the normal equilibrium is reached between capillary blood in the lungs and alveolar air. $P_{a_{CO_2}}$ particularly, if anything, tends to decrease when the exercise becomes severe as a consequence of the hyperventilation component due to the increased lactic acid concentration in the body fluids.

The changes induced by exercise on the cardiovascular function are described in Fig. 16. Cardiac output at steady state increases almost linearly in man with the O_2 uptake (Fig. 20). The $(a\text{-}\bar{v})_{O_2}$ difference increases also with increasing $\dot{V}_{O_2}$, only the rate of increase is progressively reduced. The maximal value seems to be about 15 ml for women and about 17 ml for men per 100 ml of blood (Fig. 17).

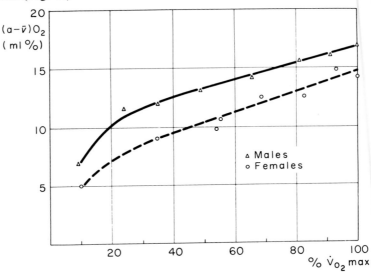

Fig. 17. Oxygen arteriovenous difference in milliliters per 100 ml of blood as a function of the work load in subjects exercising on a bicycle ergometer. (Drawn after Åstrand *et al.*, 1964.)

In the dog, Cerretelli *et al.* (1964) found that $\dot{Q}$ increases continuously with increasing $\dot{V}_{O_2}$. The maximal value of $\dot{Q}$ is reached when $\dot{V}_{O_2}$ is about 70% of the maximum. At the highest work levels, $\dot{Q}$ is constant, while the oxygen uptake still increases. Evidently in this range the increase of $\dot{V}_{O_2}$ is supported uniquely by the increase of the $(a\text{-}\bar{v})_{O_2}$ difference. This may indicate that in the dog the performance capability of the heart is one of the primary factors responsible for the limitation of the O_2 uptake.

The common observation that in both man and dog there is no substantial lactate production at work levels below that for which the maximum oxygen uptake is required, suggests that in this condition O_2 is available in an adequate amount at the tissue level. This means that the local peripheral circulatory factors are well adjusted to provide the required amount of O_2 to the active tissues. Only under certain conditions, such as when heavy work is performed by a limited group of muscles, does blood lactate increase when the $\dot{V}_{O_2}$ is sensibly below the overall maximal value. This indicates that the transport of O_2 to the working muscles is insufficient, and that the limitation of the aerobic power is due to a relatively inadequate local perfusion.

It is important, therefore, that an exercise involving great muscular masses be adopted in tests for maximum O_2 consumption or maximal minute volume of the heart, or when the production of lactic acid is to be considered as the anaerobic component of the total energy expenditure.

It has been observed (Cerretelli *et al.*, 1968) that treadmill exercise (walking or running at top speed on a given grade) meets these requirements, and that an additional work load on the arms does not increase significantly the O_2 consumption.

Taylor *et al.* (1955) found a slight increase, of about 200–250 ml/min, in subjects running on a treadmill at speeds and grades requiring a maximum O_2 uptake when they were operating at the same time a hand ergometer.

Christensen and Högberg (1950), on the other hand, report that one of their subjects was able to attain a significantly higher $\dot{V}_{O_2}$ while skiing than when cycling or running. It is difficult to establish whether this increase can be attributed to a further increase of cardiac output or to a higher desaturation of the mixed venous blood due to an increased work load on the lower limbs when skiing.

The tissue factor includes both the diffusion of O_2 from the blood capillary to the cell ($D_{t_{O_2}}$) and the chemical utilization of the oxygen inside the cells. Venous blood, collected from the isolated gastrocnemius muscle of the dog (di Prampero and Piiper, 1966), stimulated to perform submaximal and maximal work loads, contains very low O_2 concentrations (occasionally down to 1 vol %, or less) so that no margin for a further desaturation is left. This seems to indicate that neither the diffusion of O_2 from the blood to the cells nor the kinetics of the cell oxidative systems may be limiting the O_2 utilization capacity by the active tissues.

C. Kinetics of the O_2 Uptake at the Onset of Exercise and during the Recovery Phase

At the onset of an exercise of a given intensity, $\dot{V}_{O_2}$ increases gradually following a definite time course until a steady state is reached in 2–5 min, depending on the intensity of the exercise. If the exercise is interrupted abruptly, $\dot{V}_{O_2}$ decreases slowly, reaching the rest value in several minutes, also depending on the intensity of the exercise.

The recovery curve of O_2 consumption has been analyzed long ago by Margaria *et al.* (1933) and found to be an exponential function when the work load is light or moderate, or a more complex curve when the work load is very severe and lactic acid production occurs. The first process has been found to be a fast one, having a half reaction time of 30 sec; it has been called "alact-acid" as no lactic acid production was involved.

The recovery curve from an intense exercise has been analyzed and found to be composed of at least 2 components, the first of which had the same characteristics of the simple recovery curve typical of moderate exercise, while the second was indicative of a process also of an exponential type, having the same time constant of the lactic acid disappearance from the blood, i.e., about 15 min. It was therefore interpreted as the O_2 consumption required for the resynthesis of lactic acid to glycogen. Also this process has the significance of an O_2 debt payment, and this component was called "lactacid."

The kinetics of the O_2 uptake at the beginning of exercise has been investigated by De Moor (1954) and by Henry and De Moor (1956) and found to be also of an exponential type, the half reaction time being generally somewhat smaller than that of the recovery process. Cerretelli and Brambilla (1958) showed that the half reaction time is about the same ($t_{1/2} = 30$ sec) for both the initial and the recovery processes. Only at very high work levels does the speed of the O_2 uptake process appear to increase with the intensity of the exercise, in spite of the fact that the maximal O_2 consumption level is the same in all experiments. More recently, Margaria et al. (1965), assuming that

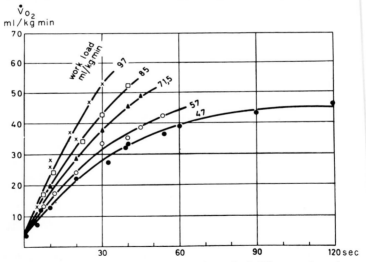

Fig. 18. O_2 consumption from the onset to the end of different exhausting exercises (running on a treadmill at different speed and inclines). The work load expressed in O_2 consumption per minute and per kilogram of body weight was calculated after Margaria et al. (1963a). The data are the average of 4 experiments on four different subjects. The lines appear to be exponential curves of the type $\dot{V}_{O_2} = 10^a (1 - 10^{-bt})$, where $\dot{V}_{O_2}$ is the O_2 consumption over the rest value, and 10^a the O_2 requirement for the work involved, b the speed constant and t the time in seconds. (From Margaria et al., 1965.)

the kinetics of O_2 consumption in the muscles is not a function of the O_2 consumption level actually reached, but of the energy expenditure (work load), this being expressed as O_2 requirement, found that the O_2 consumption curve at the onset of the exercise is an exponential function, independent of the work load, the half reaction time being in all cases 30 sec (Figs. 18 and 19).

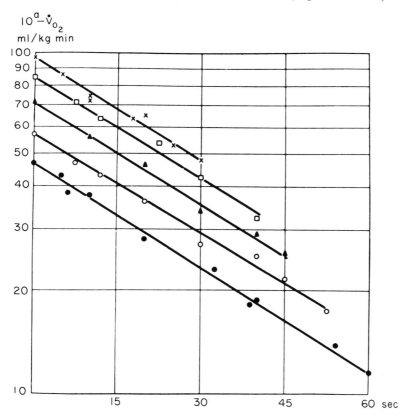

Fig. 19. The same data of Fig. 18 are plotted on a semilog scale, showing that for all work loads the function may be satisfactorily described by the formula given above, rearranged: $\log (10^a - \dot{V}_{O_2}) = a - bt$.

This result seems to indicate that the kinetics of the O_2 uptake is directly related to the rate of splitting of the high energy phosphate in the muscles. This process is directly related to work intensity. It indicates also that while the intracellular oxidative reactions can be started at a rate dictated by the energy requirement of the working muscles, the upper limit of the O_2 consumption is set by other factors, probably by the availability of O_2 at the tissue level, or by the transport capacity of O_2 to the tissues.

The kinetics of the O_2 uptake at the onset and at the end of the exercise has been studied also on the isolated gastrocnemius muscle of the dog by di Prampero and Piiper (1966). Here again both processes are of the exponential type, only they seem to proceed at a higher rate, the half reaction time appearing to be only 15–20 sec. A faster rate is not surprising if one considers that the O_2 debt as measured on the body as a whole includes not only the chemical energy stored in the muscles as high energy phosphate compounds, or as glycogen, but also the O_2 uptake from the O_2 stores of the body, as given by the lower O_2 saturation of the venous blood, of the myoglobin, etc., in exercise as compared to rest. This last fraction has not, obviously, the significance of a true muscular O_2 debt. When measuring the whole body O_2 debt, however, this appears greater than the true muscular one, as it can be measured directly on the isolated muscle. Its kinetics is also presumably slower, because respiratory and cardiovascular adaptations are required, and because the O_2 transport from the lungs to the active muscles requires a considerable time. The whole process of O_2 transport and utilization is, so to speak, buffered when the whole body is considered, and, therefore, its kinetics appears slower than when it is measured on the isolated muscle (Margaria, 1967).

D. Readjustment of the Cardiovascular and Respiratory Function to Exercise

If the minute volume of the heart measured at steady state is plotted as a function of the work load in terms of O_2 requirement, a straight line is obtained (Fig. 20). The minute volume, measured at the onset of exercise before a steady state is reached, is given in the same figure by the dots and triangles,

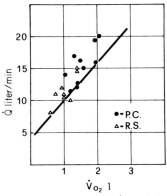

Fig. 20. Relationship between cardiac output ($\dot{Q}$) and O_2 uptake ($\dot{V}_{O_2}$) in exercising man. The line refers to data obtained at steady state. The dots and triangles are data obtained at the onset of exercise before a steady state was reached. (Modified after Cerretelli *et al.*, 1967.)

showing that in this condition the rise in the minute volume of the heart anticipates the rise of the O_2 consumption (Cerretelli *et al.*, 1967).

The line of Fig. 20 indicates that the minute volume of the heart is possibly adjusted to the metabolic needs of the working subject. At the onset of exercise, however, some extra stimulus to cardiac activity, presumably neurogenic, seems to be added.

In Fig. 21 the adjustments of some respiratory and cardiovascular functions at the onset of exercise are shown. The time course of the CO_2 output adjustment is about 30% slower than that of the O_2 uptake. Berg (1947) has

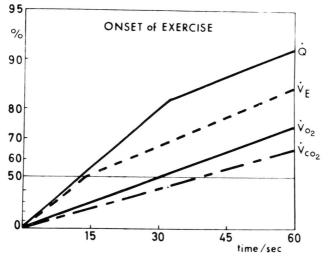

Fig. 21. Relative increase of $\dot{V}_{CO_2}$, $\dot{V}_{O_2}$, $\dot{V}_E$, and $\dot{Q}$ at the onset of exercise in percentage of the equilibrium levels. The ordinate is on a logarithmic scale. (Modified after Cerretelli *et al.*, 1967.)

shown essentially the same difference in moderate exercise during the transition from exercise to recovery. The time lag in the CO_2 elimination as compared to the O_2 uptake leads necessarily at the onset of the exercise to a relative retention of CO_2. The body stores of CO_2 increase; certainly the O_2 stores under these conditions decrease because of the lower O_2 saturation of the venous blood pool. A possible increase of the CO_2 stores may be related either to an increase of P_{CO_2}, or to a transient increase of the alkali reserve of the body. The alveolar P_{CO_2} falls appreciably in the first few seconds from the beginning of the exercise, and therefore no increase of CO_2 in the body can take place by way of P_{CO_2} increase. An increase of the alkali reserve, on the other hand, may well be brought about by the splitting of creatine phosphate. The products of the splitting are more alkaline than the unsplit creatine phosphate, and their concentration in the muscle increases leading to an alkalization of the muscle (Margaria, 1934; Dubuisson, 1937). These increased alkali may accommodate some of the CO_2 produced, which then escapes elimination through the lungs.

When a steady state in muscular exercise is reached, the ratio of split to unsplit phosphagen in the muscle is constant, and the alkali reserve of the body does not increase further. The CO_2 output must then keep pace with the O_2 consumption, as dictated by the well-known chemical factors on which the R.Q. value depends.

While both $\dot{V}_{O_2}$ and $\dot{V}_{CO_2}$ increase exponentially at the onset of exercise (the corresponding line of Fig. 21 plotted on logarithmic scale being straight), the lines for both $\dot{Q}$ and $\dot{V}_E$ are more complex; the first portion of these lines is steeper, showing that the kinetics of these 2 processes at the very beginning of the exercise is redundant as related to the gas exchange process.

The functional significance of this behavior for $\dot{Q}$ has been discussed above. The higher ventilation taking place at the onset of the exercise is evidenced by the drop of $P_{A_{CO_2}}$, and will be discussed further in Section III.

E. Diffusion of the Respiratory Gases through the Alveolocapillary Membrane

The diffusing capacity of the lung (D_L) gives an index of the dimensions and the other characteristics of the pulmonary membrane, which is made by all the tissue systems separating the blood in the lung capillaries from the air in the alveoli.

It has been found that D_L for O_2 averages 25 ml O_2 per mm Hg pressure gradient per minute at rest; it increases in exercise up to about 80.

According to Shepard et al. (1955), a maximal value for the diffusing capacity for O_2 is attained at work levels which are only half the maximal. When the diffusing capacity was measured for CO instead of for O_2, an increase up to the maximal work levels was found.

No conclusive evidence, however, is available at present concerning the possibility that the diffusion of the respiratory gases through the alveolocapillary membrane may limit the uptake of O_2 by the blood even at maximal work levels.

It has been shown that the arterial O_2 tension, even in the most severe exercise, does not undergo any significant change when compared to normal resting values. Evidently the diffusion of oxygen through the alveolocapillary membrane in the normal fit subject is sufficient to meet the demand.

The increased diffusing capacity of the lung as found at exercise is probably related to an increase of the number of pervious capillaries. Only a fraction of them in fact is open at rest. The opening of a number of capillaries in the lung, together with their dilation, gives a basis also for the relatively slight increase of blood pressure in the pulmonary bed at exercise in spite of the very considerable increase of cardiac output. Evidently this can be explained only with a decreased resistance to blood flow, and this can only take place through an increased cross-sectional area of the lung vessels.

This opening of the capillaries at exercise is particularly noticeable in the apex of the lungs. It seems that at rest capillaries in the upper portion of the lungs are in part collapsed because of gravitational factors. During work, a better perfusion of these regions is secured (see Fig. 22), as shown by West (1962).

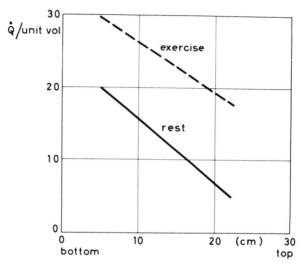

Fig. 22. Blood flow in different sections of the lung from the apex (top) to the base (bottom), in rest and at exercise. (Redrawn from West and Dollery, 1960.)

F. Ventilation–Perfusion Ratio at Exercise and the Alveoloarterious Gradient

The overall ventilation–perfusion ratio of the lung, which has a value of the order of magnitude of 0.8, approximately triples during exercise (see Fig. 15). In fact, while the ventilation increases up to about 15 times, the cardiac output increases only about 5 times.

The average $\dot{V}_A/\dot{Q}$ value is the result of the $\dot{V}_A/\dot{Q}$ values for all the individual gas exchanging units of the lung. In the single unit this ratio may vary from 0 (when the alveolus is only perfused and not ventilated) to ∞ when the alveolus is ventilated and not perfused. The composition of the mean alveolar gas is the result of the statistical distribution of the gas exchange in all the population of the gas exchanging units of the lung.

In an ideal lung in which $\dot{V}_A/\dot{Q}$ has the same value for all alveoli, if a diffusion equilibrium is reached between blood and alveolar air, the pressure of the gases at equilibrium is the same in the alveoli as in the blood capillaries. The possible existence of an alveoloarterial O_2 or CO_2 gradient would then be explained only by venous admixture (true shunt).

If, on the contrary, the ventilation–perfusion ratio is different for the different alveoli, the average gas tension in the alveoli will not have the same value as the capillary blood leaving them. The greater the variance of $\dot{V}_A/\dot{Q}$ from the mean value, the larger will be the difference in gas composition between alveoli and arterial blood.

A change of $\dot{V}_A/\dot{Q}$ at the level of each gas exchanger (alveolus) may be brought about by either a change in ventilation or a change in perfusion. Changes in ventilation occur during exercise, but they do not seem to affect appreciably the relative distribution within the lung. On the contrary, significant changes in perfusion in different sections of the lung have been recently shown to take place as an effect of exercise, as shown in Fig. 22 (data from West and Dollery, 1960).

In a normal lung, the P_{O_2} alveoloarterial difference amounts to 10–15mm Hg at rest. This includes both factors, the arteriovenous shunt and the ventilation–perfusion inequalities. It increases with exercise as shown in Fig. 23, where the work load is given as O_2 uptake (Asmussen and Nielsen, 1960).

As $P_{a_{O_2}}$ remains practically unchanged with increasing work load, the increased $(A-a)O_2$ gradient must be related to an increased $P_{A_{O_2}}$ value due to the hyperventilation that takes place, particularly at the highest work levels.

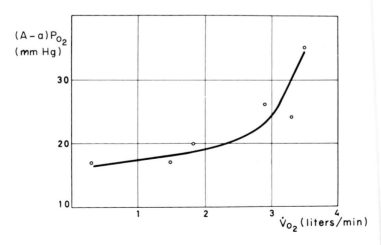

Fig. 23. Alveoloarterial P_{O_2} gradient as a function of $\dot{V}_{O_2}$ when breathing air (drawn from Asmussen and Nielsen data, 1960).

The O_2 saturation of the arterial blood does not decrease even at the maximal levels of exercise and this seems to support the view that in spite of the shorter time of equilibrium in the lung capillary, a diffusion equilibrium between blood and gas in the lungs is usually reached, as discussed above. It may well be that the alveoloarterial gradient tends to decrease in exercise as an effect of the lesser variance of the ventilation–perfusion ratio of the population of alveoli, but this effect is compensated at least in part by the smaller, insufficient diffusion time required for an equilibrium between capillary blood and alveolar air. This second effect may be predominant, and this is probably the reason for the overall *A-a* gradient increase in strenuous exercise, as shown in Fig. 23.

Also the shunt effect tends to decrease in exercise because its absolute value should be fairly constant, or at least it should not increase as much as the amount of blood flowing through the lungs. Its magnitude is therefore certainly not greater in exercise than at rest.

III. Control of Pulmonary Ventilation in Exercise

In 1796, Sausurre reported that at altitude the breathing pattern is different than at sea level. This was attributed to a reaction of the body to the changes of the surrounding medium, such that a constancy of the internal medium could be maintained. The O_2 content of the inspired gas was then the first mechanism considered responsible for changes of ventilation. About a century later, CO_2 (Pflüger, 1868) and the (H^+) concentration (Walter, 1877) were recognized as important respiratory stimulants.

The initial approach to the study of the problem of the regulation of respiration was for a great many years bound to the analysis of relatively simple mechanisms, and the control of respiration during exercise was dealt with in terms of a decrease of the arterial O_2 or of an increased CO_2. Much time was spent in discussing whether the stimulation of the respiratory center was due to the CO_2 as such or the H^+ ions released by carbonic acid, H_2CO_3, the hydrated form of CO_2.

The exercise hyperpnea mechanism being simply interpreted in terms of chemical changes in the blood or at the respiratory center level appeared unsatisfactory to many authors. In fact, neither CO_2, nor anoxia, even combined, lead to such ventilation values that are observed in exercise. The possibility that, besides the chemical, other stimuli of a different nature originating from active muscles may affect respiration has therefore been raised, and will be discussed below.

A. Humoral Theories

The chemical substances transported by the blood stream that may be responsible for the hyperpnea of exercise are as follows.

1. Carbon dioxide

The CO_2 production is largely increased in muscular exercise, and this should lead to an increased concentration of CO_2 in the blood sufficient to stimulate the respiratory center, The hyperventilation that follows would lead to a decreased blood CO_2 content, so that the whole process of the regulation of respiration could be considered as a simple feedback system, well apt to regulate the CO_2 output according to its production and to maintain a reasonable level of CO_2 in the blood.

The blood CO_2 increase during exercise, however, is very small as compared to the CO_2 increase obtained by administration of CO_2 that is required to bring about the same ventilation response when the subject is at rest.

2. Increase of H^+ Ion Concentration

The increased H^+ ion concentration of the arterial blood (acidification of the blood) due to CO_2 accumulation (Winterstein, 1911) has never been observed in mild or even in sustained exercise. Only during strenuous exercise when significant amounts of lactic acid are produced does the H^+ ion concentration of the arterial blood increase (Fig. 13). To give reason for the lack of an evident relation between blood pH and respiratory activity, Winterstein in his late years put forward the hypothesis that even if a blood pH decrease cannot be detected, a change in this direction may take place in the intracellular fluid of the responsible cells of the respiratory center. This assumption, however, is not very plausible, as the increased H^+ ion concentration in the respiratory center cells should be the result of their activity, i.e., it should follow the hyperpnea and, therefore, it cannot be responsible for eliciting the increased ventilation.

3. Decrease of Arterial P_{O_2}

A possible decrease of arterial P_{O_2} during exercise may take place as discussed above (see Section II). This, however, cannot amount to more than a few mm Hg, as the saturation of the arterial blood with O_2 is not appreciably affected in strenuous exercise. Anoxia affects respiration by eliciting a chemoreflexogenic drive from the chemoceptors located in the carotic bodies or in the aortic arch. The threshold for a sizable effect of this type is however very low, at about $P_{aO_2} = 60$ mm Hg, a value which is not reached breathing air at sea level.

The existence of other specific chemical receptors affecting respiration, located possibly in the internal jugular vein (Lambertsen et al., 1959), in the vena cava, in the right atrium (Riley and Ross, 1961), or in the pulmonary artery (Armstrong, 1961) has also been postulated.

4. Nonsubstantiated Theories

The release of substances formed in the muscles during activity and having some effects on respiration, such as the hypothetical "hyperpnein" (Y. Henderson) or "respiratory X factor," has been postulated to give a basis for the hyperpnea. Such substances, however, have never been identified, and no evidence for their existence has ever been collected.

In conclusion, all the humoral mechanisms postulated, even if considered to be at work at the same time, do not seem to give the basis for an effective regulation of the ventilation such as takes place in exercise. Ventilation increases linearly with O_2 uptake within the limits of aerobic metabolism,

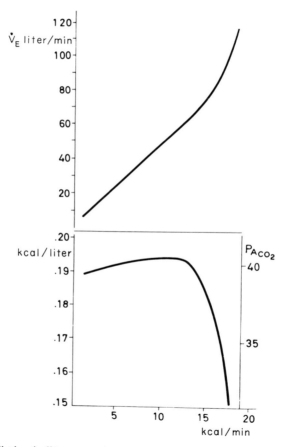

Fig. 24. Ventilation in liters per minute as a function of metabolism (upper diagram) and the tangent of this line (lower diagram) being equivalent to the efficiency of ventilation in kilocalories per liter (scale at left) or in $P_{A_{CO_2}}$ (scale at right).

independent of any chemical change in the blood. Only when oxidation become insufficient, an additional stimulus to ventilation is evident (see Fig. 24), and the slope of the line, i.e., dV_E/dV_{O_2}, increases. However, this increase is small when compared to the overall ventilation due to exercise and considering the relevancy of the chemical changes occurring at that level evidenced by the consistent increase of the lactic acid and of the H^+ ion concentration of the blood. This last factor particularly seems to have been greatly overemphasized in view of the data of the experiment of Fig. 13.

B. Neurogenic Theories

Krogh and Lindhard (1913, 1917) were the first to interpret the sudden increase of ventilation at the onset of exercise on nervous grounds; impulses arising in the motor cortex and radiating to the respiratory center would increase the respiratory activity.

Later, Harrison et al. (1932) evidenced a ventilatory response to passive movements of the limbs. The impulses would presumably originate in the mechanoceptors of the muscle, joints, and tendons, and they would be carried through afferent fibers to the respiratory center. This effect is abolished by deafferentation, which shows its reflex nature. Comroe and Schmidt (1943), however, found that the mechanoceptors involved are limited to the joints, while those of the muscle or tendons do not seem to take any part in this action.

Kao (1963) in cross-circulation experiments on dogs showed that the hyperventilation accompanying muscular activity is limited to the exercising dog (neural). In the other dog (humoral), whose head was perfused by blood coming from the active limbs of the neural dog, the ventilation remained constant. The hyperventilation in the neural dog was obviously not due to the chemical stimulation of the respiratory center, as no chemical changes took place in the blood of the humoral dog.

Also Asmussen and Nielsen (1950) showed that if the venous return from the exercising legs is blocked by an inflated cuff applied to the limbs so that the metabolically produced CO_2 does not reach the lung, $P_{A_{CO_2}}$ tends to decrease. This seems to indicate that the respiratory center was affected only by impulses reaching it through the only possible way, the nervous one, all chemical substances produced in the limbs as an effect of the exercise being unable to reach the centers.

On the other hand it is well known that at the onset of exercise pulmonary ventilation increases abruptly in a much shorter time than the circulation time, i.e., before chemical substances formed in the muscles as a consequence of their activity can reach the respiratory center.

Furthermore this leads to an initial fall of $P_{A_{CO_2}}$, thus indicating that the chemical stimulus of the R.C. decreases in that short time, possibly masking in part the neurogenic stimulation effect. Although some of this effect has been shown to be due to a conditional reflex, for a consistent fraction of it at least other nervous mechanisms are responsible, presumably impulses arising from the exercising limbs (Torelli and Brandi, 1961).

The ventilatory response to exercise cannot, however, be explained only on neurogenic grounds, particularly if consideration is taken of its very high level of adequacy in maintaining the chemical composition of the blood the same as at rest in relation to CO_2, arterial O_2, and H^+ ion concentration.

Presumably, therefore, both humoral and neurogenic mechanisms are involved for the most effective control of respiration in muscular exercise.

C. NEUROHUMORAL THEORIES

Dejours (1959, 1963, 1964) recorded ventilation and $P_{A_{CO_2}}$ on a single breath to detect the very fast changes of ventilation at the onset and at the end of exercise. The ventilation increases abruptly at the onset of the exercise, this causing a fall of $P_{A_{CO_2}}$. The ventilation thereafter increases more slowly, reaching a steady state in a few minutes, while $P_{A_{CO_2}}$ increases to reach the pre-exercise or a somewhat higher level. Corresponding changes take place when the work is abruptly stopped. A sudden fall of $\dot{V}_E$, accompanied by a transitory increase of $P_{A_{CO_2}}$, is followed by a more slow return to the rest value.

The fast changes taking place at the transition of the activity levels are interpreted as neurogenic, while the following slower processes may be interpreted on a humoral basis.

According to Dejours, a quantitative evaluation of both nervous and humoral components of the ventilatory response to exercise can be done by

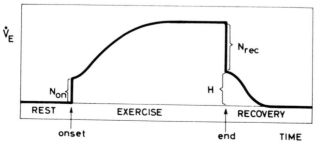

Fig. 25. Changes of pulmonary ventilation as an effect of exercise. The abrupt change indicated by N at the beginning and at the end of exercise has been attributed to a neural stimulus to the respiratory center; the slow change of ventilation (H) to humoral factors.

measuring the nervous (N) and the humoral (H) components of the change of ventilation at the end of the exercise, calculated on the assumption given above, and illustrated schematically in Fig. 25. However, such evaluation is difficult, as the results of different authors show some discrepancies. It is perhaps not too far from reality to consider as a first approximation that the neurogenic and the humoral mechanisms contribute to about the same extent to the increase of pulmonary ventilation in muscular exercise.

Fenn (1963) thinks that the contribution of the neurogenic component is appreciably more sizable than the chemical one, and that it consists mainly in the gross regulation of the ventilation. The function of the humoral component seems to be limited to the fine adjustment of the $P_{A_{CO_2}}$, such that its variations from the rest value to exercise are kept very small. This conclusion

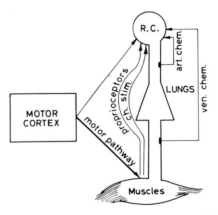

Fig. 26. Schematic representation of the mechanisms controlling breathing at exercise. For explanation see text. (Modified after Dejours, 1964.)

was reached on the basis of the observation that no gross change of $P_{A_{CO_2}}$ can be observed at exercise, while a great change of $P_{A_{CO_2}}$ must take place to give the same ventilation value when CO_2 is administered.

Figure 26 summarizes all the mechanisms that have been postulated as acting on the respiratory center in muscular exercise. They are

1. Impulses irradiating from the motor cortex
2. Impulses originated in the peripheral mechanoceptors
3. Chemical substances produced in muscle as a consequence of their activity and being transported to the respiratory center by the blood stream
4. Impulses arising from the presso- and chemoceptors of the arterial section, and of the venous section of the vascular bed

REFERENCES

Agostoni, E. (1961). *J. Appl. Physiol.* **16**, 1055.

Agostoni, E. (1963). *Med. Sport (Turin)* **3**, 635.

Agostoni, E., Sant'Ambrogio, G., and Del Portillo Carrasco, G. H. (1960). *J. Appl. Physiol.* **15**, 1093.

Armstrong, B. W. (1961). *Science* **133**, 1897.

Asmussen, E., and Nielsen, M. (1950). *Acta Physiol. Scand.* **20**, 79.

Asmussen, E., and Nielsen, M. (1960). *Acta Physiol. Scand.* **50**, 153.

Åstrand, P. O., Cuddy, T. E., Saltin, B., and Stenberg, J. (1964). *J. Appl. Physiol.* **19**, 268.

Berg, W. E. (1947). *Am. J. Physiol.* **149**, 597.

Brambilla, I., Cerretelli, P., and Brandi, G. (1958). *Boll. Soc. Ital. Biol. Sper.* **34**, 1820.

Campbell, E. J. M. (1958). "The Respiratory Muscle and the Mechanics of Breathing." Lloyd Luke, London.

Cerretelli, P., and Brambilla, I. (1958). *Boll. Soc. Ital. Biol. Sper.* **34**, 679.

Cerretelli, P., and Margaria, R. (1961). *Intern. Z. Angew. Physiol.* **18**, 460.

Cerretelli, P., di Prampero, P. E., and Sassi, G. In preparation. (1968).

Cerretelli, P., Piiper, J., Mangili, F., Cuttica, F., and Ricci, B. (1964). *J. Appl. Physiol.* **19**, 29.

Cerretelli, P., Sikand, R., and Farhi, L. E. (1967). *J. Appl. Physiol.* **21**, 1345.

Christensen, E. H., and Högberg, P. (1950). *Arbeitsphysiol.* **14**, 292.

Comroe, J. H., Jr., and Schmidt, C. F. (1943). *Am. J. Physiol.* **138**, 546.

Cuttica, F., Cerretelli, P., Mangili, F., and Piiper, J. (1965). *Boll. Soc. Ital. Biol. Sper.* **41**, 1556.

Dejours, P. (1959). *J. Physiol. (Paris)* **51**, 163.

Dejours, P. (1963). *In* "Regulation of Human Respiration" (D. J. C. Cunningham and B. B. Lloyd, eds.), pp. 535–548. Blackwell, Oxford.

Dejours, P. (1964). *In* "Handbook of Physiology" (Am. Physiol. Soc., J. Field, ed.), Sect. 3, Vol. 1, pp. 631–649. Williams & Wilkins, Baltimore, Maryland.

De Moor, J. (1954). *J. Appl. Physiol.* **6**, 460.

di Prampero, P. E., and Piiper, J. (1966). Personal Communication.

Dubuisson, M. (1937). *Proc. Soc. Exptl. Biol. Med.* **35**, 609.

Elsner, R. W., Bolstad, A., and Forno, C. (1964). *In* "The Physiological Effects of High Altitude" (W. H. Weihe, ed.), pp. 217–223. Pergamon Press, Oxford.

Fenn, W. O. (1951). "Studies in Respiratory Physiology," Wright Patterson Air Force Tech. Rept. No. 6528, p. 156.

Fenn, W. O. (1963). *Atti Accad. Med. Lombarda* **18**, 1.

Harrison, W. G., Calhoun, J. A., and Harrison, T. R. (1932). *Am. J. Physiol.* **100**, 68.

Henry, F. M., and De Moor, J. (1956). *J. Appl. Physiol.* **8**, 608.

Kao, F. F. (1963). *In* "Regulation of Human Respiration" (D. J. C. Cunningham and B. B. Lloyd, eds.), pp. 461–502. Blackwell, Oxford.

Krogh, A., and Lindhard, J. (1913). *J. Physiol. (London)* **47**, 112.

Krogh, A., and Lindhard, J. (1917). *J. Physiol. (London)* **51**, 182.

Lambertsen, C. J., Owen, S. G., Wendel, H., Stroud, M. W., Lurie, A. A., Lochner, W., and Clark, G. F. (1959). *J. Appl. Physiol.* **14**, 966.

Margaria, R. (1934). *J. Physiol. (London)* **82**, 496.

Margaria, R. (1937). *Arch. Sci. Biol. (Bologna)*, **23**, 266.

Margaria, R. (1966). *Arch. Fisiol.* **64**, 45.

Margaria, R. (1967). *In* "Exercise at Altitude" (R. Margaria, ed.), pp. 15–32. Excerpta Medica Foundation.

Margaria, R., and Marro, F. (1955). *Exptl. Med. Surg.* **13**, 249.

Margaria, R., and Talenti, C. (1933). *Arch. Fisiol.* **32**, 165.

Margaria, R., Edwards, H. T., and Dill, D. B. (1933). *Am. J. Physiol.* **106**, 689.

Margaria, R., Milic-Emili, G., Petit, J. M., and Cavagna, G. (1960). *J. Appl. Physiol.* **15**, 354.

Margaria, R., Cerretelli, P., Aghemo, P., and Sassi, G. (1963a). *J. Appl. Physiol.* **18**, 367.

Margaria, R., Cerretelli, P., di Prampero, P. E., Massari, C., and Torelli, G. (1963b). *J. Appl. Physiol.* **18**, 371.

Margaria, R., Mangili, F., Cuttica, F., and Cerretelli, P. (1965). *Ergonomics* **8**, 49.

Mead, J. (1960). *J. Appl. Physiol.* **15**, 325.

Milic-Emili, G., and Petit, J. M. (1959). *Arch. Sci. Biol.* (*Bologna*) **43**, 326.

Petit, J. M., Milic-Emili, G., and Koch, R. (1959). *Arch. Intern. Physiol. Biochim.* **67**, 350.

Petit, J. M., Milic-Emili, G., and Delhez, L. (1960). *J. Appl. Physiol.* **15**, 1101.

Pflüger, E. (1868). *Arch. Ges. Physiol.* **1**, 61.

Rahn, H., Otis, A. B., Chadwick, L. E., and Fenn, W. O. (1946). *J. Physiol.* (*London*) **146**, 161.

Riley, R. L., and Ross, R. S. (1961). *Federation Proc.* **20**, 131.

Saibene, F., Mognoni, P., and Sant'Ambrogio, G. (1965). *Boll. Soc. Ital. Biol. Sper.* **41**, 1550.

Shepard, R. H., Cohn, J. E., Cohen, G., Armstrong, B. W., Carroll, D. G., Donoso, H., and Riley, R. L. (1955). *Am. Rev. Tuberc. Pulmonary Diseases* **71**, 249.

Taylor, H. L., Buskirk, E., and Henschel, A. (1955). *J. Appl. Physiol.* **8**, 73.

Torelli, G., and Brandi, G. (1961). *Intern. Z. Angew. Physiol.* **19**, 134.

Walter, F. (1877). *Arch. Exptl. Pathol. Pharmakol.* **7**, 148.

West, J. B. (1962). *J. Appl. Physiol.* **17**, 893.

West, J. B., and Dollery, C. T. (1960). *J. Appl. Physiol.* **15**, 405.

Winterstein, H. (1911). *Arch. Ges. Physiol.* **138**, 167.

3

THE CARDIOVASCULAR SYSTEM IN EXERCISE

K. Lange Andersen

I. Introduction

The function of the circulatory system is to provide a proper environment for the functioning of the cells. The exchange of metabolic material and respiratory gases takes place in the capillaries which are thus the focal point of activity in the circulatory system. Because of continuous cell activity a proper cellular environment can only be maintained by an uninterrupted flow of blood to the tissues. The rate of tissue metabolism is not constant, but varies, sometimes rather drastically. The demand of blood flowing through the tissue varies accordingly and the blood flow rate is, in general, closely related to the state of tissue metabolism. A change in the rate of metabolism in one organ usually requires adjustments, which involve the whole cardio-vascular system.

Muscle contraction is the activity which may cause the largest increase in metabolism of any tissue. The muscles are also by far the largest organs of the body, amounting to about 40% of the total body weight. During exercise the blood flow to the muscles is primarily adjusted to cover the needs of the increased muscle metabolism, and may increase manyfold above that at rest. In addition the regulation of body temperature puts extra strain on the circulatory system during work, because the extra heat produced by the contracting muscles must be eliminated. Consequently, muscular exercise requires a drastic adjustment of the circulatory functioning with increased cardiac output in addition to a scrupulous regulation of regional blood flow.

A proper understanding of the circulatory system's response to exercise and its adaptation to training can not be gained without knowledge of the fundamental functional properties of this system. Detailed information of this subject can be read in standard textbooks of physiology; only a brief summary will be presented here.

II. General Features of the Function of the Cardiovascular System

A. THE MICROCIRCULATION

The cross sectional area of the aorta is approximately 2.5 cm², and the combined cross sectional area of all the capillaries together is estimated to be 1700 cm². This means that the velocity of blood flow in the capillaries is much less than in the aorta, at rest approximately 0.5 cm/sec against 24 cm/sec in the aorta. The capillaries have a length of 1 to 2 mm. Therefore, blood remains in the capillaries only 1 to 2 sec.

Figure 1 shows schematically the structure of a unit capillary bed. Blood enters the unit through an arteriole and leaves it by way of a venule. Blood from an arteriole passes into a series of metarterioles before it enters the capillaries. The arterioles are highly muscular, and their diameter can change manyfold by contraction and relaxation of the muscles. The metarterioles have fewer muscle fibers. At the origin of the true capillaries a smooth muscle fiber usually encircles the capillary and is named the precapillary sphincter. The venules are larger than the arterioles and are less supported with muscle fibers, but functionally they may act as postcapillary resistance vessels.

The capillary tubes consist of a single layer of endothelial cells, which rest on a thin continuous membrane. The physiological evidence accumulated to date indicates that the capillary wall contains pores through which constituents of plasma and extracellular fluid may pass. So far, the electron microscope has failed to locate such pores, but on the basis of the size of molecules which are known to pass the membrane by diffusion, it has been estimated that the diameter of the pores is 30–50 Å.

Microscopic examinations of a capillary unit have revealed that not all capillary networks contain blood at the same time. The proportion of active to inactive capillaries varies in accordance with the level of tissue metabolism. These variations are caused by contraction and relaxation of metarterioles and precapillary sphincters.

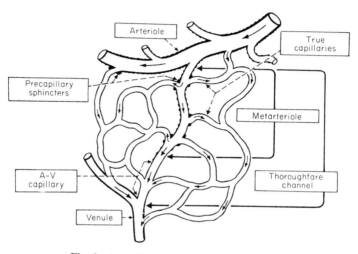

Fig. 1. A capillary unit (from Selkurt, 1962).

Molecules pass through the pores of the capillary membranes; large amounts of water, respiratory gases, and material can diffuse back and forth between the blood and the extracellular spaces, and hence between the extra- and intracellular fluid. This process of diffusion is caused by kinetic motion of molecules in both the plasma and the extra- and intracellular fluids, and is regulated to maintain static conditions in the extracellular fluid, or the homeostasis of the "millieu interne."

The transcapillary exchange of water depends upon the relationship between the forces which move molecules from the blood (filtration), and the forces which move water from the extracellular fluid into the blood (absorption). The total filtration pressure for water movement is the sum of the hydrostatic capillary pressure and the colloidosmotic pressure exerted by the concentration of proteins in the extracellular fluids. The total absorption pressure is the combined force of the hydrostatic extracellular fluid pressure and the osmotic pressure exerted by the plasma proteins.

The capillary hydrostatic pressure undergoes significant changes from the arterial to the venous end of the vessels. The pressure at the arterial end is estimated to be about 35 mm Hg at rest which is raised during exercise because the arterial pressure increases, and that at the venous end about 15 mm Hg which is not much changed by muscle contractions. Mean capillary pressure at rest is about 25 mm.

The hydrostatic pressure of the extracellular fluid is normally very low, 1 to 2 mm, but may be raised considerably in the muscle tissue during contraction, probably exceeding the intracapillary hydrostatic pressure at the peak of contraction.

Since the proteins mainly are restricted to the circulatory compartment, and since the electrolytes are osmotically ineffective across the capillary wall because they rapidly equilibrate between the two compartments by diffusion, the effective osmotic pressure is provided by the proteins of the plasma. The plasma colloid osmotic pressure is 28 mm Hg, the plasma albumins exerting the major effect. Due to hemoconcentration the plasma colloid osmotic pressure is raised in muscular exercise.

Total diffusion across the capillary membrane depends greatly upon the size of the surface area available for diffusion. Capillary surface area is determined by the luminal diameter of the vessels and of the number of active capillaries. Capillary surface area is directly related to the capillary blood volume, which is related to the inflow and outflow of blood. Consequently factors which influence the capillary pressures may also affect capillary surface area.

Regulation of capillary pressure and surface area is by means of two mechanisms. For the first, capillary dynamics and volume are altered by changes in arterial and venous pressure. The second mechanism is an autoregulation which tends to maintain adequate capillary pressure and normal relationship between filtration and absorption despite variation in capillary blood flow and infusion pressure.

B. THE HEART

1. Structural Properties

The heart is a hollow muscular pump subdivided internally into 4 chambers, the right and left auricles (or atria) and the right and left ventricles. From a functional standpoint the heart may be divided into the right part, which receives blood from the veins and pumps it out through the lungs (the pulmonary circulation), and the left part which receives the oxygenated blood from the lungs and pumps it through the aorta and into the systemic arteries and further into all the tissues of the body (the systemic circulation).

The auricles are thin walled chambers and they can only exert little contractile power. They serve primarily to collect and store the blood brought to them from the veins, and then pass this blood into the ventricles during their period of relaxation or diastole. The ventricles, on the other hand, are thick walled chambers that are able to exert a considerable force during contraction or systole.

The cardiac muscle, the myocardium, is composed of 3 major types of fibers, the atrial and ventricular muscles, and the specialized excitatory and conductive structures.

The atrial and ventricular muscles are striated in the same typical manner as skeletal muscles; the myofibrils contain actin and myosin filaments embedded in sarcoplasma. A reticular structure, the sarcoplasmatic reticulum, envelops the myofibrils and probably transmits the action potential from the outside membrane of the fiber to the interior. The actin and myosin filaments interdigitate and slide along each other during the process of contraction.

The cardiac muscle fibers are in reality muscle cells connected in series. The action potential, wherever it begins, travels through the cardiac muscle and spreads to all the fibers at much the same speed and without significant hindrance through the fiber connections. Therefore, cardiac muscle is a functional syncytium, and when one of the cells becomes excited the action potential spreads to all of them, causing a single contraction. In this process the cardiac muscle follows the all-or-nothing principle. The heart beat is thus a myocardial twitch. Since the refractory period of the myocardial muscle fibers is prolonged compared to that of the skeletal muscle, temporal and normal summation cannot be obtained, which prevents tetanization.

The atrial and ventricular syncytium are connected by the conducting fibers of the A-V bundle, which are specialized muscle fibers with few contractile elements. Other than for this connection the atrial and ventricular muscles are separated from each other by the fibrous tissue surrounding the valvular ring.

The excitatory and conductive system that controls the cardiac contractions is schematically illustrated in Fig. 2. The sino-atrial (S-A) node is a small specialized section of the atrial muscle, approximately 3 mm wide and 1 cm long. The S-A fibers are connected in series with the other atrial fibers so that action potential that begins in the S-A node travels inevitably into the atrium.

The resting membrane potential of the S-A fibers is low, only 55–60 mV compared to 80–90 mV for the other cardiac muscle fibers. This low resting potential is probably related to a high conductivity of sodium through the membrane, and this feature could account for the rhythmic self-excitation.

The S-A nodal fibers, when not stimulated from any outside sources, discharge at an intrinsic rhythmic rate of 70–80/min, and is the normal pacemaker of the heart. The impulse excites the atrial muscles and a contraction follows. The action potential spreads via the A-V node through the A-V bundle and Purkinje fibers into the ventricles which become excited and contract.

The depolarization and repolarization of the cardiac muscle is reflected in the electrocardiogram.

The heart is well supplied with both sympathetic and parasympathetic (vagal) nerve fibers. Stimulation of the vagi releases the hormone acetylcholine from the nerve endings. Acetylcholine decreases the rate of rhythmic excitation from the S-A node, and retards the speed by which the impulses travel into the ventricles.

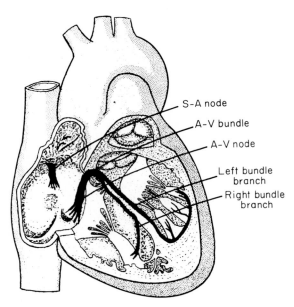

Fig. 2. The excitatory and conductive system of the heart (from Guyton, 1966).

Sympathetic stimulation releases noradrenaline from the nerve endings which has the opposite effect on the heart to that caused by vagal stimulation. Noradrenaline or norepinephrine increases the rate of S-A discharge, increases the excitability of all portions of the heart, and increases greatly the force of contraction.

2. Cardiac Output

From a functional standpoint cardiac output is the most important aspect of heart function. Cardiac output is the volume of blood pumped by each ventricle per minute, and is the product of stroke volume and heart rate as expressed in the following equation:

$$Q = S.V. \times f \tag{1}$$

where

   Q = Volume of blood in liters per minute
$S.V.$ = Volume of each stroke in liters (or milliliters)
  f = Number of beats per minute

It follows from the formula that cardiac output may be raised either by increasing the stroke volume, the heart rate, or both.

The cardiac output is regulated by two basic mechanisms: (1) intrinsic autoregulation in response to the amount of venous return of blood to the heart, and (2) control by the autonomic nervous system.

One of the major factors determining the amount of blood which the heart pumps out each minute is the rate of blood flow into the heart, the venous return. As each peripheral tissue of the body to a large extent controls its own blood flow, this implies that the total venous return is controlled by the peripheral tissue. That the heart in turn has the ability automatically to pump the incoming blood into the arteries, so that it can flow around the system again, means that cardiac output is controlled by the peripheral tissue, and that the level of cardiac output is set and regulated by the total metabolic activity of the body. This intrinsic ability of the heart to adapt itself to increasing loads of inflowing blood is called Starling's law of the heart.

Basically Starling's law states that the greater the ventricles are filled during diastole, the greater will be the amount of blood pumped into aorta. Or in other words: The heart pumps, within physiological limits, all the blood that flows into it.

Humeral factors play a minor role in the regulation of cardiac output, but cathecolamines affect the heart in the same direction as sympathetic stimulation.

C. HEMODYNAMICS OF SYSTEMIC AND PULMONARY CIRCULATION

1. Pressures

At its simplest the circulation consists of a pump feeding a high pressure system, and a low pressure capacity system, or venous compartment which in turn drives the pump.

When blood is pumped from the heart, the arteries are distended and pressure is developed in the arterial system. At rest the systolic pressure of the systemic arteries is normally 120–140 mm Hg, the diastolic pressure 70–90 mm Hg, and mean pressure about 100 mm Hg. These figures refer to young adult healthy subjects. The resting arterial pressure becomes increased with age.

The pulmonary circulation is a low pressure and low resistance system. At rest systolic pulmonary arterial pressure is about 20–22 mm Hg, diastolic pulmonary arterial pressure 5 mm Hg and mean pulmonary arterial pressure 14 mm Hg. As the blood flows through the circulatory system, the pressure falls approximately to 0 by the time it reaches the atria.

The veins including venous sinuses contain at rest approximately 50% of the total blood volume, the heart and pulmonary vessels about 30%, and only 15% remains in the arteries. The volume of blood in the capillaries is about 5% of the total blood volume. These figures demonstrate the significance of the blood storing function of the veins. During exercise the veins contract, the blood depots thus become reduced and the effective amount of circulating blood is increased.

The systemic arterial pressure is normally regulated to a level much higher than needed to assure adequate flow of blood to the peripheral tissues. This high inflow pressure allows the tissues to increase their blood flow immediately, simply by means of dilating their resistance vessels. During muscular exercise and in other stresses which demand a high perfusion rate of blood, the blood flow cannot be increased sufficiently by the dilatation of the arterioles. In addition the arterial pressure is increased to provide better conditions for blood flow.

There are three basic mechanisms which normally regulate the arterial blood pressure: (1) regulations by the autonomic nervous system, (2) regulation by the kidneys, and (3) humeral regulation by endocrine glands.

The blood pressure is sensed by pressoreceptors or mechanoreceptors which primarily are located in the arch of the aorta and in the carotid body, but also may be found in the large veins, in the cardiac chambers and in the pulmonary artery. The impulses from the mechanoreceptors travel along different nerves to the cardiovascular centers or stations located in the brain stem where the signals are integrated and by means of interneurons connected to the effector neurons. The cardial neurons in the brain stem are powerfully influenced by an impulse flow along the corticohypothalamic pathway.

The effector mechanism is dual. Blood pressure is changed by variation in either cardiac ouput (vagal or sympathetic stimulation) or by variation of peripheral resistance (by changing the sympathetic vasoconstrictor tone).

When the blood flow to the kidneys is restricted, the arterial pressure progressively increases over a period of days. The mechanism for this increase is not well understood.

At least 3 hormones may influence the arterial blood pressure. These are the vasopressin of the posterior hypophysis, the catecholamines from the adrenal medulla, and the aldosterone of the adrenal cortex.

2. Resistance and Conductance

A pressure gradient between 2 ends of a vessel causes blood to flow from the high pressure area toward the low pressure area while resistance impedes the flow. This can be expressed mathematically as follows:

$$Q = \frac{\Delta P}{R} \qquad (2)$$

where

Q = Blood flow (in liters or ml/min)
ΔP = Pressure gradient (mm Hg) between the 2 ends
R = Resistance

The formula may also be written in two other forms:

$$\Delta P = Q \times R \qquad (3)$$

$$R = \frac{\Delta P}{Q} \qquad (4)$$

Resistance is the impediment to blood flow in a vessel. It cannot be measured by any direct means, but must be calculated on a basis of the measurement of flow and pressure gradient. If the pressure gradient between 2 points in a vessel is 1 mm Hg, and the flow is 1 ml/sec, then the resistance is said to be 1 peripheral resistance unit. In the CGS system the unit of resistance is expressed in dynes sec/cms^5, and is calculated according to the following formula:

$$R \left(\text{in } \frac{\text{dynes sec}}{\text{cm}^5} \right) = \frac{1333 \times \text{mm Hg}}{\text{ml/sec}} \qquad (5)$$

Conductance is the reciprocal of resistance in accordance with the following equation:

$$\text{Conductance} = \frac{1}{\text{Resistance}} \qquad (6)$$

The cardiac output at rest (basal state) is close to 100 ml/sec and the pressure gradient from the systemic arteries to the veins is about 100 mm Hg. Therefore, the total peripheral resistance of the entire systemic circulation is approximately 1 peripheral resistance unit, or in CGS units 1333 dynes sec cm^{-5}.

In the pulmonary system the mean arterial pressure is 14 mm Hg and the mean left atrial pressure about 4 mm Hg, giving a pressure gradient of 10 mm Hg. The total pulmonary resistance is calculated to be about 0.12 peripheral resistance unit.

D. PERIPHERAL CIRCULATION AND REGULATION OF TISSUE BLOOD FLOW

The circulatory system is a closed circuit, and the blood circulates continuously through this circuit, propelled by the pumping action of the heart.

The peripheral circulatory system is divided into the distributory vessels which are the aorta, the branching arteries and the arterioles, the exchange vessels or capillaries, and the collecting system of venules and veins. Since the distributing vessels are elastic structures, they serve to change the rate of blood flow in the arterial system. In this way the rhythmic outflow from the heart is converted into a fairly smooth flow of blood in the arterioles and capillaries (Wind-Kessel-Effect).

The blood flows easily in all parts of the circulatory system except in the resistance vessels, which comprise a major precapillary section (small arteries, arterioles, precapillary section of the capillary unit, and also venules and small veins).

In the resistance vessels the pressure drop is considerable and can be altered by changing the luminal diameter of these vessels by the action of smooth muscles. The changes in the luminal diameter are responsible for variation in the regional blood flow, which is regulated by intrinsic and extrinsic mechanisms. The resistance in an organ is usually regulated so that the adequate amount of blood flow is assured according to the need set by the metabolic activity. This regulation is mainly an autoregulation by intrinsic mechanisms. Local metabolities or a drop in oxygen tension may produce a vasodilatation effect, but the nature of the local process governing the vasodilatation is not known.

Normal blood pressure could hardly be maintained if local needs were allowed to dominate the activity of the resistance vessels. The nervous system exerts a strong influence by means of sympathetic nerve fibers which generally carry vasoconstrictor activity. Sympathetic nerve fibers to the skeletal and cardiac muscles also carry vasodilator activity. Thus, the nervous system is allowed a control of vascular resistance always appropriate to provide adequate pressures in the arterial system, mainly by means of the mechanoreceptor reflex control system. This extrinsic nervous control of the resistance vessels means that local blood supply may temporarily be reduced below the demand level in order to provide sufficient blood to organs when the organism as a whole requires such an adjustment. An example of this principle is the temporary reduction of the blood flow to the skin in the beginning of muscular exercise. The vasomotor centers in the brain stem are under the influence of an impulse flow from higher brain structures coming along the corticohypothalamic pathway.

Besides functioning as collecting tubes the veins also play an important role as capacitance vessels. The venous compartment is rather voluminous and may contain large quantities of blood. Changes in luminal diameter of the veins do not affect the resistance to flow, but they have a profound effect on the capacity for storing blood in the veins; and hence on the return of blood, the filling of the heart by means of the "venous pump," and consequently on the output from the heart. The capacitance vessels may thus be considered as a functional part of the pump besides serving to collect and return to the heart the blood which has passed through the tissues. The constrictor activity of the capacitance vessels is very little influenced by the intrinsic factors, but is mainly regulated by the central nervous system through sympathetic nerves.

III. The Cardiovascular Responses to Muscular Exercise in Man

A. MICROCIRCULATION IN EXERCISE

The entire capillary surface that is available for exchange of material within the muscles cannot be measured, but a rough estimate gives a possible figure of 300–600 m² in the adult man, or close to the size of the pulmonary alveolar surface area.

The famous Danish physiologist and Nobel prize winner, August Krogh, made the classical observations on the capillary circulation. After injection of India ink into the circulation of experimental animals, he counted 5 capillaries per square millimeter in the resting muscles, and 190 per square millimeter after stimulation. It was estimated that only 1/20–1/50 of the capillary bed is open in the resting state (Krogh, 1922).

As the increase in active capillaries and in blood flow is approximately the same, about 20 times that at rest, it follows that the velocity of flow in the capillaries is much the same in exercise as at rest, and the time each blood corpuscle spends in the capillaries is not much changed by activity.

The activation of capillaries increases the capillary surface area and shortens considerably the distance of diffusion which the molecules have to travel from the blood to the mitochondria of the cells, which is the main site of the metabolic activity. Thus the activation of the capillaries of the muscles facilitates greatly the transfer of metabolic material across the capillary cellular membrane barrier.

The functional state of the capillary membrane is determined by the permeability (i.e., the dimensions and number of pores per unit of capillary surface area). Capillary permeability is not ordinarily affected by the produced vasodilatator substances in muscular exercise. Consequently, the capillary filtration coefficient, which is defined as the amount of fluid filtered across the capillary membrane per minute per 100 gm tissue for each mm Hg transcapillary membrane pressure, is determined by the capillary surface area or the number of active capillaries.

The systolic arterial pressure of the systemic circulation augments during exercise in order to improve blood flow through the working muscles. The pressure in the venous compartment, however, is little affected. Thus the hydrostatic capillary pressure increases considerably, and as a consequence, the filtering forces enlarge, and exceed the absorption forces. The dynamic equilibrium state of out- and inflowing water is outbalanced, and fluid leaves the blood.

The rise in the mean capillary pressure may amount to as much as 10 mm Hg during heavy exercise. The consequence of this increase upon the blood volume would be drastic if the filtering forces were not counteracted. Assuming a maximal filtration coefficient of 0.04 ml/mm Hg/min/100 ml tissue a mean capillary pressure rise of 10 mm Hg within a muscle mass of 10 kg (which probably is the muscle mass activated in running) would reduce the circulating blood volume by about 1 liter or close to 20% during the course of 10 min.

The increased filtration is, however, met by compensation. As the extracellular fluid increases in amount, the hydrostatic pressure of this compartment rises. A hemoconcentration takes place, the concentration of plasma proteins rises, and increases the plasma colloid pressure. These changes tend to increase the absorption forces resulting in larger inflow of fluid to the blood. Further, the lymphatic system promptly returns to the circulatory compartment the greater part of the filtrated fluid, facilitated by the massaging effect of the muscle contractions. Consequently, the lymphatic drainage is increased in exercise.

The loss of fluid into the extracellular space reduces the circulating blood volume. The water loss by sweating, which during heavy exercise may amount to as much as 1–2 liters per hour, adds to this effect, and a serious dehydration associated with a drastic reduction of the circulating blood volume may develop during prolonged exercise if not compensated by consumption of water.

The counter actions to the increased filtration do not provide full compensation, and a new dynamic equilibration level is established with larger amounts of fluids in the extracellular compartments.

This shift in the size of the water compartments of the body during performance of muscular exercise can easily be demonstrated by measurements of blood hemotocrit. During short exposure to exercise the hemotocrit values increase in rough relation to the intensity of work.

The hemoconcentration during exercise may amount to as much as 20%. During prolonged work, there seems to be no further change in the blood volume after the first few minutes.

The reduction of the circulating blood volume in exercise is met by mainly two compensating adjustments: (1) by increased absorption of fluid in tissues other than the active muscles. The reduced output of urine does not account for much in this situation, because the amount of fluid which normally leaves the kidney is only 1–2 ml/min, and (2) by adjustments of the capacitance vessels of the vascular bed. The capacitance vessels of the systemic and pulmonary circulation are able to constrict and dilatate under the influence of sympathetic stimulation. In this way the volume of the capacity vessels can be regulated, and the volume set at a level appropriate to secure adequate filling of the pump. In exercise the capacitance vessels become constricted.

The reduced blood volume is known to be associated with higher heart rate and lower stroke volume than in normal conditions, cardiac output being little changed. The hemoconcentration also implies other functional consequences.

The capacity of the blood to carry oxygen is raised due to increased concentration of red blood corpuscles. The acid buffering capacity of the blood is also increased, due to increased concentration of proteins. These adjustments may be considered as beneficial in the exercise situation. On the other hand, hemoconcentration tends to increase the viscosity of the blood, which implies inhibition of the conductance of blood through the vessels. Also other functional properties of the blood become changed by the hemoconcentration, such as the clotting time, the number of white blood cells, etc.

The physiological significance of the shift in the filling level of the water compartments of the body during muscular exercise can thus be stated, but much experimental work remains to be done in order to evaluate the quantitative aspects of this shift.

B. CARDIAC OUTPUT IN EXERCISE

1. Cardiac Output

At rest the rate of blood flow from the heart depends upon the position of the body because gravity exerts an effect upon the circulation. When the body changes from horizontal to upright, there is a tendency for blood to pool in the lower extremities, and the central blood volume and the venous return become diminished resulting in lower stroke volume and lower cardiac output (Table I). The cardiac output at rest is thus a highly variable function, also inasmuch as the output is greatly influenced by excitement and emotional disturbances, influencing the cardiac performance by impulse flow along the corticohypothalamic pathway to the stations on the brain stem, which control the rate of heart beat and the vasconstrictor tone of resistance and capacitance vessels.

The position of the body also influences cardiac output during muscular exercise, the stroke volume and cardiac output are lower in the upright position than in the supine position. It is therefore necessary to take the body position into consideration in the analysis of cardiac function at work.

TABLE I

HEMODYNAMICS AT REST AND DURING EXERCISE IN RELATION TO BODY POSITION[a]

Function	Rest (supine upright)		Moderate exercise (supine upright)		Heavy exercise (supine upright)	
Cardiac output (liters/min)	9.18	6.61	18.98	16.89	26.26	24.50
Stroke volume (ml)	141	103	163	149	164	155
Heart rate (beats/min)	65	64	116	113	160	158
A-V O_2 difference (ml/liter)	38.5	60.7	94.3	110.3	128.2	138.4
Systemic systolic arterial pressure	123	132	162	175	211	202
Pulmonary systolic arterial pressure	20.6	19.1	36.0	33.1	47.0	46.3
O_2 uptake (ml/min)	345	384	1765	1864	3364	3387

[a] From Bevegaard *et al.* (1963).

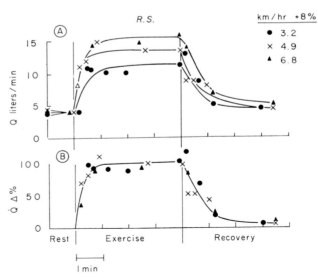

Fig. 3. The kinetics of adaptation of cardiac output to exercise. From Cerretelli (1966).

Under basal conditions the cardiac output is most stable in the lying position and is about 4–5 liters per minute, or expressed on the basis of surface area (cardiac index) 3–3.5 liters per minute per square meter surface area.

In the transition from rest to exercise the cardiovascular function undergoes remarkable changes. During the initial stage of rhythmic muscular work, the cardiac output increases, first rapidly and then more gradually from the resting state and up to a niveau ("steady state"), the level of which is set by the intensity of work. The steady state niveau is reached at about the same time as the oxygen uptake levels off at its "steady state" (Fig. 3).

Thus there are two components in the kinetic adjustment of cardiac output to rhythmic muscular exercise, a fast one caused by a centrally induced nervous drive, and a slower secondary phase which may be a result of some unknown reflex mechanisms. The final level of cardiac output is closely related to the intensity of work.

In light and moderate work the duration of the adaption phase lasts for 1–2 min, but is related to the intensity of work and becomes longer in heavy exercise. Fit subjects adapt quicker to exercise than unfit subjects. It is this lag in the circulatory adjustment that causes the partly anaerobic conditions of the muscles at the beginning of work and which results in an oxygen deficit, which at the end of exercise manifests itself as an oxygen debt. After cessation of exercise, cardiac output does not promptly return, but decreases

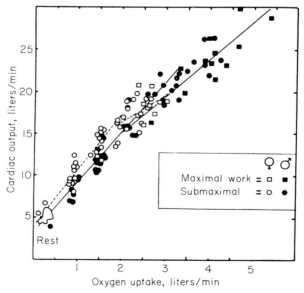

Fig. 4. Cardiac output at rest and during work in the sitting position. From Åstrand *et al.* (1964).

gradually toward the resting level. The recovery curve is closely exponential in shape.

The steady state values for cardiac output are closely related to the metabolic rate as shown in Fig. 4. The relationship is not exactly linear as the increase in cardiac output with increasing oxygen uptake becomes less. This tendency to a curvilinear relationship is probably related to the extra demand for blood flow to the skin as exercise progresses. If the blood flow to the skin had been the same at all levels of exercise as at rest, a close linear relation would likely have appeared.

2. Stroke volume

The cardiac output is determined by the stroke volume and the heart rate. At rest and in the supine position the stroke volume of an adult nonathletic man is 70–90 ml depending upon the body size. In females the stroke volume is usually 25% less. As a result of the greater venous return which occurs in transition from rest to exercise in the upright position, the stroke volume increases rapidly, reaching a level which is maintained constant during exercise of 5–10 min duration. With exercise which lasts for hours the stroke volume is known to decrease. There has been reported a 16% reduction in stroke volume measured an hour after the start of exercise compared to that measured in the first few minutes. Even at moderate work loads there is a tendency for the stroke volume to decrease after a few minutes of work, but cardiac output remains fairly constant due to an increase of the heart rate. The mechanism for this tendency of the stroke volume to decrease as exercise

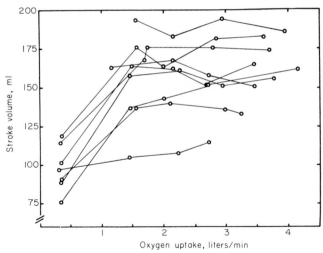

Fig. 5. Stroke volume in relation to oxygen uptake in the sitting position. From Grimby *et al.* (1966).

progresses is not fully understood. It might be related to the reduction of the circulating blood volume, or to a redistribution of the blood with a reduction of the central blood volume.

Maximal stroke volumes are usually reached at exercise levels requiring an oxygen uptake of 30–40% of the maximal, Fig. 5. In the upright position the increase in stroke volume from the resting to the maximal value may be up to 40–50%, and no differences have been observed between men and women. When exercise is performed in the supine position, stroke volume increases only slightly. Even at maximal exercises in which the heart rate may reach 200 beats per minute, the stroke volume is maintained at its maximal value. This indicates that the time available for the filling of the ventricles at heart rates up to 200 is sufficient to secure maximal stroke volumes.

3. Heart rate

During light exercise the first increase in the heart rate may be exaggerated, and it therefore subsequently diminishes to a lower level which is maintained throughout the period of exercise. However, during prolonged work and particularly if the load is heavy, there is a tendency for the heart rate to increase as exercise progresses in order to achieve adequate cardiac output when the stroke volume decreases (Fig. 6).

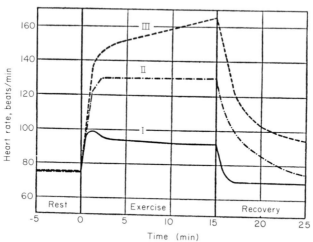

Fig. 6. Heart rate response to exercise of different degree. I, light exercise; II, moderate exercise; III, heavy exercise. From Brouha (1960).

During heavy and "hypermaximal" work the heart rate tends to increase until the state of exhaustion is reached. In this situation the heart rate recorded at the end of the exercise period is considered as the "maximal" attainable heart rate.

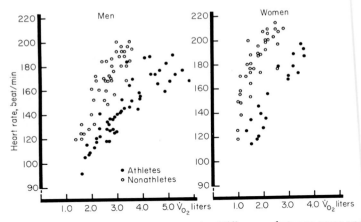

Fig. 7. Heart rate in relation to oxygen uptake. Differences between sexes and degree of physical training.

Heart rate at steady state or taken at the end of a few minutes exercise period is closely and linearly related to the oxygen uptake (Fig. 7). This characteristic is different in men and women, and changes with training. In a homogeneous group of sedentary subjects of the same sex, the relationship is remarkably similar (Fig. 8), and not much affected by age. The higher maximal cardiac output and maximal oxygen uptake achieved in young compared to old subjects is brought about by a higher maximal heart rate in young subjects.

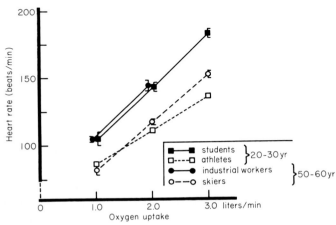

Fig. 8. Heart rate in relation to oxygen uptake in different ages.

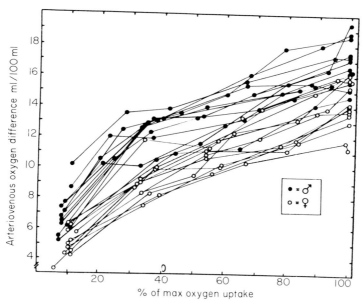

Fig. 9. A-V oxygen differences in relation to oxygen uptake. From Åstrand *et al.* (1964).

In many subjects, particularly in unfit people unaccustomed to severe exercise, the heart rate approaches the ceiling level in an asymptotic manner. It is probable that this asymptotic approach reflects the inability of the heart to produce larger cardiac output, and that in this situation, a larger oxygen uptake and consumption is achieved by a greater extraction of oxygen from the blood. That A-V differences increase with increasing work load has been observed by many workers (Fig. 9).

The highest attainable heart rate during performance of heavy muscular work depends upon age and state of training, Fig. 10 (and Table VII). At the age of 20 the maximal heart rate is about 200 which is reduced to 155 at the age of 70. That this rate becomes lower with training does not necessarily imply a reduction of the heart's capability to raise its rate of contractions. It may be that there is no need for maximal activation during exhaustive exercise of a heart, which is strengthened by training. If this concept is correct, it implies that the trained heart, even during maximal work by the muscles, operates with a functional reserve.

That the maximal heart rate becomes lower with increasing age can be considered as one sign of the inevitable and general reduction of biological functions which comes with age. The precise mechanism involved in this age reduced maximal heart rate is not understood.

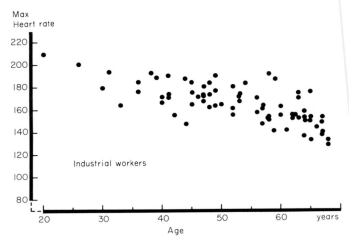

Fig. 10. Maximal heart rate in relation to age

C. Pressures in Exercise

1. Systemic Circulation

Despite an immediate and drastic dilatation of the resistance vessels of the working muscles at the transition from rest to exercise, the systemic arterial pressure is not only maintained, but actually increases. This observation rejects the hypotheses advanced by earlier workers, that the circulatory adjustment to exercise is elicited by an arterial pressure drop which activates the high pressoreceptor control system.

The initial period of increasing arterial pressure during performance of rhythmic exercise lasts for 1–2 min, after which a fairly constant value is reached and maintained, the level of which depends upon the intensity of exercise. When the work stops, there is an immediate pressure drop to sub-resting values, the minimum reached 5–10 sec after cessation of work. Subsequently, pressure rises to a little above the pre-exercise level.

The diastolic systemic pressure remains practically unchanged by light and moderate heavy exercise, but may increase slightly during heavy exercise following a course similar to that described for the systolic arterial pressure. As a consequence of the differential rise in systolic and diastolic pressure, the pulse pressure increases greatly.

The systolic pressure taken at the apparently steady state level is roughly proportional to the intensity of work, Fig. 11. At maximal exercise systolic pressure may reach levels well above 200 mm Hg or 50% higher than at rest. Holmgren (1956) who made a comprehensive study of the arterial blood pressure during bicycle riding found that for fit persons the increase in systolic pressure was about 8 mm Hg for each 0.5 liter increase in oxygen uptake. Considerably higher values are reported for unfit subjects and for older subjects, but the final maximal value seems to be much the same and about 200 mm Hg.

The total peripheral resistance falls considerably during work, especially in transition from rest to light exercise. This fall illustrates the drastic vasodilatation which occurs in the contracting muscles and also in the skin as exercise progresses.

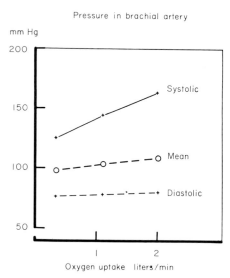

Fig. 11. Pressures in brachial artery during exercise. From Bevegaard *et al.* (1960).

The pressure in the peripheral veins is usually found to increase slightly at the beginning of exercise, subsequently followed by a drop almost to resting levels. The increase varies considerably in the investigations purporting to study this problem. Increases of up to 10–15 mm Hg in the peripheral veins during heavy exercise are reported. The measurements of peripheral venous pressure and the interpretation of this finding may be quite difficult, because the pressure varies with the position of the measuring point in relation to the level of the heart, and the peripheral venous pressure is also affected by the activity of the "venous pump" and by the abdomino-thoracic pump. The central venous pressure, e.g., in the right atrium, is better defined and exerts great influence, because it affects the filling pressure of the right ventricle.

The pressure curves in the right atrium have recently been studied quite intensively by means of heart catheterization, and it has been firmly established that the central venous pressure responds only slightly to exercise. The enlargement of the stroke volume in exercise is thus not related to the increased pressure in the right atrium.

The attainment and maintenance of a high cardiac output depends on adequate filling of the ventricles in the brief interval between their contractions. Man has the handicap during upright exercises of having to overcome increased hydrostatic forces. In fact, at any given work load there is a slight but significantly lower cardiac output than in the performance of supine leg exercise. The muscle pump, the venous valves, and the abdomino-thoracic pump help in aiding venous return and hence in the ventricular filling. In addition, an increased constriction of the venous compartment contributes an important aid to the ventricular filling. Bevegaard and Shepherd (1965) measured the forearm volume during supine leg exercise and noticed a considerable drop in the volume, increasing with exercise intensity. This indicates a definite increase in venoconstrictor tone, which increases abruptly in close linear relation to the rate of work performed.

2. Pulmonary Circulation

In the pulmonary circuit the balance between the pre- and postcapillary resistance has to be adjusted so that capillary pressure does not increase to the critical level of the plasma colloid osmotic pressure in order to prevent outward filtration of water which would create the serious condition of pulmonary edema.

At rest and in the upright position the systolic pressure in the pulmonary arteries is 15–20 mm Hg, the diastolic 5–8 mm Hg, and mean pressure 8–12 mm Hg. In the supine position pressures are somewhat higher. The pressure in the left atrium is a little higher than in the right atrium. The mean capillary pressure is estimated to be about 8–10 mm Hg. The lung vessels normally offer very slight resistance to flow. At rest the pulmonary vascular resistance is 0.12 peripheral resistance units in young men. In older men a greater total pulmonary resistance has been measured.

During work the pulmonary arterial pressure increases in relation to the increase in cardiac output, Fig. 12. Despite this rise in pulmonary arterial pressure, the total vascular resistance changes little.

The arterioles of the pulmonary circuit have smooth muscles which contract and relax in much the same way as the resistance vessels of the systemic circulation. They are innervated by sympathetic nerve fibers which carry constrictor activity. However, it seems that the pulmonary resistance vessels mainly are affected by physical factors related to the pumping activity of the heart and factors of the systemic circulation, and that nervous and humeral regulation plays only a minor role. At rest and in the upright position most of the blood passes through the lower levels of the lungs, and the middle and upper part is less circulated. During exercises in the upright position, which may increase the cardiac output up to 4–5 times the resting level, there occurs an activation of the resting capillaries. The size of the capillary bed of the lungs during maximal exercise is raised by a factor of 2–3. This means that the velocity of the blood flow increases in the capillaries during work. It has been estimated that at rest a red blood cell remains in the pulmonary capillaries for 1 sec, while in heavy exercise the time is reduced to 0.5 sec.

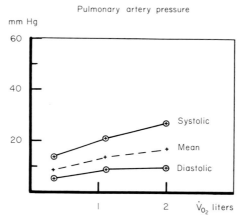

Fig. 12. Pressures in pulmonary artery during exercise. From Bevegaard *et al.* (1960).

At rest the pulmonary capillary bed contains about 70–100 ml blood, an amount which may be doubled during performance of heavy exercise. The blood content of the total pulmonary circuit at rest is about 700–900 ml. This amount of blood is important for the output from the left ventricle, because it can be considered as a blood reservoir.

D. REGIONAL BLOOD FLOW IN EXERCISE

In addition to increased cardiac output and a greater force exerted by the cardiac muscle in exercise resulting in higher perfusion pressure of the systemic circulation, the adjustment to exercise makes necessary a redistribution of cardiac output. Some of the changes which take place in the rate of blood flow to the various organs of the body are given in Table II.

1. Muscle Blood Flow

The blood flow through the muscle tissue has been studied by means of occlusion plethysmography, and recently also by the "clearance" technique, using injections of radioactive Xenon as the tracer substance. The rate of blood flowing through the resting muscles is 4–7 ml/min/100 mil of tissue. During strenuous rhythmic contractions the flow increases manyfold, reaching rates of more than 100 ml/min/100 ml tissue or 15–20 times above the resting value.

The flow of blood increases and decreases with each muscle contraction, becomes reduced during contraction and increases in the relaxation phase (Fig. 13). This change in the rate of flow is caused by variation in the intra-

TABLE II

DISTRIBUTION OF CARDIAC OUTPUT AT REST AND IN EXERCISE[a]

Circulation	Rest (ml/min, %)		Exercise (ml/min, %)					
			Light		Moderate		Maximal	
Splanchnic	1,400	24	1,100	12	600	3	300	1
Renal	1,100	19	900	10	600	3	250	1
Cerebral	750	13	750	8	750	4	750	3
Coronary	250	4	350	4	750	4	1,000	4
Skeletal muscle	1,200	21	4,500	47	12,500	71	22,000	88
Skin	500	9	1,500	15	1,900	12	600	2
Other organs	600	10	400	4	400	3	100	1
	5,800	100	9,400	100	17,500	100	25,000	100

[a] Estimated figures.

muscular pressure which during maximal or near maximal contraction may be so great that it exceeds the intracapillary pressure, and the minute vessels become closed. The extent of this hindrance varies in different muscles; it is much less in the forearm than in the calf. It presumably depends on the pressure developed within the muscles, and the way in which the vessels are distributed.

At the onset of exercise or even in anticipation of exertion the blood flow becomes immediately increased, and continues to increase until a plateau—a steady state between inflow and outflow—is reached. This period of adaptation usually takes 1–2 min at light and moderately heavy exercise, possibly longer in maximal exercise. The apparent "steady state" level is closely related to the intensity of work or to the aerobic metabolic activity of the tissue. After cessation of work, blood flow gradually decreases.

The decline of blood flow is very nearly exponential for periods of exercises up to 5–10 min. After exercise of long duration an additional slower component becomes apparent. The blood flow during recovery is related to the payment of the oyxgen debt and to the restoration of normal tissue homeostasis.

Even if blood flow during activity may be raised fifteen- to twentyfold above that at rest, the volume of blood in the muscles only increases by 50%. This relatively small increase is due to the massaging influence of the muscle contractions upon the flow of blood in the veins.

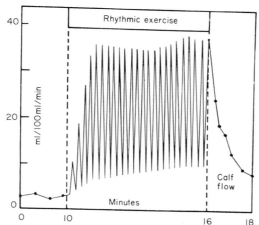

Fig. 13. Changes in blood flow in the calf muscles of the human leg during rhythmic contraction. From Barcroft (1963a).

The aerobic metabolism of muscle fibers may increase up to a hundred times above that at rest while the blood flow rate may only increase by a factor of 15–20. This implies a greater extraction of oxygen from the blood passing the tissue. While normal utilization is only 20–25% in most organs, the muscle is capable of extracting up to 80% of the oxygen offered to it by the blood, and the oxygen tension of blood coming from active muscles may be close to zero.

That the muscle blood flow may increase manyfold during contraction implies that the resistance vessels are greatly constricted in the resting muscles. This vasoconstrictor activity appears to be an inherent activity of the smooth muscle coat surrounding the precapillary arterioles supported by a sympathetic vasoconstrictor tone. The vasoconstrictor activity is modified by a variety of stimuli, mainly by reflex impulses originating in the peripheral pressoreceptors of the high and low pressured vessels inside the thoracic cavity.

During exercise there is an increase in vasoconstrictor tone in muscles not involved in the exercise. For example, blood flow in the forearm muscles suffers a small fall during leg exercise. The increase in vasoconstrictor tone seems to be related to the degree of exercise, because the decrease in blood flow is found to be greater during heavy than during light exercise.

2. Blood Flow in Visceral Organs

In a normal resting man with a cardiac output of 5 liters per minute the visceral organs (liver, kidneys, spleen, and gastrointestinal tract) receive about 2.5 liters per minute or 50% of the cardiac output.

During muscular exercise the resistance and capacitance vessels of the visceral organs become greatly constricted, so that the blood flowing to these organs is diminished and the volume of blood in the splanchnic area is reduced. Most drastic is the reduction which takes place in the blood flow to the kidneys. At rest the volume of blood flowing through the kidneys is great, about 1200 ml/min, or 20–25% of the cardiac output. During exercise the kidneys may suffer a reduction of 50–80%; the decrease is roughly related to the intensity of work. Even zero values for kidney blood flow have been estimated during short spells of heavy exercise (Fig. 14).

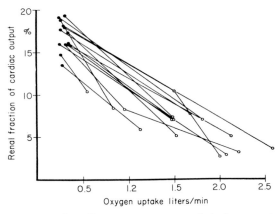

Fig. 14. Renal fraction of cardiac output at rest and during exercise in the supine position at different work levels. From Carlsten and Grimby (1966).

A large share of the cardiac output flows through the vessels of the intestines and the spleen, and then into the portal venous system and through the liver. The portal circulatory system plus the arterial blood flow into the liver is the splanchnic circulation. The splanchnic blood flow is about 1500 ml/min at rest or 30% of the cardiac output. One hundred ml/min circulate through the portal system. We have little detailed knowledge about the splanchnic circulation during work. The redistribution of blood in the splanchnic area and especially the behavior of the spleen has drawn great interest. In experiments on animals it has been shown that the spleen contracts during exercise, and its content of blood diminishes. All evidence available indicates that splanchnic blood flow is reduced during work. During light leg exercise in the supine position a reduction of the order of 350–500 ml/min has been reported. Rowell *et al.* (1965) have studied hepatic blood flow during exercise by means of injecting a tracer substance into the circulation and which is cleared from the blood by the liver cells. The clearance rate was found to be inversely proportional to the metabolic rate (Fig. 15), not for the

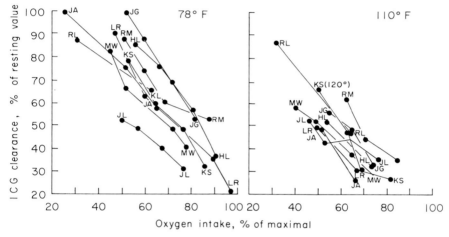

Fig. 15. Percentage decrements in ICG clearance at different work levels, where oxygen uptake is expressed as percent of maximal O_2 intake. Data from experiments in a cool (78°F) and a hot (110°F) environment. From Rowell *et al.* (1965).

absolute values, but relative to the maximum, which indicates a similar reduction in the splanchnic blood flow.

It thus seems to be a general principle that the degree of vasoconstriction of the visceral organs induced by muscular exercise is closely related to the relative intensity of work.

3. Coronary Circulation

The rate of blood flow to the cardiac muscle during muscular exercise increases in amount and is linearly related to the increase in cardiac output. The rate of blood flow to the cardiac tissue at rest is about 60–70 ml/min/100 ml tissue, which may increase at least fivefold above this level. The oxygen extraction is very high in the myocardium, even at rest, about 70–80% of the oxygen of the blood entering the cardiac muscle is utilized. This indicates that increased demand for oxygen must be met by increased rate of coronary blood flow, an important phenomenon inasmuch as the cardiac muscle cannot utilize the anaerobic glycogenolysis as an exergenic source for energy supply to the contractile process.

The resistance of the myocardium is under sympathetic nervous influence. The catecholamines cause a vasodilatation of the myocardium's resistance vessels which is the opposite effect to that normally exerted. Sympathetic stimulation, which increases the force of contraction and raises the heart rate and cardiac output, results in vasodilatation of the coronary circulation, a very beneficial reaction in this situation. However, all available evidence indicates that the nervous vasomotor control of the coronary blood flow plays a minor role in the regulation of intracardial circulation. The control mechanism is an autoregulation, and mainly two factors set the rate of coronary blood flow; the rate of myocardial metabolism and the pressure in the aorta.

4. Skin Blood Flow

Circulation through the skin has two major functions; to provide transportation of metabolic material to the tissue and to conduct heat from the inside of the body to the surface for heat exchange with the environment.

The vessels of the skin are constructed to serve this function. The vessels which primarily serve the temperature regulation consist of subcutaneous venous plexus and atriovenous anastomoses. The walls of these anastomoses have strong muscular coats innervated by sympathetic vasoconstrictor nerve fibers.

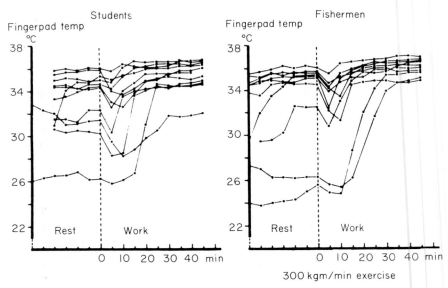

Fig. 16. Finger temperature during leg exercise of moderate intensity. From Strömme *et al.* (1963).

The rate of blood flow through the skin is highly variable. The flow required under different conditions changes variably under the influence of the cooling power of the surrounding air and the overall metabolic rate of the body. Although excitement and emotional disturbances may be reflected in highly variable skin blood flow.

Under ordinary conditions the total blood flow to the skin is about 400 ml/min in the average adult man. When the skin vessels are fully dilated the vessels may conduct at least up to 7 times as much blood as at rest or 3 liters/min.

In transition from rest to exercise, blood flow through the skin becomes first diminished. Continuous exercise results subsequently in vasodilatation (Fig. 16). During prolonged and heavy exercise the raised heat production imposes a thermal stress on the organism, and the vessels of the skin become fully dilated. Also the sweating requires large amounts of blood to the sweat glands. This implies that about 3 liters or 15–20% of the cardiac output is diverted to the skin during heavy exercise.

E. Circulatory Adjustment to Static Muscle Work

Static exercise involves isometric contractions of muscles, and the force exerted can be exactly monitored. The maximal isometric force measured in standardized positions varies considerably between individuals, and defines the strength of the muscles. The endurance time, which is the duration of contractions held to fatigue, depends upon the force exerted. The maximal voluntary contraction (M.V.C.) can only be held for a few seconds, while 25% M.V.C. can be held for many minutes.

The blood flow during sustained contraction of the forearm (grip strength) has been studied quite intensively. At 5% and 10% M.V.C., which are contractions that can be held for a very long time, the blood flow reaches a steady state, and after cessation blood flow falls immediately to resting levels (Fig. 17). In contrast, at 20% M.V.C. and above, tensions that quickly result in fatigue, the pattern of response is quite different. The flow increases continuously throughout the contraction, and rises after the contraction before returning to resting levels.

Lind et al. (1966) have calculated the "blood debt" during sustained contractions. In the case of nonfatiguing contraction no blood debt occurs. A contraction of about 15% M.V.C. is the upper limit for nonfatiguing activity, and at tensions above this limit, the blood debt increases rapidly with tension.

The central circulation is also involved in the response to static work (Fig. 18). Cardiac output, heart rate, and systemic arterial blood pressures follow response patterns which are not unlike the local blood flow response. At nonfatiguing tensions a steady state is usually established, but a continuous rise is observed in all the parameters during fatiguing contractions.

The interaction and regulation of the circulation during sustained contractions involve mechanisms other than those operating during dynamic work. The pressor response to sustained contractions seems to be initiated by some peripheral processes of the active muscles which activate receptors, resulting in a pressor reflex mechanism. The use of such a reflex mechanism is readily understood. When tension increases, the receptors discharge at a higher rate

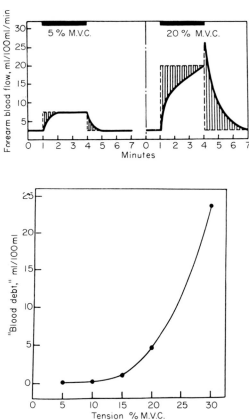

Fig. 17. In the upper part of the diagram: Forearm blood flow before, during and after 3-min contraction at tension of 5% and 20% of maximal voluntary contraction (M.V.C.). At 5% M.V.C. the shaded area above the curve during the contraction equals the postexercise hyperemia (shaded area below the curve). During fatiguing contractions (20% M.V.C.) the shaded area above the curve is less than the postexercise hyperemia because the blood flow during the contraction is never sufficient for the muscles' metabolic needs, and therefore a "blood debt" is created. In the lower part of the curve the "blood debt" (the difference between the postexercise hyperemia and the blood deficit during exercise) is shown for contractions held for 3 min at tensions from 3 to 30% M.V.C. At nonfatiguing contractions there is no blood debt. From Lind *et al.* (1966).

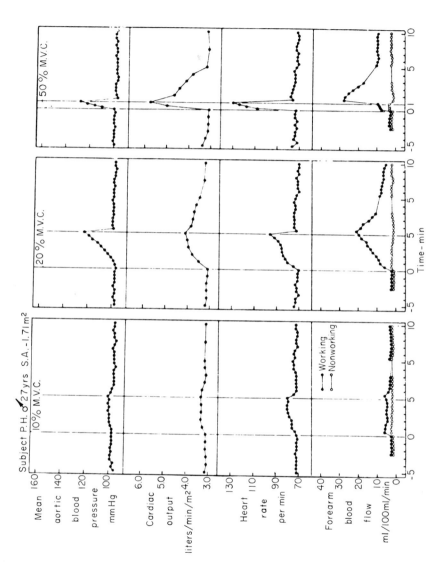

Fig. 18. Hemodynamic response to sustained contractions. From Lind *et al.* (1966).

and blood pressure tends to increase in order to facilitate blood flow through the active muscles. The rise of blood pressure is caused partly by cardio-acceleration, partly by peripheral vasoconstriction. The receptors and the nature of the factors which stimulate the receptors are not known.

F. Circulatory Responses to Daily Life Activities

Muscular performance in the body may take the form of static and dynamic work. All daily life activities are maintained by a continuous shift or combinations of these kinds of muscular performance.

In the preceding chapter the basic principles in the circulatory adjustment to static and dynamic work have been described. This knowledge may be applied in the investigation of the loads placed upon the cardiovascular system in daily life.

Since hemodynamics are closely related to the overall metabolic rate, an evaluation of daily life responses must include measurements of oxygen uptake of the various work tasks. By using conventional methods of sampling expired gas in Douglas bags or in respirometers with subsequent gas analysis, the oxygen uptake is easily determined in most human activities. Chapter 10 presents the caloric expenditure of some common activities.

When the energy consumption data are interpreted, it should be borne in mind that the strain placed on the cardiovascular system depends, not upon the absolute values, but more importantly upon the relative load, e.g., the caloric cost in relation to the maximal aerobic power. An energy load which is easy for a fit man may become extremely heavy for an unfit man. According to this concept the strain or stress of any activity can only be properly evaluated in an individual when the maximal aerobic power (the maximal oxygen uptake) is also known.

The use of heart rate recordings throughout a working day offer a possibility to evaluate the stress placed upon the cardiovascular system, because heart rate with certain exceptions follows closely the oxygen uptake and the cardiac output. The use of telemetric equipment or miniature tape recorders has greatly facilitated the ease by which heart rate may be recorded continuously without disturbing the subjects. Figure 19 gives examples of patterns of responses throughout a working day. When these responses are related to the resting and maximal heart rate, evidence of the stress placed on the organism may be evaluated.

G. Regulation of Circulation in Exercise

The complex interrelation of all the mechanisms concerned in the regulation of circulation makes it extremely difficult to analyze the significance of individual components in exercise. The mechanisms involve autoregulation and nervous activity; the latter comprises many different nervous reflexes. Hormonal influence plays only a minor role in cardiovascular behavior in exercise, and is mainly limited to adrenal cathecolamine liberation, which becomes increased as part of the "alarm" reaction, and which to a minor degree superimposes the effect exerted by the powerful sympathetic drive in exercise.

The finding of areas in higher brain structures which upon stimulation produce cardioacceleration, vasodilatation in the skeletal muscles, etc., has given evidence to the concept that the initial cardiovascular adjustments to muscular exercise are caused by a central excitatory impulse flow to the vasomotor neurones in the brain stem resulting in a powerful mass sympathetic discharge, which increases cardiac performance, dilates skeletal and cardiac muscle vessels, constricts resistance vessels of inactive organs, and mobilizes extra energy through an effect upon the metabolism. This centrally induced excitement of sympathetics is one component of the "alarm" or "stress" reaction to environmental physical stimuli, bringing the body into a state of alertness. It is reasonable to assume that the intensity of these centrally induced cardiovascular adjustments depends upon the mental engagement which precedes or accompanies the motor activity. The degree of mental engagement is largely a result of the situation and the subject's experience in the situation. Habitual muscular activity where only few and minor muscle groups are engaged is likely to bring about only a mild, if any, central drive, because the locally induced hyperemia will be sufficient. It is important to realize that the initial nervous drive in exercise, which may even anticipate motor activity, provides a means to adjust the circulation to a situation of increased metabolic demand ahead of the events. Even if this aspect may have lost much of its importance for the ordinary civilized man, it certainly is of significance, e.g., for successful performances in athletics. Daily life of many animal species, where survival governed by flight or hunt often depends upon narrow time margins, could not be performed without this mechanism.

The close relationship between cardiovascular performance and metabolism in muscular work strongly suggests a functional interplay. The classic concept, that the regulation of cardiac output in exercise is mainly an effect of Starling's law, is not supported by recent findings. In the supine position stroke volume and heart volume are little affected during exercise as they would be if Starling's law governed the increased output in exercise. Starling's law would also imply a raised pressure in the right atrium, which does not occur in exercise.

During exercise there is evidence that the sympathetic excitatory drive continues, e.g., constricted vessels in inactive organs, increased venomotor tone, increased cardiac performance (Asmussen and Nielsen, 1955). This drive may during prolonged exercise emanate from the highest levels of the central nervous system, which in that case also has to be continued after exercise has

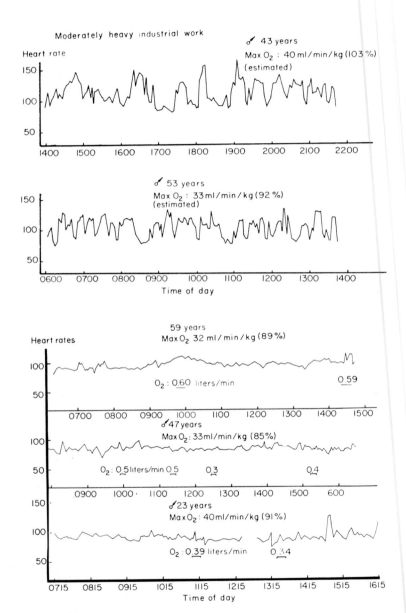

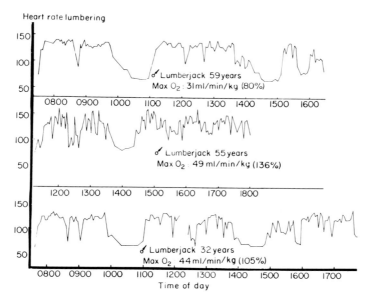

Fig. 19. Heart rate response throughout a working day in three occupations: industrial work, office work, and lumbering.

stopped in order to explain the high cardiac performance observed in the recovery period. However, this is highly unlikely. Many workers have suggested that the exact and fine adjustment of the cardiovascular system to the steady state level cannot be explained without the existence and operation of a chemoreceptor control system, which drives the excitation of the cardiovascular center in exercise in addition to the baroreceptor supervision of the pressure level. Since the pressures in the systemic and pulmonary circulation are considerably raised in exercise, the baroreceptor control reflex system acts mainly as a brake on the system, preventing abnormally high pressure levels.

The chemoreceptors of the circulatory system are situated at the arterial side. This implies that these receptors do not receive information before the blood has eliminated excess carbon dioxide and is filled up with oxygen. The carbon dioxide tension in the arterial blood may vary considerably during exercise, sometimes being raised, sometimes being lowered, depending upon the pulmonary ventilation and the amount of lactate in the blood. If the carbon dioxide tension of arterial blood should drive the circulation in exercise, a highly variable response would be the result. Also oxygen would be a poor trigger substance, because the oxygen tension of arterial blood is not much changed by exercise. Only if lactate, or some other metabolites not eliminated in the lungs, appears in the blood stream in increased amounts, does the activation of the arterial chemoreceptors become possible. However, blood lactate becomes elevated only in heavy exercise. Some workers suggest that unidentified metabolites not eliminated in the lungs may be the stimuli for the arterial chemoreceptors. Another hypothesis is that unknown chemo-receptors are situated in the muscle tissue to sense the chemical environment, and that these provide the excitatory drive to the cardiovascular centers (Folkow *et al.*, 1963).

IV. Adaptation of the Cardiovascular System to Physical Training

Most of the available information about the cardiovascular system's adap-tation to physical training is gained from comparative studies of athletic and nonathletic populations, and relatively few training experiments have been carried out. This is a drawback, because differences between 2 populations are apt to be influenced by many factors other than variations in the degree of physical activity. Furthermore, the extremely heavy training program which is undertaken by motivated athletes, cannot be applied on ordinary people who for medical or other reasons need to improve their fitness. Scientific work directed toward the effect of physical training on subjects of various ages and fitness levels is thus highly desirable.

A. Maximal Oxygen Uptake

An increased fitness for work is manifested in a rise in the maximal powers and capacities of the energy delivering mechanisms. The maximal power of the aerobic metabolism is measured by the maximal oxygen uptake (Fig. 20). Maximal oxygen uptake in work which engages the larger muscles of the body depends on the functional dimension of the oxygen transporting system which includes the lungs, the cardiac muscles, the size of the capillary bed of the skeletal muscles, and the capacity of the blood to carry oxygen. In the normal man pulmonary function is seldom a limiting factor. Maximal oxygen uptake may therefore be considered as a measure of maximal cardiovascular per-formance (Åstrand, 1956).

Maximal oxygen uptake in exercises which engage the larger muscles of the body is in ordinary sedentary men about 40–50 ml/min/kg body weight, but in athletes of international standard may reach values up to 80 ml/min/kg body weight (Table III), a difference which at least partly is attributed to the athletic training regimen.

The trainability of maximal oxygen uptake depends upon age and fitness level at the start of the training period. Athletes of endurance sports, who have reached peak performance, do not change their maximal oxygen uptake much, despite engagement in extremely heavy physical activities over many years.

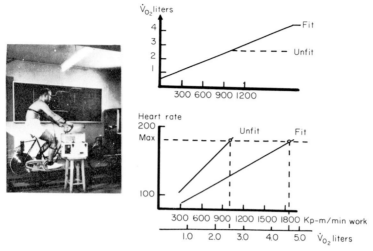

Fig. 20. The measurement of maximal oxygen uptake. Oxygen uptake at steady state exercise in relation to work output is established at submaximal intensities, and the level of work found at which a further increase in work output does not bring about any further increase in oxygen uptake. This leveling off of oxygen uptake is used as a criterion that the true maximal level is established.

When ordinary sedentary subjects who have reached their full growth as measured by height are conditioned by strenuous training regimen, only small increments in maximal oxygen uptake are found, amounting to 10–20% in training periods of several months duration. On the other hand, subjects who have lost their normal optimal level of fitness by inactivity associated with bedrest, etc., are able to improve the oxygen uptake power quite impressively during the course of a few weeks. In old age, training does not seem

TABLE III

MAXIMAL OXYGEN UPTAKE IN YOUNG ATHLETES AND NONATHLETES[a]

Subjects	Max O_2 (liters/min)	$\dot{V}_{O_2}$ (ml/min/kg)	STPD (mets[b])	Max heart rate (beats/min)	Max O_2 pulse
♂ Athletes	4.8	7.1	19.8	178	27.2
♂ Sedentary	3.2	44	12.3	189	17.0
♀ Athletes	3.3	55	15.3	186	17.8
♀ Sedentary	2.3	38	10.7	203	11.3

[a] Data from Hermansen and Andersen (1965).
[b] Multiple of basal metabolic rate.

to produce any increment in maximal oxygen uptake, but more studies are needed to fully answer this problem (Andersen, 1967).

Considerations such as the above lead to the suggestion that the size of the maximal oxygen uptake more or less is established when the individual reaches full growth. How much of a large maximal oxygen uptake is attributed to genetical constitution, and how much is attributed to adaptation to physical activity during growth, is not known (Grande and Taylor, 1965).

B. STRUCTURAL ADAPTATION TO PHYSICAL TRAINING IN ANIMALS

1. Capillarization of the Muscles

Petren *et al.* (1936) made the classic observation on the influence of training upon the capillaries in skeletal muscles. They observed an increase in the number of capillaries per unit of muscle mass (Fig. 21) in those muscles

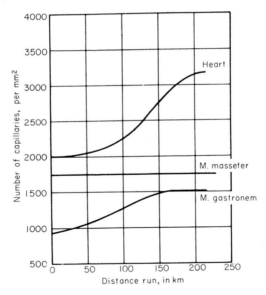

Fig. 21. The capillarization of muscles as increased by training. From Petren *et al.* (1936).

which were engaged in training, but no effect upon muscles not activated by training. Other training studies on animals have failed to confirm this observation. However, since "athletic" animals have been shown to have a markedly larger density of capillaries in the skeletal muscle than "nonathletic" animals, there is no doubt that the muscle tissue may adapt to increased activity by the formation of new capillaries. It is an open question what type, intensity, and duration of training is necessary to produce structural changes, and also the mechanism involved in this adaptation process is poorly understood.

An increased density of capillaries of the muscles contributes to increased fitness for work inasmuch as it makes possible a greater blood flow capacity of the muscles, and facilitates the transfer of metabolic material across the capillary–cellular membrane by increasing the area available for diffusion and shortens the distance the molecules have to travel.

2. The Heart

The maximal oxygen uptake in running has been established in wild and domesticated rats (Rattus Norwegicus); it appears that the wild rats average 107 ml/min/kg body weight, and the domesticated rats average 80 ml/min/kg.

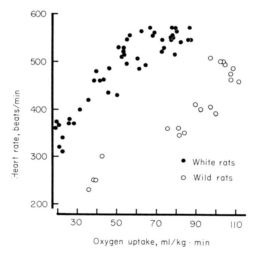

Fig. 22. The heart rate in relation to oxygen uptake in running rats. Data by Segrem and Andersen (1968).

This is a magnitude of differences comparable to that found between champion athletes and untrained subjects. Furthermore, the differences in heart rate at rest and during submaximal and maximal exercise are similar to those observed in man (Fig. 22). A comparison between "athletic" and "non-

TABLE IV

<small>SIZE AND CAPILLARIZATION OF THE HEART MUSCLE IN WILD AND DOMESTICATED RATS</small>

A. Data according to Poupa and Rakusane (1966)

Animal	Body wt (gm)	Heart wt (mg)	Heart ratio	Right vent. (mg)	Left vent. (mg)	Cells (per mm²)	Capillaries (per mm²)
Rattus norwegicus (wild)	322	1061	0.34	242	652	3332	3332
Domesticated rats (albino)	309	797	0.26	160	481	2262	2666

B. Data according to Segrem and Andersen (1968)

Animal	Body wt (gm)	Heart wt (mg)	Heart ratio	Capillaries (per mm²)	Max $\dot{V}_{O_2}$ (ml/min/ kg)	Heart rate Rest	Heart rate Max
Rattus norwegicus	243	962	0.40	2160	107	258	491
Domesticated rats	345	1040	0.30	1400	80	358	559

athletic" rats forms therefore a good basis for the evaluation of what structural changes may take place in response to increased physical activity in man.

The size of the heart is greater in the athletic animals. The ratio of heart weight to total body weight is 0.34 for wild animals compared to 0.26 for domesticated animals. Both the right and left ventricles are larger in the athletic animals (Table IV). Training experiments performed on rats also give evidence to the suggestion that the larger hearts of athletic animals are related to the degree of their physical activity (Fig. 23).

The effect of physical activity on the density of capillaries in the heart muscle has been much disputed since Petren *et al.* (1936) reported that the capillary density increases with training. Recent studies by Poupa and Rakusane (1966) and by Segrem and Andersen (1968) support the finding by Petren *et al.* (1936).

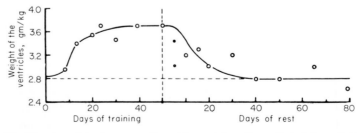

Fig. 23. The size of the heart as affected by training. From Reindell *et al.* (1960).

Poupa has summarized his important findings as follows:

1. In wild or athletic animals the heart is larger relative to the body than in nonathletic or domesticated ones.
2. The capillary density in the hearts of athletic or wild animals is larger than in nonathletic or domesticated ones.
3. The number of muscle cells per unit heart mass in athletic or wild animals is larger than in nonathletic or domesticated ones.
4. The cardiac cells in athletic or wild animals are smaller than in non-athletic or domesticated ones.

It thus seems that the construction of the systems which supply oxygen and those utilizing oxygen becomes better adapted to heavy physical efforts in animals with high levels of daily physical activity than in animals with a sedentary living pattern.

C. The Size of the Heart in Man

Reliable data about the heart weight of individuals in relation to the degree of physical activity are not numerous. Reindell *et al.* (1960) have summarized German literature on this problem. The weights of the athletes' hearts are well above the average for the sedentary population (Fig. 24).

The heart has been much studied by the x-ray method. With this procedure the heart shadow is shown in two planes during diastole, and the volume of the heart is calculated based upon measurements of length and breadth of the heart shadow.

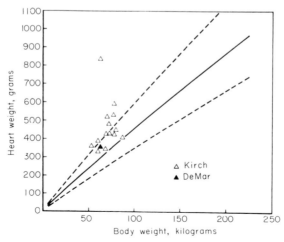

Fig. 24. The weight of the heart of athletes in relation to body weight. Data from Reindell *et al.* (1960). △ and ▲ represent athletes. Cross lines represent averages and ranges of normal subjects.

In normal sedentary men mean heart volume is about 800 ml; it is considerably higher in athletes (Table V).

TABLE V

HEART VOLUME ESTIMATED FROM AREAS OF HEART SHADOW[a, b]

Subjects	N	Heart volume (ml)	
		$\overline{X}$	Range
Normals	67	790	490–1080
Wrestlers and high jumpers	30	782	610–920
Swimmers, soccer players, and tennis players	86	876	605–1130
Skiers, long distance runners, and swimmers	66	923	645–1180
Professional cyclists	18	1104	880–1460

    [a] Data from Reindell et al. (1960).
    [b] N, number of subjects; $\overline{X}$, average.

The heart volume increases by training. Andersen and Wilson (1966) found on average a 15% increase during the course of 5-weeks strenuous training in 20 young, healthy adults. In the same period maximal oxygen uptake only increased by 6%. The volume of the heart has been shown to be related to the maximal oxygen uptake, but this relationship changes with training (Fig. 25).

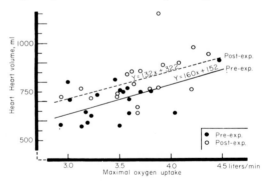

Fig. 25. Volume of the heart in relation to maximal oxygen uptake before and after a 5-week training period. From Andersen and Wilson (1966).

This implies that a few weeks of training produces a larger effect on the size of the heart than on the power of the muscle metabolism. The enlargement of the heart which comes with a few weeks of training is associated with a larger stroke volume, and is probably a dilatation rather than a hypertrophy.

Reindell *et al.* (1967) have found a high correlation between the volume of the heart and the maximal oxygen pulse. The regression line relating these 2 parameters is different in athletes and nonathletes (Fig. 26), which is another indication that training improves stroke volume more than it improves maximal oxygen uptake.

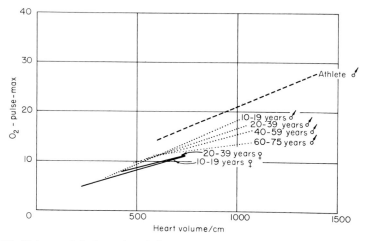

Fig. 26. Volume of the heart in relation to maximal oxygen pulse in athletes and non-athletes. From Reindell *et al.* (1967).

Kjellberg *et al.* (1949) found a high correlation between heart size, total hemoglobin, and total blood volume, which subsequently has been verified by many other workers.

D. CARDIAC OUTPUT

The oxygen uptake at rest tends to increase with training, 10–15% increase is usually found during the course of 5–6 weeks of heavy physical exertion. Also well-trained athletes possess a 10–20% higher basal metabolic rate than nonathletes. The somewhat higher cardiac output at rest found in athletes compared to nonathletes is probably related to this elevation of basal metabolism.

Ekblom (1966) reports that training tends to lower the cardiac output during performance of submaximal exercises, compensated by an increased peripheral utilization of oxygen. However, comparative studies of well-trained athletes and nonathletes have shown a somewhat hyperkinetic circulation in athletes during moderate exercise with a tendency to larger cardiac outputs for a given metabolic rate. It is therefore likely that physical training exerts little influence upon the cardiac output during exercises of submaximal intensities.

The maximal cardiac output becomes increased with training demonstrating the allover effect of training in improving the efficiency of the heart as a pump. A 4-month hard training period conducted by Ekblom (1966) raised the maximal cardiac output by 6%. Well-trained athletes may achieve maximal cardiac outputs well above 30 liters per minute compared to about 20 liters for sedentary subjects (Table VI). Also middle-aged active athletes in cross-country running and skiing are able to produce cardiac outputs of up to 30 liters per minute. The better efficiency of the heart as a pump which comes with training is also manifested in the well-known increase of stroke volume and a corresponding reduction of the heart rate.

TABLE VI

MAXIMAL CIRCULATORY VALUES IN ATHLETES AND SEDENTARY SUBJECTS[a, b]

Subjects (N)	Age (years)	Mean maximal values in upright leg exercise				
		$\dot{V}_{O_2}$ (liters/min)	$\dot{Q}$ (liters/min)	HR beats/min	SV (ml)	A-V differences (ml/liter)
Sedentary (8)	19–27	3.10	22.8	198	116	136
Athletes (6)	23–30	4.93	28.9	185	161	171
Athletes (9)	45–55	3.56	26.9	171	163	133

[a] Data from Carlsten and Grimby (1966).
[b] N, number of subjects; HR, heart rate; SV, stroke volume.

At rest and in the upright position the stroke volume is found to be about 105 ml in well-trained athletes compared to 60–70 ml in nonathletes (Table VII). In transition from rest to exercise the stroke volume increases, both in athletes and nonathletes, reaching their maximal values at a work rate corresponding to 30–40% of the maximal aerobic power. Further increase in rate affects the stroke volume little, but during prolonged exercises it tends to decrease it, this is compensated by increased rate. The maximal stroke volume in the upright position averages 150–160 ml in athletes, and about 50 ml less in nonathletes (Table VI).

Heart rate diminishes with training. The well-known sports bradycardia may be as low as 30 beats per minute, but values around 40 beats per minute are usually observed under true basal conditions in well-trained athletes.

TABLE VII

CIRCULATORY VALUES AT REST IN ATHLETES AND SEDENTARY SUBJECTS[a]

Function	Sedentary		Athletes	
	Supine	Upright	Supine	Upright
O$_2$ uptake (ml/min)	289	348	345	384
Cardiac ouput (liters/min)	7.89	5.85	9.18	6.61
Stroke volume (ml)	116	70	141	103
Heart rate (beats/min)	78	84	65	64
Mean systemic arterial pressure (mm/Hg)	93	98	85.2	99.7
Mean pulmonary arterial pressure (mm/Hg)	12.4	8.7	13.6	13.0
A-V O$_2$ difference (ml/liter)	37	60	39	61
O$_2$ saturation in mixed venous blood (%)	77	67	77	67
Blood volume (liters)	5.7		7.5	
Total Hb of body wt (gm/kg body wt)	10.3		14.0	
Heart volume (ml)	887		1087	

[a] Data from Bevegaard et al. (1960, 1963).

During performance of exercise the heart rate is much lower for a given oxygen uptake in athletes than in nonathletes.

The effect of training upon the heart rate is demonstrated in Fig. 27, which gives pre- and post-training data for heart rate in relation to oxygen uptake. The effect of training upon the heart rate may be summarized as follows:

1. The heart rate becomes lower at all metabolic rates, including the maximal aerobic rate.
2. A certain increase in metabolic rate brings about a smaller increase in the heart rate after training.
3. Before training the heart rate approached its maximal value, asymptotic in most subjects. In the trained state this is changed to a closer linear relationship.

The highest attainable rates during performance of exhaustive exercises are taken as "maximal" heart rate values. Athletes usually have a lower "maximal" heart rate in several types of exercises than nonathletes (see Table III).

In the training experiment referred to above, maximal heart rate before training averaged 196 and after training 187. It is difficult to understand that the trained heart muscle has a reduced ability and increases its rate of contractions. It is more reasonable to relate the reduced maximal heart rate with training to an increased pumping capacity, so that even during maximal exercise involving the larger part of the muscle mass there is no need for maximal activation of the cardiac pump.

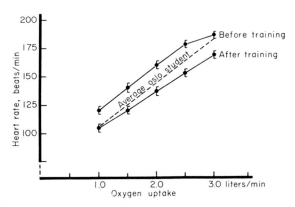

Fig. 27. Effect of training on the heart rate. From Andersen and Wilson (1966).

The effect of training upon the functioning of the heart comes quickly. In the above-mentioned experiment the bradycardia at rest and during exercise was fully established within 2 weeks after the start of training, and was associated with an increase in the volume of the heart amounting to 15%. Despite these marked effects upon the functioning of the heart the maximal oxygen uptake was little affected. Similar findings have also been reported by Hollmann and Venrath (1963).

It thus seems that physical training produces a quick adaptation in the functioning of the heart. The changes are in a direction which makes the heart a more efficient pump (increased stroke volume and reduced rate in producing the same cardiac output and possibly an increased pumping capacity). These changes are apparently not dependent upon structural changes, as they appear before there is any evidence of such adjustment.

The dominant effect upon the heart during the initial adjustment to training is the bradycardia and the increased stroke volume. The blood volume tends to increase with training (values up to 10% have been reported), but this increase is not sufficient to explain the greatly reduced heart rate during exercise.

The mechanisms involved in the development of a training bradycardia are not fully understood. The common experience that a few days of strenuous muscular exercise result in a feeling of emotional relaxation and well-being and a feeling of greatly reduced stress during performance of an exercise task may be explained by a "habituation" process involving brain structures. This process may well be associated with a reduction in the corticohypothalamic impulse flow or a shift in the cerebral stimulation formation which controls and regulates cardiac performance through the stations in the brain stem. The result may either be increased vagal stimulation or an inhibition of the sympathic drive on the heart muscle.

Other signs of a high vagal tone or inhibited sympathetic activity are frequently found in well-trained athletes. In addition to bradycardia, high T-waves are found in the electrocardiogram, and even prolonged atrioventricular conduction time or rarely partial A-V block of the Wenckebach type is noted.

The possibility also exists that the mechanism for the bradycardia may be provoked by peripheral factors such as—on the effector side—a reduced sensitivity of the excitatory structures for noradrenaline, or a reduced output of catecholamines from the adrenal cortex.

Whatever the true mechanism of the training induced bradycardia without any related metabolic effect may be, this phenomenon should always be borne in mind when heart rate is used as an index in studying fitness improvement by physical training. If fitness for work is defined as the maximal aerobic power, a reduction of the heart rate does not necessarily imply a similar increased maximal oxygen uptake.

E. Pressures as Affected by Physical Training

The pressure and dynamics at rest in the systemic and pulmonary circulation are not much affected by physical training. Slightly lower pressure in the arterial systemic circulation has frequently been found in athletes compared to a nonathletic population, and training experiments (Andersen and Elvik, 1956) have also indicated this effect which is likely related to a generally reduced sympathetic activity which tends to decrease peripheral resistance by a lessening of the sympathetic vasoconstrictor tone of the resistance vessels (Mellerowicz, 1962).

During work at apparently steady state, pressure and resistance are found to be slightly different in athletes and nonathletes (Fig. 28). The systolic arterial pressure increases more in athletes than in nonathletes, reaching in athletes values of well above 200 mm Hg during heavy exercises. Also the pressure in the pulmonary artery increases more in athletes than in nonathletes, and their mean pulmonary capillary pressure tends to be larger.

The increased pressure in the pulmonary circulation during heavy exercises indicates that the athletes' lungs contain more blood during exercise than non-athletes. A larger central blood volume tends to facilitate cardiac performance, helping to maintain a large stroke volume during heavy exercise when the effective filling time is short (Holmgren *et al.*, 1960).

That physical training increases the pressure in the arterial system during performance of exercise, has been verified by Ekblom (1966). He reports that cardiac output at a given oxygen uptake was slightly reduced after training, but the intra-arterial blood pressures, systolic and diastolic, as well as integrated mean pressure, showed a marked increase at all levels of exercise after the training period.

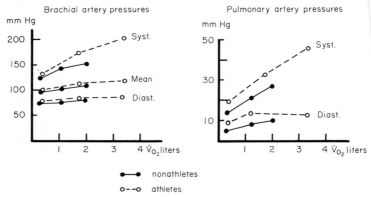

Fig. 28. Pressures in systemic and pulmonary arterial system in athletes and non-athletes. Data from Bevegaard *et al.* (1960, 1963).

The increased arterial pressure of the systemic circulation during exercise, which comes with training, facilitates the flow of blood through working muscles and also through the skin because the perfusion pressure increases.

That arterial blood pressure during work becomes greater despite a tremendous dilatation of the minute vessels of the working muscles implies probably that blood flow in inactive areas becomes more restricted in the trained state. Physical training provides thus a more adequate regulation of peripheral blood flow, involving an increased vasoconstriction in organs and tissues not activated by exercise, a better utilization of blood oxygen and an improved cardiac performance. Physical training of adequate intensity but of short duration (weeks) may improve cardiac performance and alter the regulation of peripheral circulation during muscular exercise without measurable changes in the structural basis and functional dimensions. Long periods of training (months and years) give rise to morphological changes which probably are necessary for improving the power of the aerobic metabolism.

F. Kinetics of Recovery Affected by Training

The kinetics of recovery from exercise is affected by training inasmuch as the recovery processes take place at a quicker rate in the trained state.

The blood flow through muscles which have been activated in exercise, falls quicker to resting levels in athletes than in nonathletes (Elsner and Carlson, 1962). Numerous investigations of heart rate and arterial blood pressure recovery from standard exercise tests have also revealed that the central circulation recovers much quicker in the trained than in the nontrained state.

Less well studied are the metabolism during the recovery phase and the functional relationship between metabolism and circulation. Andersen (1959) found that in brief exercises not involving lactate formation, the recovery of circulation and payment of the oxygen debt followed each other closely, which indicates a functional relationship. The elimination of excess carbon dioxide lagged behind, and therefore carbon dioxide does not govern the circulation in recovery. Respiratory recovery took place at a much quicker rate in athletes than in nonathletes. When lactate is formed, the recovery time for circulation is more irregular, usually quicker than for respiratory recovery which is greatly influenced by the pattern of lactate elimination.

The kinetics of circulatory recovery from exercise, and the time taken before resting values are reached, is thus related to the restoration of normal metabolic tissue homeostasis. The metabolism is, however, not the only mechanism which governs the pattern of circulatory recovery from exercise. The oxygen debt after exercise equals the deficit occurring in the beginning of exercise, the latter depending upon the lag in circulatory adaptation to exercise. The kinetics of adaptation to exercise is mainly a result of a nervous regulatory mechanism which also has an influence upon the behavior of circulation in recovery from exercise.

REFERENCES

Andersen, K. L. (1959). "Respiratory Recovery from Muscular Exercise of Short Duration." Oslo Univ. Press, Oslo.

Andersen, K. L. (1967). *In* "Physical Activity and the Heart" (W. Raab, ed.), pp. 5–20. Thomas, Springfield, Illinois.

Andersen, K. L., and Elvik, A. (1956). *Acta Med. Scand.* **153**, 367.

Andersen, K. L., and Wilson, O. (1966). *Acta Univ. Lundensis*, 11–20.

Asmussen, E., and Nielsen, M. (1955). *Physiol. Rev.* **35**, 778.

Åstrand, P. O. (1956). *Physiol. Rev.* **36**, 307.

Åstrand, P. O., Cuddy, T. E., Saltin, B., and Stenberg, J. (1964). *J. Appl. Physiol.* **19**, 268.

Barcroft, B. (1965). *In* "Handbook of Physiology" (Am. Physiol. Soc., J. Field, ed.) Sect. 2, Vol. II. Williams & Wilkins, Baltimore, Maryland.

Barcroft, H. (1963a). *In* "Handbook of Physiology" (Am. Physiol. Soc., J. Field, ed.), Sect. 2, Vol. II, pp. 1353–1385. Williams & Wilkins, Baltimore, Maryland.

Barcroft, H. (1963b). *Brit. Med. Bull.* **19**, 97.

Bevegaard, S., Holmgren, A., and Jonsson, B. (1960). *Acta Physiol. Scand.* **49**, 279.

Bevegaard, S., Holmgren, A., and Jonsson, B. (1963). *Acta Physiol. Scand.* **57**, 26.

Bevegaard, S., and Shepherd, J. T. (1965). *J. Appl. Physiol.* **20**, 1.

Brouha, L. (1960) "Physiology in Industry." Pergamon Press, Oxford.

Carlsten, A., and Grimby, G. (1966). "The Circulatory Response to Muscular Exercise in Man." Thomas, Springfield, Illinois.

Cerretelli, P. (1966). *In* "Physical Activity in Health and Disease" (K. L. Andersen, ed.), pp. 64–73. Universitetsforlaget, Oslo.

Ekblom, B. (1966). *In* "Physical Activity in Health and Disease" (K. L. Andersen, ed.), pp. 15–18. Universitetsforlaget, Oslo.

Elsner, R. W., and Carlson, L. (1962). *J. Appl. Physiol.* **17**, 436.

Folkow, B., Heymans, C., and Neil, E. (1963). *In* "Handbook of Physiology" (Am. Physiol. Soc., J. Field, ed.), Sect. 2, Vol. III, pp. 1787–1823. Williams & Wilkins, Baltimore, Maryland.

Grande, F., and Taylor, H. L. (1965). *In* "Handbook of Physiology" (Am. Physiol. Soc., J. Field, ed.), Sect. 2, Vol. III, pp. 2615–2677. Williams & Wilkins, Baltimore, Maryland.

Grimby, G., Nilsson, N. J., and Saltin, B. (1966). *J. Appl. Physiol.* **21**, 1150.

Guyton, A. C. (1966). "Textbook of Medical Physiology." Saunders, Philadelphia, Pennsylvania.

Hermansen, L., and Andersen, K. L. (1965). *J. Appl. Physiol.* **20**, 425.

Hollmann, W., and Venrath, H. (1963). *Sportartzt* **9**, 189.

Holmgren, A. (1956). *Scand. J. Clin. & Lab. Invest.* **8**, Suppl. 24, 1.

Holmgren, A., Mossfeldt, F., Sjöstrand, T., and Strom, G. (1960). *Acta Physiol. Scand.* **50**, 72.

Kjellberg, S. R., Rudke, V., and Sjöstrand, T. (1949). *Acta Physiol. Scand.* **19**, 152.

Krogh, A. (1922). "The Anatomy and Physiology of the Capillaries." Yale Univ. Press, New Haven, Connecticut.

Lind, A. R., McNicol, G. W., and Donald, K. W. (1966). *In* "Physical Activity in Health and Disease" (K. L. Andersen, ed.), pp. 38–63. Oslo Univ. Press, Oslo.

Mellerowicz, H. (1962). "Ergometrie." Urban & Schwarzenberg, Munich.

Petren, T., Sjöstrand, T., and Sylven, B. (1936). *Arbeitsphysiol.* **9**, 376.

Poupa, O., and Rakusane, K. (1966). *In* "Physical Activity in Health and Disease" (K. L. Andersen, ed.), pp. 18–29. Oslo Univ. Press, Oslo.

Reindell, H., Klepzig, H., Steim, H., Musshoff, K., Roskamm, H., and Schildge, E. (1960). "Herz, Kreislaufkrankheiten und Sport." Barth, Munich.

Reindell, H., Konig, K., and Roskamm, H. (1967). "Funktionsdiagnostik des gesunden und kranken Herzens." Thieme, Stuttgart.

Robinson, S. (1938). *Arbeitsphysiol.* **10**, 251.

Rowell, L. B., Blackmon, J. R., Martin, R. H., Mazzarella, J. A., and Bruce, R. (1965). *J. Appl. Physiol.* **20**, 384.

Segrem, N., and Andersen, K. L. (1968). Unpublished data.

Selkurt, E. (1962). "Physiology." Churchill, London.

Strömme, S., Andersen, K. L., and Elsner, R. W. (1963). *J. Appl. Physiol.* **18**, 756.

4

OTHER BODY SYSTEMS AND EXERCISE

P. J. Rasch and I. Dodd Wilson

I. Introduction

The physiology and biochemistry of the systems covered in this chapter are complex, confusing, and often controversial. In some cases the data submitted by researchers are susceptible to a different interpretation than that placed upon them by the original author. In other instances we found it impossible to decide between conflicting evidence. Since the authors believe it necessary to present both sides, a certain amount of inherently contradictory writing has inevitably resulted. No attempt has been made to describe the variability which may be exhibited in the functioning of apparently "normal" biological systems, nor has any effort been made to present the effects of exertion upon pathological conditions. Our sole aim has been to set forth what happens, or what is believed to happen (which may be something quite different), when certain body systems are subjected to the stresses of physical exertion. Neither is this chapter designed for the specialist in the field. Every effort has been made to keep the presentation as simple as possible without the sacrifice of accuracy in the hope that the material will be found informative and helpful by readers whose backgrounds and areas of specialization may differ widely.

II. The Kidney

A. General Considerations

The adult human kidney is composed of approximately 1,000,000 separate functional units termed nephrons. Each nephron consists of a tortuous tubule which is dilated at its origin to form a Bowman's capsule. This in turn encloses a cluster of capillaries termed a glomerulus. According to Wakim, "The kidney is the organ on which depends the dynamic stability of the internal environment of the body and the subsequent maintenance of a steady state. The kidney is mainly responsible for the regulation and maintenance of fluid, electrolyte, osmotic and acid–base balance . . . urine is a by-product of the regulatory functions of the kidney" (Smith, 1963). Under normal conditions about 1300 ml of blood (25% of the resting cardiac output) flow through the average male kidneys each minute. In women, who are physically smaller, the quantity is about 80% of this figure. There are, however, large individual differences.

The secretion of urine is of great importance in maintaining the homeostasis of the body; consequently it has been a subject of considerable interest to exercise physiologists for over 200 years. Of the 1300 ml renal blood flow per minute, about 700 ml are plasma. The process of urine formation begins with the formation of approximately 120 ml of glomerular filtrate every minute. Thus, the filtrate forms at the rate of about 170–180 liters per day. The unfiltered blood passes out of the glomeruli into a set of capillaries which surround the tubules. As the filtrate proceeds through the tubules of the nephron, about 99% of the water, all of the glucose, and perhaps 90% of the sodium, calcium, chloride, and bicarbonate may be reabsorbed through the walls of the tubules and accepted back into the blood stream. This reabsorption process controls the electrolyte balance and maintains a constant hydrostatic pressure, which has led to Smith's often quoted dictum, "The kidney is not so important in what it excretes as in what it retains" (Wakim, 1958). Additional substances may be added to the fluid as it proceeds through the tubules, so that the composition of urine is not identical with that of the filtrate.

When other conditions remain constant, there is a distinct diurnal rhythm in the excretion of water and electrolytes. There is a fall during the night hours and an increase in the morning. This is remarkably persistent under experimentally altered conditions, but its basic cause is uncertain. Urea secretion is depressed during the first hour after rising. This is followed by a regular increase, which continues during the morning. After lunch a definite drop occurs, followed by a rise during the later afternoon. During normal waking hours changes of posture affect the picture. Normally, lying down results in an increase of urine flow and of sodium and chloride excretion. Potassium excretion and acidity of the urine are reduced. These are reversed when the individual again stands. In part this can be attributed to changes in the distribution of the blood volume, but some specific action on the tubules is also believed to be involved (MacKay, 1928; Van Slyke *et al.*, 1932).

The actual mechanisms involved in the functioning of the kidney are extremely complex and beyond the scope of this chapter. From the standpoint of those concerned principally with the physiology of activity, any discussion of the effect of exercise on the kidney may be resolved into two subproblems: (1) the effect of the exercise per se on the kidneys, and (2) the effects of the trauma to the kidneys sustained during the exercise. Separation of these two aspects in some cases presents considerable difficulty.

B. Effects of Exercise

1. Physiology

Severe exercise appears to have three principal effects upon the kidney: transient proteinuria, diminished urine flow, and diminished renal blood flow. As early as 1906, Collier (1907) made repeated observations of the urine of college crews. He reported that practically every oarsman displayed albuminuria (protein in the urine) at one time or another, the quantity being proportional to the severity of the work done. It disappeared the following day, from which he concluded that its presence was not a sign of renal disease. Four years afterwards Barach (1910) found albumin, hyaline and granular casts, and red blood cells in the urine of marathon runners. After less severe exercise the subjects showed increased urinary acidity, but the albumin and casts did not seem to be quantitatively related to the pH of the urine. Later he demonstrated similar findings in baseball players and trackmen (Barach, 1920). The more severe the exercise, the more marked the evidence of disturbance of the renal function.

It is now generally conceded that perfectly healthy athletes may display both albuminuria and cylindruria following severe exercise regardless of whether bodily contact is involved (Morgan *et al.*, 1957). These conditions usually subside within a short time, but their mechanism is not well understood. Normally 18 to 360 gm of plasma protein pass through the glomeruli with the filtrate daily and are reabsorbed by the renal tubules so that no protein is detectable in the urine. Cantone and Cerretelli (1960) have demonstrated an increase in the albumin globulin ratio in urine from 0.57 to about

1.59 with exertion. Leakage of plasma proteins through abnormally permeable glomerular capillaries, a failure in tubular reabsorption, and increased time of contact between blood and renal tissue may be important to the appearance of protein in the urine. Suggested explanations for these changes resulting from exercise have included mechanical trauma to the kidneys (Barach, 1910), damage to the glomeruli due to ischemia during exercise (Christensen *et al.*, 1934; White and Rolf, 1948; Chesley *et al.*, 1939), increased blood acidity (Nedbal and Seliger, 1958), possibly affecting the permeability of the glomerular intracellular cement (Javitt and Miller, 1952), decreased tubular reabsorption of protein (Cantone and Cerretelli, 1960), and changes in renal circulation (Taylor, 1960; Starr, 1926).

It is still a matter of dispute whether the observations made result from the partial shutdown of all nephrons or are due to a complete shutdown of some of them. Hellebrandt (1932) and Hellebrandt *et al.* (1932) consider that the experimental evidence is consistent with the theory that strenuous exercise shunts the blood to the working muscles and the skin, affecting the circulation of the blood to an extent that causes asphyxiation of the renal cells beyond that seen in normal functioning. The evidence indicates that at work below a certain critical level [about 1000 kgm/m according to Christensen *et al.* (1934)] there is vasoconstriction in all channels; above this level glomeruli begin dropping out. The occurrence of postexercise proteinuria may be an index of this. Protein does not occur in urine formed during exercise, but appears in that formed after exercise. This suggests that when the flow and filtration are re-established after exercise, protein appears in the filtrate of the glomeruli which had dropped out. Since the critical level of work is higher than can be maintained for more than a few minutes, the kidneys are protected against the damage that might result from any prolonged period of ischemia. The picture is complicated by the fact that two types of postexercise albuminuria may exist. One occurs a relatively long time after the cessation of moderate, prolonged exercise. The other appears during rapid exhausting effort and seems related to the speed of doing work (Chesley *et al.*, 1939). Norepinephrine is believed by some to play a role in the transient proteinuria of exercise (Cantone and Cerretelli, 1960; King and Baldwin, 1956). As an athletic training season progresses, the amount of postexertion proteinuria decreases, suggesting that training and physical fitness may be factors (Light and Warren, 1936). It may also mean that the trained man responds to strenuous activity with a more controlled output of norepinephrine than does the untrained individual. Taylor (1960) found that the coefficient of correlation between postexercise proteinuria and pulse count was 0.70, and a decrease in pulse count following training would be expected.

Proteinuria has also been found in those who swim in cold water. This has been attributed both to vasoconstriction in the glomerular and preglomerular blood vessels of the kidneys, with a consequent anoxia, and to the markedly lordotic position assumed in swimming (Chesley *et al.*, 1939). It is of interest in this connection that Hellebrandt (1932) found that sufferers from albuminuria frequently had an exaggerated lumbar lordosis.

During exercise there is a marked fall in renal plasma flow and in glomerular filtration rate (Barclay *et al.*, 1947). The reduction in the renal blood flow is progressive for at least 30 min after the start of exercise and is directly related to the severity of the exercise. It reaches a stable value during the first 40–60 min of exercise, and the return to normal is not complete approximately 40 min after its cessation (Chapman *et al.*, 1948a, b). The diversion of blood to the working muscles presumably explains the drop in renal blood flow during exercise. Recovery of renal plasma flow is considerably slower than is recovery in pulse rate or in blood pressure (Chapman *et al.*, 1948a,b). The decrease in renal blood flow may not be responsible for the decrease in urine secretion, as the volume and composition of the urine appear largely independent of the blood flow. The resting kidney has such a large inbuilt safety margin that the renal blood flow can be altered significantly without any appreciable effect on the volume of glomerular filtrate produced (Berlinger, 1963).

It is generally agreed that exercise exerts an antidiuretic effect. This appears to be independent of the nerve supply to the kidney, as denervation of this organ is apparently without effect on this response. One suggestion is that the pituitary gland controls this function of the kidneys through an antidiuretic hormone. However, Eggelton (1942) observed that the urine flow decreased even though the subject ingested water during the activity. This suggested a temporary renal vasoconstriction to her but is also compatible with other interpretations. In any given instance the reaction of the right kidney may precede or follow that of the left (Klisiecki *et al.*, 1933a).

In mild exercise the inhibition of water diuresis is accompanied by a rise in the percentage of chloride in the urine (Klisiecki *et al.*, 1933b). In a short burst of violent exercise there is a fall in the rate of excretion of chloride, which lasts for about half an hour after the exercise has ended. During the postexercise period the excretion rate of (1) water is about the resting value; (2) of phosphates and ammonia is over twice the resting rate; and (3) of chloride is sometimes less than during the activity. Part of the fall in chloride excretion may be due to an increased secretion of this substance in the sweat, but not all of it can be accounted for on this basis. It may be connected with acidosis due to the excess of lactic acid in the blood. This temporary acidosis is responsible for the rise in the excretion of phosphates and ammonia (Havard, 1937).

During severe exercise the rise in body temperature causes increased sweat and respiratory loss of water, so that the kidney changes are intensified. Such changes may be still further accentuated by the fact that the athlete is already dehydrated as a result of "making weight," or is being trained by a coach who disapproves of the consumption of water during activity.

Addis and Drury (1923) reported that urea clearance (a rough measure of renal function) during strenuous exercise is about 70% of the value observed during rest. MacKay (1928) found a drop of about 50% of the standard clearance. A study of football players indicated that clearance values are roughly inversely proportional to the playing time. This was attributed to the demands of the heavily working muscles and the possible dehydration of the blood by sweating (Edwards et al., 1937). The decline in urea clearance has been interpreted as indicating that something happens to the walls of the tubules which increases their permeability to urea. The sweat excreted during work contains from 300 to 600 mg urea per liter, thus compensating to a considerable extent for the decrease in excretion of this substance through the kidneys.

2. Athletic Pseudonephritis

In the years following the studies of Collier and of Barach, interest in the effects of exercise on the kidneys had largely centered around the physiological aspects of the problem. Renewed interest in the effects of possible sports trauma on the kidneys date largely from an important paper by Amelar and Solomon (1954). Disturbed by the fact that boxing is considered the most dangerous trade, they undertook a study of the trauma of the kidneys incurred by those participating in it. Urine specimens were taken from 139 professional boxers, and an effort was made to estimate the number and severity of blows received in the region of the kidney during the fight. It was found that 46% of the fighters' urine changed from clear before the fight to turbid immediately afterwards; the urinary specific gravity increased in 80%; traces of acetone were observed in 14%; the urinary pH decreased in 39%; sugar spilled into the urine in 9%; albuminuria was present in 68%; red blood cells were found in significant pathological amounts in 73%; granular or hyaline casts were present in 73%; crystals, mostly calcium oxalate, were seen in 20%. The extent of these urinary changes appeared to be positively correlated with the number of rounds fought. The authors modestly claimed only that they had proved the obvious, that exercise affected the kidneys, that there was an additional effect resulting from trauma, and that the more severe the exercise, the greater these effects. One difficulty, of course, is that the boxers who fought the most rounds had the greater amount of exercise, as well as the greater exposure to possible trauma. Their recommendation was that a routine urinalysis should be a part of each prefight examination and a boxer should not be allowed to fight unless his findings were normal. This suggestion has received the editorial support of the *Journal of the American Medical Association* (Editorial, 1954).

Inspired by Amelar and Solomon's investigation, Boone *et al.* (1955) undertook a study of the varsity football squad at a major college. They found that nearly all samples were normal when the players reported to the training camp. Preliminary conditioning exercises produced albuminuria, casts, and microscopic hematuria in many of the players. With the beginning of body contact work, urinary abnormalities increased, reaching a peak after the Saturday games. During the season all of the players bled intermittently, hematuria sufficient to grossly discolor the urine being noted in 6 men. Both gross and microscopic bleeding promptly disappeared following rest. The authors suggested that microscopic hematuria was not a reason to restrict activity.

In one study of football players, 70% of the paired samples changed from a pregame clear to a postgame turbid appearance; 92% developed proteinuria; 81% exhibited hyaline and/or granular casts after the games. Only an insignificant incidence of hematuria was seen. The investigators concluded that the evidence did not indicate that football playing is likely to be any more injurious to the kidneys than is a comparable exercise which does not involve physical contact (Selman and Gualano, 1955).

Additional information was obtained from research conducted on 47 University of Pennsylvania varsity players. Of the 424 specimens obtained over a 12-day period, 44.8% were considered to be abnormal. On no day did every member of the squad submit a completely normal sample. This study served to re-emphasize the fact that,

Elements heretofore considered almost pathognomonic of parenchymal renal disease may appear in the urine of a player during the athletic season without other evidence of glomerular nephritis. These elements most frequently are protein, hyaline and granular casts, and red blood cells; however, red blood cell, epithelial, broad, and white blood cell casts may also be found. . . . Formed elements usually held to be indicative of nephritis may be found in the urinary sediment obtained from an athlete during the season of his active participation in a sport. Under such circumstances, however, these elements usually do not indicate serious disease, for their disappearance from the urinary sediment is prompt when the athlete is withdrawn from daily exertion. . . . The name "athletic pseudonephritis" is proposed for this phenomenon . . . (Gardner, 1956).

The only way of distinguishing the urinary findings in football players from those of acute glomerulonephritis is that those resulting from exercise disappear within a week after the activity has been discontinued. As a result of these studies attention was again focused on the problem of whether it was the exercise per se or the contact involved in the sport which was responsible for the observed changes. In general, the results have tended to confirm the results obtained by earlier investigators.

Perhaps the definitive studies in this respect, however, are those made by Alyea and his associates (Alyea and Boone, 1957; Alyea and Parish, 1958). Their first step was to examine oarsmen, as crew is an activity in which the kidneys are not likely to sustain trauma. Of the 31 crewmen examined, none of whom had albumin, casts, or red blood cells in his urine before exercise, 71% showed albumin, 84% showed casts, and 55% showed red blood cells after the first practice. These urines became normal within a week. The authors believed that the findings were the same as in acute glomerular nephritis and probably are due to a similar injury.

Their second step was to compare the urinary findings of sports considered nontraumatic to the kidneys—crew, track, and swimming with those considered traumatic—football and lacrosse. The striking thing about the results was their similarity. Regardless of the sport, 50% to 80% of the contestants showed albumin, casts, and red blood cells in the urine. The exception was distance runners who showed albuminuria in 100% of the cases. Abnormal findings were also extremely high among long-distance swimmers. The amount of blood in the urine was higher in football players than in other sports, probably due to contact trauma of the kidneys. These conditions do not appear to be related to the nervous tension experienced by the athlete. They raise the question of whether any insult of this kind to the kidney can be truly benign and suggest that it may be inadvisable for those who have a history of definite renal disease, such as glomerulonephritis or pyelonephritis, to participate in severe exercise. Perhaps one thing that is needed here is a study of athletes to determine whether they display a higher incidence of renal disease than is true in a sedentary population.

Of all sports, boxing is generally assumed to be the most damaging to the kidneys. Particularly important, therefore, is Kleiman's (1958, 1960) 3-year study involving 764 professional boxers. This included clinical and laboratory examinations before their bouts, observations during the bouts, roentgenographic examinations of the urinary tract in 100 boxers with significant hematuria, and supplementary clinical studies of other individuals. Significant hematuria was demonstrated in 27% of the 1518 postbout urinalyses. The incidence was twice as high in the white as in the nonwhite boxers, which suggests the possibility that the perirenal fascial support is stronger in the latter. Hematuria was not ordinarily elicited by emotional stress or by exercise alone. Roentgenographic findings included hydronephrosis in 26 of 100 boxers studied.

The kidneys may develop a pericalyceal deformity, with particular involvement of the right upper calyx. Kleiman attributes this deformity to repeated traumatization. Significant impairment of renal function was not associated with this abnormality and progressive renal deformity was uncommon. Kleiman (1958) has proposed the term "athlete's kidney" to designate this condition. He has theorized that the crouch position predisposes to anterior displacement of the kidney, tending to dislocate it from its fossa and causing excessive strain on its fascial envelope.

The loss of perirenal fat as a result of training may be a factor. The resultant renal mobility may result in interference with the venous return, producing venostasis. The distended veins of the pyramids thus become more easily prone to trauma. Forced crouching may also mechanically compress the vessels and viscera, inducing renal hypoxia followed by tubular or cortical necrosis. Hydrostatic processes within the kidney when it is compressed by a forceful blow may contribute to the pathological process. The most important factor in treatment is rest, which may require 30 to 60 days. Coupled with this is appropriate chemotherapy and, if indicated, a forced fluid regimen. If complications are involved there may be no alternative to retiring from competition.

Athlete's kidney is far less common among professional wrestlers, basketball players, and hockey players than among boxers (Kleiman, 1960). Amateur wrestling is accompanied by the usual increases in acidity and the number of casts, and the appearance of albumin, red blood cells, and sugar. After a rest period these tend to return to precompetition levels. None of these transient signs appear to be of sufficient severity or duration to indicate that permanent damage to the kidneys may result from the sport (Rasch *et al.*, 1958).

3. March Hemoglobinuria

March hemoglobinuria has been defined as "a condition in which physical exertion gives rise to the passage of a red urine containing hemoglobin in solution" (Gilligan and Blumgart, 1941). The basic abnormality actually is intravascular breakdown of red blood cells during exercise, the hemoglobin appearing in the urine only after the plasma haptoglobins have been saturated. The syndrome was first reported by Fleischer in 1881. Since then, a relatively large literature has grown up around it. Gilligan and Blumgart reviewed 40 case reports, mainly in the German literature, and added three more of their own. By 1953, a total of 75 cases was reported in the literature (Stahl, 1957). In the last few years this total has increased considerably, reflecting in part, at least, the great number of men in the military services.

Although the exact pathogenesis of the condition has not been completely elucidated, certain salient features can be described:

1. It usually occurs after vigorous exercise in the upright position. Conditions associated with the entity may have either brisk walking or running in common. Equal or more vigorous work found in sawing wood, calisthenics, or other physical activities does not produce hemoglobinuria, but it has been reported following "squat jumps," deep knee bends, and push-ups, or such

exercises as swimming or crawling (Chaiken *et al.*, 1953; Witts, 1936; Howenstine, 1960).

2. Constitutional symptoms are absent or mild.

3. The condition is benign, and usually of short duration.

4. Hemoglobinemia is present at the time of hemoglobinuria. Somewhat less exercise than necessary to produce hemoglobinuria may be associated with hemoglobinemia. Gilligan and Blumgart (1941) found elevated plasma hemoglobin values in 18 of 22 marathon runners after a race of greater than 26 mi. Only three of these men had hemoglobinuria.

5. The greatest part of the hemolysis must occur during the exercise since the plasma hemoglobin levels are greatest at the termination of exertion.

6. No definite evidence of intrinsic red blood cell defects or abnormal plasma hemolytic systems has been elucidated. Flatmark (1963) did note a slight postexertional susceptibility of the erythrocyte to increased spontaneous hemolysis which he termed "transitory acquired erythropathia."

7. There is some evidence that march hemoglobinuria is related to lumbar lordosis or to the assumption of a lordotic position during exercise. It is sometimes inhibited if the patient is placed into a jacket which forces him to assume a kyphotic position.

8. There is evidence that running on a hard surface is of paramount importance in producing the syndrome. Using 2 patients and 2 control runners, Davidson (1964) has shown that running 3 mi on a hard roadway produced a greater rise in plasma hemoglobin than did the same distance run on grass. He also presented evidence which suggested that the patient with march hemoglobinuria had a much heavier stride than the control runners. Buckle (1965) was able to extend this data by reducing the severity of the hemolysis with the use of sorbo-rubber insoles to cushion the foot. Thus, there is a reasonably strong suggestion that mechanical trauma to the erythrocyte as it passes through the foot may be the prime factor in the pathogenesis of march hemoglobinuria.

4. Myoglobinuria

Stahl (1957) draws a distinction between "march hemoglobinuria," in which blood appears in the urine 1 to 3 hr after exercise, and "exercise myoglobinuria," in which dark urine appears 24 to 48 hr after exercise. He believes that the latter is due to breakdown of muscle fibers from excessive exercise, so that myoglobin is released into the blood plasma and then excreted through the kidneys. The initial findings may closely resemble those of acute glomerulonephritis (Howenstine, 1960). Stahl considers the time factor in the onset of discolored urine an important differential diagnostic point in identification of myoglobinuria. Strictly speaking, this condition falls outside the limits of this chapter. It is mentioned here because the literature suggests that the two conditions have been confused in the past and may be again in the future. Those concerned with the problems of the physiology of exercise will find an extensive discussion of this particular problem in a paper by Kreisle *et al.* (1960).

III. The Gastrointestinal Tract

A. GENERAL CONSIDERATIONS

Despite rapid progress in the comprehension of gastrointestinal physiology and biochemistry, the specific effects of exertion upon this system are incompletely understood. There is a dearth of experimental data and much of the available work was done before the development of our present physiological concepts and investigational techniques.

B. EFFECTS OF EXERCISE

1. Stomach

Perhaps the best data are available regarding the acute effects of exertion upon the stomach. It appears that strenuous exercise inhibits both the motor and secretory functions of this organ. Campbell *et al.* (1928) concluded from their investigations that exercise of "moderate" intensity (i.e., running 2 or 3 mi slowly) inhibited both the secretion of gastric juice and the rate of gastric emptying of its contents into the duodenum. Lighter exercise such as walking did not change the rate of gastric secretion and actually appeared to enhance emptying of the stomach. The amount of exercise required to inhibit gastric function varied with the physical fitness of the individual. They concluded that "exercise which produced no discomfort helped digestion, and exercise which produced discomfort delayed it."

Hellebrandt *et al.* (1934a,b) confirmed and extended these observations. All types of exercise after a meal prolonged the final emptying time of the stomach more than the same activity preceding the meal. When examined fluoroscopically immediately after exertion, the stomach appeared either totally inactive or had only feeble peristaltic movements. Recovery was usually prompt, however, and emptying was greatly accelerated during the second postexercise hour.

Experimental work using dogs with surgically prepared gastric pouches has confirmed the inhibitory effect of exertion upon total acid secretion and volume after either histamine or food stimulation, or in the fasting state (Crandall, 1928; Lillehei and Wangensteen, 1948; Hammar and Öbrink, 1953). Lillehei and Wangensteen found that the exercised animals had a higher incidence of histamine-induced gastric ulceration in spite of the depressed gastric acidity. They felt that these apparently paradoxical results might be explained by the changes in blood supply produced by exertion. Hammar and Öbrink noted that the suppression of acid secretion sometimes continued after the exercise had been completed. Increasing the "dose" of exercise also appeared to further depress secretion. They postulated that a circulating blood substance was the important factor in these changes since the transfusion of blood from an exercised donor dog to a resting, stimulated recipient dog tended to decrease gastric secretion.

Although these studies pertain to acute changes in gastric function produced by exertion, they are not helpful in discerning changes associated with physical conditioning. Frenkl et al. (1962, 1964) noted that the conditioned athlete tended to have reduced acid secretion response at rest to either caffeine or histamine stimulation. They investigated this observation experimentally by using histamine stimulated, anesthetized, surgically prepared rats. Although this is a highly artificial experimental preparation, several interesting observations were made. After swimming to the point of exhaustion daily for three weeks, the gastric acid response to histamine was significantly reduced from control levels. This was even more pronounced after 6 weeks. The amount of a dose of intravenously injected radioactively labeled sulphur found within the stomach was significantly increased at 6 weeks, suggesting increased production of gastric mucin. No changes were found in pepsin content, serum chloride, gastric adenosine triphosphate, or histology of the stomach. The exercised rats were more resistant to experimental production of gastric ulcers. The effect of physical conditioning disappeared rapidly since the response to histamine administration had returned to normal by 16 days after the daily exercise was discontinued.

2. Small and Large Intestine

Very little is known about the effects of exercise upon the motor and absorptive functions of the small and large intestine. The rate at which water passes from the stomach to the small intestine is increased by exercise (Neilson and Lipsitz, 1915). Barcroft and Florey (1929) observed blanching of the exteriorized colon in dogs during exertion. This probably is a reflection of the reduction in hepatic and splanchnic blood flow discussed in Section III, B, 3.

The mechanics of the bowel are altered by exertion. Buntine and Hughes (1965) studied intrarectal pressure changes during various activities. They found that a hard cough by an athletic subject could produce intraluminal pressures as high as 200 mm Hg (normal = 10 to 15 mm Hg). Activities such as pushups, which involve contraction of the abdominal musculature, produce intrarectal pressures of approximately 50 mm Hg. DeYoung et al.

(1931) reported a sharp rise in colonic pressure and activity in dogs usually beginning one to three minutes after the start of exercise and lasting several minutes. They concluded that these changes were due to alterations in parasympathetic nervous activity. After exercise, a variable period of subnormal activity was found.

Stickney *et al.* (1956) were unable to find evidence for any significant acute effect of strenuous exercise upon the propulsive motility of the small intestine in rats and dogs. Van Liere *et al.* (1954), however, noted increased propulsive motility of the small intestine in physically conditioned rats. They were unable to explain their results but they did suggest the possibility that either changes in activity of the parasympathetic nervous system or intestinal smooth muscle hypertrophy due to increased food intake in the exercised rats might explain the results.

The effect of exertion upon the absorption of food constituents is essentially unknown. It appears that the absorption of triolein is more rapid and efficient in exercised rats (Simko *et al.*, 1963). However, in spite of the evidence that strenuous exercise elevates blood vitamin A levels (James and ElGindi, 1953; Hillman and Rosner, 1958), it appears that routine daily activity depresses vitamin A absorption from the intestine (Schjoth, 1965). Many factors, such as changes in the rate of peripheral utilization of substances and the alterations in delivery of food to the bowel from the stomach, must be considered in assessing the effects of exercise upon intestinal absorption. Much more data are required before a more definitive statement can be made on this subject.

3. Hepatic and Splanchnic Blood Flow

During severe exercise, the heart of a healthy man can increase its output to approximately 5 times its resting value. This is not enough to supply the amount of oxygen consumed by the active muscles during physical exertion. A change in the pattern of blood flow also occurs. Arterial blood is diverted from certain organs to the active skeletal muscles when the need for oxygen is acute (Chapman and Mitchell, 1965).

The hepatic and splanchnic vascular beds are well-suited for the rapid adjustment of imbalance between cardiac output and oxygen requirements. Normally the splanchnic region receives about 20 to 25% of the cardiac output but extracts only 10 to 25% of the available oxygen. Rowell *et al.* (1964) have clearly demonstrated a fall in the hepatic and splanchnic blood flow, sometimes in excess of 80%, during severe exertion. This correlated highly with oxygen intake by the subject. They also confirmed the observation that the hepatic arteriovenous oxygen difference increased during exertion (Bishop *et al.*, 1955) and noted that this change corresponded closely to the changes in hepatic blood flow.

4. Athletic Performance

The eating of light meals at times varying from 3 hr to $\frac{1}{2}$ hr before athletic events cannot be shown to affect time in sprinting (Youmans *et al.*, 1960), middle distance events (Asprey *et al.*, 1963), the mile run (Asprey *et al.*, 1964), or swimming (Ball, 1962). None of the subjects in any of these tests suffered from nausea or stomach cramps. Similarly, the ingestion of water before running or swimming does not adversely affect performance (Little *et al.*, 1949; Blank, 1959). The situation may, of course, be quite different in football or combat sports, where forceful blows or pressures might be directed at the distended abdomen.

IV. Blood Coagulation

A. GENERAL CONSIDERATIONS

Blood coagulation is an enormously complicated subject. Any statement regarding the effects of exercise upon this system requires at least a brief review of this mechanism, which is "superbly designed to permit, when needed, the ready, smooth and rapid mobilization of a series of beautifully integrated and unimaginably complicated reactions involving surface phenomena, electrostatic forces, interaction of cells with proteins, of proteins with proteins and of proteins with metals" (Alexander, 1955). As with much of the other material in this chapter, the discussion which follows is necessarily oversimplified.

The classic theory is that blood clotting takes place in three steps:

$$\text{Platelet} + \text{"foreign substance"} \longrightarrow \text{thromboplastin} \qquad (1)$$

$$\text{Prothrombin} \xrightarrow{\text{thromboplastin, Ca}^{++}} \text{thrombin} \qquad (2)$$

$$\text{Fibrinogen} \xrightarrow{\text{thrombin}} \text{fibrin} \qquad (3)$$

This scheme, although inadequate in the face of present knowledge, is a useful guide in understanding changes that occur after exercise.

Steps (2) and (3) remain relatively unaltered by present knowledge, but step (1) is now known to be much more complex. Two thromboplastin pathways are available to the body for the formation of prothrombinase, a potent substance which converts prothrombin to thrombin (Gaston, 1964). The first, or so-called intrinsic thromboplastin system, is exemplified by the coagulation of blood within a glass tube without the addition of tissue thromboplastin. This requires an intricate series of reactions involving contact with a foreign surface, calcium, platelets and factors XII (Hageman), XI (plasma thromboplastin antecedent), IX (plasma thromboplastin component), VIII (antihemophiliac), X (Stuart), and V (proaccelerin). System (2), the extrinsic thromboplastin system, requires tissue thromboplastin, calcium, and factors VII (proconvertin), X, and V.

In addition to the blood coagulation system, the body also has an elaborate process (fibrinolysis) for dissolving unwanted fibrin deposits and blood clots which form within the organism. It involves the conversion of plasminogen to plasmin, a fibrinolytic enzyme, by an activator. Plasmin then acts by lysing the fibrin clot.

B. Effects of Exercise

1. Clotting and Clotting Factors

The effect of exertion upon blood coagulation time and other tests of the intrinsic thromboplastin system has been extensively studied. Most investigators report a hypercoagulable state almost immediately after exertion (Hartman, 1927; Kalaja, 1950; Schneider and Zangari, 1951; Wachholder et al., 1957; Egeberg, 1963a,b; Ikkala et al., 1963; Iatridis and Ferguson, 1963).

As early as 1927, Hartman noted that the predominant response of cats after exertion was a shortened clotting time. In 1950, Kalaja described hypercoagulability after very mild exertion. He also found no difference between mild and strenuous exertion in shortening the clotting time. Ergotamine, an antisympathetic agent, appeared to block the effect of exercise upon blood coagulation. Epinephrine is known to simulate many of the exercise-induced clotting changes (Schneider and Zangari, 1951; Egeberg, 1963a). Schneider and Zangari, using the clotting time and dilute prothrombin time, and Wachholder et al., with thromboelastography, have also described postexertional hypercoagulability. In the latter study mild exercise produced only a transient alteration, whereas after strenuous work, the changes did not become maximal for 20 to 30 min.

In contrast to the above data, Billimoria et al. (1959), Rizza (1961), and Keeney and Laramie (1962) have found no significant change in coagulation times. Keeney and Laramie studied 32 male college students using four exercises of varying severity without adducing convincing evidence for hypercoagulability.

The most extensive data on blood clotting changes after exertion have been presented by Egeberg (1963a,b), Ikkala et al. (1963), and Iatridis and Ferguson (1963). Much of their data are similar and can be presented together. All found significant postexertional hypercoagulability as measured by tests of the intrinsic thromboplastin system. Two groups (Ikkala et al., Iatridis and Ferguson) noted elevations in factor XII. Ikkala et al. described a rise in factor V but this has not been confirmed by other investigators (Egeberg, 1963a; Billimoria et al., 1959). No significant changes in fibrinogen, prothrombin, and factors VII, IX, and X were found.

There is an elevation of antihemophiliac factor (VIII) after exertion that is remarkable both for its magnitude and duration (Egeberg, 1963a,b,c; Ikkala *et al.*, 1963; Iatridis and Ferguson, 1963; Rizza, 1961; Ikkala, 1965). Levels 2 to 3 times the control level are the rule. A significant elevation may remain after 8 hr (Egeberg, 1963b). Moreover, when administered to patients with classical hemophilia, plasma taken after exertion produced a greater and more prolonged rise in factor VIII than does normal plasma, thus confirming the *in vitro* observations. The rise in factor VIII is not due to intermediates produced by blood clotting after exercise since subjects with other clotting defects have a normal rise in factor VIII after exertion (Egeberg, 1963c). This elevation is mimicked by epinephrine administration. Repeated exercise tends to abolish the rise so that either depletion of factor VIII or some relation to physical conditioning may be postulated (Egeberg, 1963c).

Light muscular work which produces a 50 to 200% elevation in cardiac output results in an appreciable and consistent rise in platelet count (Ikkala, 1965). The leukocyte count also rises and neither of these alterations can be explained by hemoconcentration. Increased platelet adhesiveness has also been described after exertion (Wachholder *et al.*, 1957).

In addition to causing hypercoagulability, light exercise shortens the bleeding time (Egeberg, 1963a,b). The bleeding time is the time required for hemostasis after infliction of a standard wound and depends more upon vascular factors than upon clot formation. Using data on patient material, this change was attributed to a circulating factor very low in resting, unstressed individuals.

Much of the impetus for the recent studies of exercise-induced changes in blood coagulability was generated by the work of Keys and Buzina (1956). They noted a greater frequency of short whole blood clotting times in men with sedentary occupations than in physically active railroad switchmen. Their observations were confirmed experimentally in cholesterol-fed cockerels (Warnock *et al.*, 1957). An exercised group had a significantly longer clotting time than did a caged control group. Thus exercise appears paradoxically to not only produce hypercoagulability acutely but also a state of relative hypocoagulability in conditioned individuals. The significance of these changes is unknown.

2. Fibrinolysis

Enhanced fibrinolytic activity has been clearly demonstrated to occur immediately after vigorous exertion (Ikkala *et al.*, 1963; Iatridis and Ferguson, 1963; Billimoria *et al.*, 1959; Fearnley and Lackner, 1955; Sherry *et al.*, 1959; Sawyer *et al.*, 1960; Ogston and Fullerton, 1961; Jang *et al.*, 1964). It is believed that the appearance in the blood of a plasminogen activator is the mechanism for the enhanced fibrinolytic activity. No evidence for increased amounts of plasmin or decreased plasminogen or antiplasmin levels has been found (Sherry *et al.*, 1959). Epinephrine given subcutaneously also produces enhanced fibrinolytic activity (Fearnley and Lackner, 1955; Sherry *et al.*, 1959).

After prolonged, fatiguing exercise, fibrinolytic activity is decreased the following morning. Evidence suggests that this may result from activator depletion following exertion (Ogston and Fullerton, 1961).

V. The Endocrine System

A. GENERAL CONSIDERATIONS

We have not made an effort, in this chapter, to comprehensively review all aspects of the endocrine system relating to physical exertion. Due to the rapid advances in the technology of this medical subspecialty, older reports are, in many instances, outdated. Only in a few papers, such as those relating to growth hormone, have modern techniques been used in obtaining the data. With these reservations, we have tried to summarize some of the more important available information in this area in the following sections.

B. EFFECTS OF EXERCISE

1. Adrenal Cortex

More data are available regarding the effects of exercise on the adrenal cortex than on the other endocrine organs. However, as Cornil *et al.* (1965) point out, much of this work is open to criticism for the following reasons.

1. Earlier studies used nonspecific measures of adrenal cortical function such as the eosinophile count and urinary levels of 17-ketosteroids.

2. In sporting events, the emotional stress is difficult to separate from the effects of exertion. This is clearly demonstrated in a study of college oarsmen where the fall in eosinophile count after a race was comparable in both the oarsmen and the unexercised coach and coxswain (Renold *et al.*, 1951).

3. Studies have frequently been performed on anesthetized, surgically prepared experimental animals. These procedures, by themselves, are likely to stimulate secretion of adrenal cortical hormones.

4. Often, appropriate control groups were not used.

In spite of these difficulties, certain general statements can be made regarding the effects of exertion on the adrenal cortex.

1. Either a prolonged continuous exertion or a training program produces adrenal hypertrophy in experimental animals (Ingle, 1938b; Frenkl and Csalay, 1962).

2. Either adrenalectomy or hypophysectomy reduces the capacity for work in experimental animals (Ingle *et al.*, 1935; Ingle, 1938a; Winter and Flataker, 1960).

3. The administration of adrenal cortical hormones improves the work capacity in adrenalectomized or hypophysectomized animals (Hartman and Lockwood, 1931; Ingle, 1938a; Winter and Flataker, 1960).

4. Changes in the level of circulating eosinophiles, in situations of stress, are generally accepted as a rough index of adrenal cortical activity. Eosinophile levels are known to fall after exertion, suggesting increased adrenal cortical activity (Renold *et al.*, 1951; Thorn *et al.*, 1953; Hill *et al.*, 1956; Keeney, 1960; McDonald *et al.*, 1961). The relative roles of emotional stress and physical exertion in producing this change have not been clearly delineated.

5. There may be a state of increased utilization of adrenal cortical hormones during and after exercise. Exertion produces lowered plasma levels of adrenal cortical hormones, which is compatible with this interpretation (Staehelin *et al.*, 1955; Cornil *et al.*, 1965).

6. Prolonged exhaustive exercise does not appear to interfere with the functional reserve capacity of the adrenal cortex (Diczfalusy *et al.*, 1962).

2. Anterior Pituitary

Plasma growth hormone concentrations increase after muscular exertion (Roth *et al.*, 1964; Hunter and Greenwood, 1964; Hunter *et al.*, 1965). During a 2-hr treadmill walk at 6.4 km/hr, Hunter *et al.* (1965) noted a rise in fatty acid and growth hormone concentrations in the plasma, associated with a decrease in the respiratory quotient. This last observation implies increased combustion of fat to provide the required energy for muscular exercise. Peak plasma growth hormone concentrations were reached at one hour whereas the level of fatty acids continued to rise throughout the walk. No change in growth hormone levels was found in normally active physicians used as control subjects. In two subjects tested, exogenous carbohydrate suppressed both the secretion of growth hormone and the increase in plasma concentrations of fatty acids. The authors suggested that "during muscular exercise by normal human adults, unless exogenous carbohydrate is made available, the needs for fuel are increasingly met by mobilization of depot fat, and that secretion of growth hormone appears largely responsible for initiating and maintaining this process."

Other data are compatible with the preceding hypothesis. Havel *et al.* (1963) have presented evidence to suggest that free fatty acids are the major fuel delivered to working muscles in the postabsorptive state. Raben and Hollenberg (1959) have noted that "administration of growth hormone to animals has been found to reduce fat stores, to increase liver fat and to cause ketosis and a depression of respiratory quotient." They found that growth hormone elevated fasting values of plasma unesterified fatty acids in man and dog. Glucose, glucose and insulin, and food suppressed this effect. The small doses of human growth hormone needed to increase plasma fatty acid levels suggested to the authors that growth hormone has a physiological role in fat metabolism. Human growth hormone secretion in turn is responsive to alterations in glucose metabolism, stimulation being caused by hypoglycemia and suppression by glucose administration (Roth *et al.*, 1964; Hunter and Greenwood, 1964).

3. Posterior Pituitary

Current evidence suggests that the principal hormones of the posterior pituitary, antidiuretic hormone and oxytocin, are secreted by the supraoptic and paraventricular nuclei of the hypothalamus and then are transported via the neurohypophyseal tract to the posterior lobe of the pituitary. For those readers who wish a more complete description of this system, Daughaday (1962) has presented a concise review of the anatomy and physiology involved. Very little evidence is present in man to suggest what effect exercise has on these structures and their hormones. Vera and Croxatto (1954) measured blood antidiuretic activity after exercise with a bioassay method. They concluded that exercise increased blood antidiuretic activity and noted that water ingestion prevented this change.

Verney (1946) concluded that mild exercise, apart from its emotional stress, had no effect upon a water-induced diuresis in dogs. Härkönen *et al.* (1964), using histochemical methods in rats, concluded that exhaustive exercise produced no change in the amount of neurosecretory material in the paraventricular and supraoptic nuclei. However, a depletion of neurosecretory material was noted immediately after exertion in the infundibular process of the posterior pituitary gland, and also to some extent in the neurohypophyseal tract. The histology had returned to normal 4 days later.

The effect of daily exhausting swimming on oxytocin and the antidiuretic activity of the rat posterior pituitary has been assayed by Fendler *et al.* (1964). A slight decrease in oxytocin was noted on the sixth and eighth days of swimming. This was followed by a four- to sevenfold increase on day 18, and then a gradual decline thereafter till the end of the experiment on day 29. Pituitary antidiuretic activity also increased during this period.

4. Thyroid

Lashof *et al.* (1954) found that "moderate" exercise (walking 14 mi in 4 to $4\frac{1}{2}$ hr) produced no alterations in either serum thyroid hormone levels, as measured by butanol extractable iodine, or peripheral utilization of thyroid hormone, as determined by the rate of disappearance of injected radioactive thyroxine. "Severe brief" exercise (swimming at maximum speed for 15 min) did not alter the serum protein-bound iodine levels.

5. Androgens

Hettinger (1961) has examined the relationship of male hormones to "trainability" in terms of muscle strength. He noted that maximum results are obtained in the third decade in males when urinary 17-ketosteroid levels are high. In females and in older males, where androgen secretion is lower, "trainability" is decreased. The author has shown in dogs that testosterone and muscle work produce parallel effects upon muscle, namely an increase in muscle weight, fiber cross section, number of nuclei, and amount of protein. The amount of fat decreased in each instance.

In a study of older men, Hettinger found that testosterone augmented the rate of improvement in exercised muscles and improved the strength of untrained muscles. However, Samuels *et al.* (1942), using methyl testosterone, and Fowler *et al.* (1966), using an anabolic steroid, 1-methyl-Δ'-androstenolone acetate, were unable to show improvement in athletic performance in young males. This suggests that androgenic hormones already have a physiologically maximal effect in young males, and that further testosterone is not needed for optimal muscle performance. Thus it appears that critical levels of androgens may be necessary to attain maximal muscle strength.

REFERENCES

Addis, T., and Drury, D. R. (1923). *J. Biol. Chem.* **55**, 629.
Alexander, B. (1955). *New Engl. J. Med.* **252**, 432.
Alyea, E. P., and Boone, A. W. (1957). *Southern Med. J.* **50**, 905.
Alyea, E. P., and Parish, H. H., Jr. (1958). *J. Am. Med. Assoc.* **167**, 807.
Amelar, R. D., and Solomon, C. (1954). *J. Urol.* **72**, 145.
Asprey, G. M., Alley, L. E., and Tuttle, W. W. (1963). *Res. Quart.* **34**, 267.
Asprey, G. M., Alley, L. E., and Tuttle, W. W. (1964). *Res. Quart.* **35**, 227.
Ball, J. R. (1962). *Res. Quart.* **33**, 163.
Barach, J. H. (1910). *A.M.A. Arch. Internal Med.* **5**, 382.
Barach, J. H. (1920). *Am. J. Med. Sci.* **159**, 398.
Barclay, J. A., Cooke, W. T., Kenney, R. A., and Nutt, M. E. (1947). *Am. J. Physiol.* **148**, 327.
Barcroft, J., and Florey, H. (1929). *J. Physiol. (London)* **68**, 181.
Berlinger, R. W. (1963). *In* "Diseases of the Kidney" (M. B. Strauss and L. G. Welt, eds.), p. 46. Little, Brown, Boston, Massachusetts.
Billimoria, J. D., Drysdale, J., James, D. C. O., and Maclagen, N. F. (1959). *Lancet* **II**, 471.
Bishop, J. M., Donald, K. W., and Wade, O. L. (1955). *J. Clin. Invest.* **34**, 1114.
Blank, L. B. (1959). *Res. Quart.* **30**, 131.
Boone, A. W., Haltiwanger, E., and Chambers, R. L. (1955). *J. Am. Med. Assoc.* **158**, 1516.

Buckle, R. M. (1965). *Lancet* **I**, 1136.

Buntine, J. A., and Hughes, E. S. R. (1965). *Australian New Zealand J. Surg.* **34**, 218.

Campbell, J. M. H., Mitchell, G. O., and Powell, A. T. W. (1928). *Guy's Hosp. Rept.* **78**, 279.

Cantone, A., and Cerretelli, P. (1960). *Intern. Z. Angew. Physiol.* **18**, 324.

Chaiken, B. H., Whalen, E. J., Learner, N., and Smith, N. J. (1953). *Am. J. Med. Sci.* **225**, 514.

Chapman, C. B., and Mitchell, J. H. (1965). *Sci. Am.* **212**, 88.

Chapman, C. B., Henschel, A., and Forsgren, A. (1948a). *Proc. Soc. Exptl. Biol. Med.* **69**, 170.

Chapman, C. B., Henschel, A., Minckler, J., Forsgren, A., and Keys, A. (1948b). *J. Clin. Invest.* **27**, 639.

Chesley, L. C., Markowitz, I., and Wetchler, B. B. (1939). *J. Clin. Invest.* **18**, 51.

Christensen, E. H., Krogh, A., and Lindhard, J. (1934). *Quart. Bull. Health Organ. League Nations* **3**, 388.

Collier, W. (1907). *Brit. Med. J.* **I**, 4.

Cornil, A., DeCoster, A., Copinschi, G., and Franckson, J. R. M. (1965). *Acta Endocrinol.* **48**, 163.

Crandall, L. A. (1928). *Am. J. Physiol.* **84**, 48.

Daughaday, W. H. (1962). *In* "Textbook of Endocrinology" (R. H. Williams, ed.), pp. 80–88. Saunders, Philadelphia, Pennsylvania.

Davidson, R. J. L. (1964). *J. Clin. Pathol.* **17**, 536.

DeYoung, V. R., Rice, H. A., and Steinhaus, A. H. (1931). *Am. J. Physiol.* **99**, 52.

Diczfalusy, E., Cassmer, O., and Ullmark, R. (1962). *J. Clin. Endocrinol. Metab.* **22**, 78.

Editorial. (1954). *J. Am. Med. Assoc.* **156**, 45.

Edwards, H. T., Cohen, M. I., Dill, D. B., and Thorndike, A., Jr. (1937). *Arbeitsphysiol.* **9**, 610.

Egeberg, O. (1963a). *Scand. J. Clin. & Lab. Invest.* **15**, 539.

Egeberg, O. (1963b). *Scand. J. Clin. & Lab. Invest.* **15**, 8.

Egeberg, O. (1963c). *Scand. J. Clin. & Lab. Invest.* **15**, 202.

Eggelton, M. G. (1942). *J. Physiol. (London)* **101**, 1P.

Fearnley, G. R., and Lackner, R. (1955). *Brit. J. Haematol.* **1**, 189.

Fendler, K., Telegdy, G., and Endröczi, E. (1964). *Acta Physiol. Acad. Sci. Hung.* **24**, 287.

Flatmark, T. (1963). *Acta Med. Scand.* **173**, 307.

Fowler, W. M., Jr., Gardner, G. W., and Egstrom, G. H. (1966). *J. Appl. Physiol.* **20**, 1038.

Frenkl, R., and Csalay, L. (1962). *J. Sports Med. Phys. Fitness* **2**, 207.

Frenkl, R., Csalay, L., and Makara, G. (1962). *Acta Physiol. Acad. Sci. Hung.* **22**, 203.

Frenkl, R., Csalay, L., Makara, G., and Harmos, G. (1964). *Acta Physiol. Acad. Sci. Hung.* **25**, 97.

Gardner, K. D., Jr. (1956). *J. Am. Med. Assoc.* **161**, 1613.

Gaston, L. W. (1964). *New Engl. J. Med.* **270**, 236.

Gilligan, D. R., and Blumgart, H. L. (1941). *Medicine* **20**, 341.

Hammar, S., and Öbrink, K. J. (1953). *Acta Physiol. Scand.* **28**, 152.

Härkönen, M., Kormano, M., and Kontinen, E. (1964). *Ann. Med. Exptl. Biol. Fenniae (Helsinki)* **42**, 17.

Hartman, F. A. (1927). *Am. J. Physiol.* **80**, 716.

Hartman, F. A., and Lockwood, J. E. (1931). *Proc. Soc. Exptl. Biol. Med.* **29**, 141.

Havard, R. E. (1937). *J. Physiol. (London)* **90**, 90P.

Havel, R. J., Naimark, A., and Borchgrevink, C. F. (1963). *J. Clin. Invest.* **42**, 1054.

Hellebrandt, F. A. (1932). *Am. J. Physiol.* **101**, 357.

Hellebrandt, F. A., and Hoopes, S. L. (1934a). *Am. J. Physiol.* **107**, 348.

Hellebrandt, F. A., and Tepper, R. H. (1934b). *Am. J. Physiol.* **107**, 355.

Hellebrandt, F. A., Brogdon, E., and Kelso, L. E. A. (1932). *Am. J. Physiol.* **101**, 365.

Hettinger, T. (1961). "Physiology of Strength," pp. 44–53. Thomas, Springfield, Illinois.

Hill, S. R., Jr., Goetz, F. C., Fox, H. M., Murawski, B. J., Krakauer, L. J., Reifenstein, R. W., Gray, S. J., Reddy, W. J., Hedberg, S. E., St. Marc. J. R., and Thorn, G. W. (1956). *A.M.A. Arch. Internal Med.* **97**, 269.

Hillman, R. W., and Rosner, M. C. (1958). *J. Nutr.* **64**, 605.

Howenstine, J. A. (1960). *J. Am. Med. Assoc.* **173**, 493.

Hunter, W. M., and Greenwood, F. C. (1964). *Brit. Med. J.* **I**, 804.

Hunter, W. M., Fonseka, C. C., and Passmore, R. (1965). *Science* **150**, 1053.

Iatridis, S. G., and Ferguson, J. H. (1963). *J. Appl. Physiol.* **18**, 337.

Ikkala, E. (1965). *Ann. Med. Exptl. Biol. Fenniae (Helsinki)* **43**, 1.

Ikkala, E., Myllyla, G., and Sarajas, H. S. S. (1963). *Nature* **199**, 459.

Ingle, D. J. (1938a). *Am. J. Physiol.* **122**, 302.

Ingle, D. J. (1938b). *Am. J. Physiol.* **124**, 627.

Ingle, D. J., Hales, W. M., and Haslerud, G. M. (1935). *Am. J. Physiol.* **113**, 200.

James, W. H., and ElGindi, I. M. (1953). *Science* **118**, 629.

Jang, E., Taylor, F. B., and Bickford, A. F. (1964). *Clin. Sci.* **27**, 9.

Javitt, N. B., and Miller, A. T., Jr. (1952). *J. Appl. Physiol.* **4**, 834.

Kalaja, L. (1950). *Acta Med. Scand.* Suppl. 239, 296.

Keeney, C. E. (1960). *J. Appl. Physiol.* **15**, 1046.

Keeney, C. E., and Laramie, D. W. (1962). *Circulation Res.* **10**, 691.

Keys, A., and Buzina, R. (1956). *Circulation* **14**, 479.

King, S. E., and Baldwin, D. S. (1956). *Am. J. Med.* **20**, 217.

Kleiman, A. H. (1958). *J. Am. Med. Assoc.* **168**, 1633.

Kleiman, A. H. (1960). *J. Urol.* **83**, 321.

Klisiecki, A., Pickford, M., Rothschild, P., and Verney, E. B. (1933a). *Proc. Roy. Soc.* **B112**, 496.

Klisiecki, A., Pickford, M., Rothschild, P., and Verney, E. B. (1933b). *Proc. Roy. Soc.* **B112**, 521.

Kreisle, J. B., Queen, D. M., and Bowman, B. H. (1960). *Texas State J. Med.* **56**, 421.

Lashof, J. C., Bondy, P. K., Sterling, K., and Man, E. B. (1954). *Proc. Soc. Exptl. Biol. Med.* **86**, 233.

Light, A. B., and Warren, C. R. (1936). *Am. J. Physiol.* **117**, 658.

Lillehei, C. W., and Wangensteen, O. H. (1948). *Proc. Soc. Exptl. Biol. Med.* **67**, 49.

Little, C. C., Strayhorn, H., and Miller, A. T., Jr. (1949). *Res. Quart.* **20**, 398.

MacKay, E. M. (1928). *J. Clin. Invest.* **6**, 505.

McDonald, R. D., Yagi, K., and Stockton, E. (1961). *Psychosomat. Med.* **23**, 63.

Morgan, J. L., Tidwell, B. D., and Ryan, E. J. (1957). *J. Lab. Clin. Med.* **50**, 935.

Nedbal, J., and Seliger, V. (1958). *J. Appl. Physiol.* **13**, 244.

Neilson, C. H., and Lipsitz, S. T. (1915). *J. Am. Med. Assoc.* **64**, 1052.

Ogston, D., and Fullerton, H. W. (1961). *Lancet* **II**, 730.

Raben, M. S., and Hollenberg, C. H. (1959). *J. Clin. Invest.* **38**, 484.

Rasch, P. J., Faires, L. B., and Hunt, M. B. (1958). *Res. Quart.* **29**, 54.

Renold, A. E., Quigley, T. B., Kennard, H. E., and Thorn, G. W. (1951). *New Engl. J. Med.* **244**, 754.

Rizza, C. R. (1961). *J. Physiol. (London)* **156**, 128.

Roth, J., Glick, S. M., Yalow, R. S., and Berson, S. A. (1964). *Diabetes* **13**, 355.

Rowell, L. B., Blackmon, J. R., and Bruce, R. A. (1964). *J. Clin. Invest.* **43**, 1677.

Samuels, L. T., Henschel, A. F., and Keys, A. (1942). *J. Clin. Endocrinol.* **2**, 649.

Sawyer, W. D., Fletcher, A. P., Alkjaersig, N., and Sherry, S. (1960). *J. Clin. Invest.* **39**, 426.

Schjoth, A. E. (1965). *Scand. J. Clin. & Lab. Invest.* **17**, 275.

Schneider, R. A., and Zangari, V. M. (1951). *Psychosomat. Med.* **13**, 289.

Selman, D., and Gualano, C. (1955). *N.Y. State J. Med.* **55**, 3120.

Sherry, S., Lindemeyer, R. I., Fletcher, A. P., and Alkjaersig, N. (1959). *J. Clin. Invest.* **38**, 810.

Simko, V., Ginter, E., and Cerven, J. (1963). *Med. Exptl.* **8**, 156.

Smith, H. (1963). *In* "Diuretics" (G. deStevens, ed.), p. 8. Academic Press, New York.

Staehelin, D., Labhart, A., Froesch, R., and Kägi, H. R. (1955). *Acta Endocrinol.* **18**, 521.

Stahl, W. G. (1957). *J. Am. Med. Assoc.* **164**, 1458.

Starr, I., Jr. (1926). *J. Exptl. Med.* **43**, 31.

Stickney, J. C., Northup, D. W., and Van Liere, E. J. (1956). *J. Appl. Physiol.* **9**, 484.

Taylor, A. (1960). *Clin. Sci.* **19**, 209.

Thorn, G. W., Jenkins, D., and Laidlaw, J. C. (1953). *Recent Progr. Hormone Res.* **8**, 171.

Van Liere, E. J., Hess, H. H., and Edwards, J. E. (1954). *J. Appl. Physiol.* **7**, 186.

Van Slyke, D. D., Alving, A., and Rose, W. C. (1932). *J. Clin. Invest.* **11**, 1053.

Vera, R., and Croxatto, H. (1954). *J. Appl. Physiol.* **7**, 172.

Verney, E. B. (1946). *Lancet* **II**, 739.

Wachholder, V. K., Parchwitz, E., Egli, H., and Kesseler, K. (1957). *Acta Haematol.* **18**, 59.

Wakim, K. G. (1958). *J. Urol.* **79**, 560.

Warnock, N. H., Clarkson, T. B., and Stevenson, R. (1957). *Circulation Res.* **5**, 478.

White, H. L., and Rolf, D. (1948). *Am. J. Physiol.* **152**, 505.

Winter, C. A., and Flataker, L. (1960). *Am. J. Physiol.* **199**, 863.

Witts, L. J. (1936). *Lancet* **II**, 115.

Youmans, E., Alley, L. E., and Tuttle, W. W. (1960). *Scholastic Coach* **30**, 24.

PART 2: **SPECIAL PROBLEMS**

5

NUTRITION AND EXERCISE

Geoffrey H. Bourne

I. Historical

Organized athletics is said to have first appeared in history with the Olympic games which were held in Greece in 776 BC. Thereafter, every 4 years, whether there was war or peace, the Olympic games continued to be held for the next thousand years. However, according to Dr. H. A. Harris, there is evidence that the first Olympics were not really the beginning of organized sport, because athletic events are referred to in the poems of Homer, indicating an origin of even 5 centuries earlier.

The Greek world at the beginning of the Olympic games consisted only of a number of city states which were scattered on mainland Greece, the Aegean Islands, and the West Coast of Asia Minor. During the next 200 years, the Greeks extended and colonized areas in many parts of the Mediterranean, including North Africa, Sicily, Italy, France and Spain; later on, most of Asia Minor, Syria, Egypt, Mesopotamia, Persia, and part of India were incorporated into the Greek Empire. The colonists spread the Greek infatuation with athletics over the whole of the area which they had colonized.

Dr. Harris points out that the Greeks had a monopoly in the field of sport and that the only other sports of any magnitude were horse racing and chariot racing. He also points out that the program of events of Greek athletic meetings was very restricted. They had 3 events in which individuals fought each other; these were boxing, wrestling, and a special type of wrestling called pankration. They had 4 races, one 200 yd, one 400 yd, one which was approximately 3 mi, and another race extending 400 yd in which the participants were clad in armor. The final event was the pentathlon in which the contestants threw the javelin, threw the discus, made a long jump, took part in the 200-yd race, and wrestled. Dr. Harris points out that among the most popular events for the spectators were boxing and wrestling, and most Greek writers when they write about athletes often refer only to this type of athletics. He says that a great deal of attention should be paid to this when we are considering the diet of the athletes of the Greek period, because much of the evidence we see in the Greek literature of the time regarding the eating habits of athletes refers, in fact, to boxers or wrestlers, and as he very rightly points out the needs of these are probably very different from those of sprinters or long jumpers.

Dr. Harris indicates that there was a considerable insistence by Greek doctors on the importance of diet in general; this is probably due to their interest originally in the diet of athletes. The basic food consumed by the normal Greek population was some form of cereal, such as barley or wheat, which was eaten either as bread or in the form of a kind of porridge. There was very little meat, and wild animals or birds were eaten whenever they were obtained. Meat in most cases was eaten only at religious festivals, and eggs were obtained from the domestic fowl, kept by a number of households. Fish was plentiful because most Greek cities were close to the sea. Vegetables such as onions, carrots, cucumbers, marrow, beans, and various green leaves were eaten. Fruit was abundant, especially grapes and figs. Apples, pears, and nuts were eaten, and, as Dr. Harris points out, they appeared curiously to prize the pomegranate highly. Goat's milk was the usual type of milk, and owing to the difficulties in keeping it fresh, most of it was made into cheese. Olive oil was used in cooking, and by the athletes as an embrocation for massage. Honey was also plentiful and was made into sweet cakes. Large quantities of wine were consumed, usually diluted with water, but there were no spirits.

Dr. Harris says that the earliest Greek athlete about whose diet we have any special information was Charmis from Sparta. Dried figs appear to have been his standby in training for athletics. If this is true, it seems a very effective diet since he won the 200 yd in the Olympic games of 668 BC. Dr. Harris suggests that this may be due to the extra sugar, particularly in the form of glucose, which is present in dried figs.

Dromeus of Stymphalus (480 BC) was a long distance runner and was the first recorded athlete to train on a diet largely composed of meat, although there are reports that Eurymenes of Samos trained largely on meat a century before. Dr. Harris draws attention to the interesting fact that the trainer of

Eurymenes was Pythagoras, better known as a mathematician and philosopher than as a trainer of athletes; and it is even more interesting that he should be the trainer of a meat-eating athlete, since Pythagoras was said to have been a vegetarian.

Dr. Harris reminds us that the eating of meat by athletes goes back a lot earlier than the cases mentioned, and he quotes the reports of Milo of Croton. Milo won the wrestling at seven successive Olympiads and had 26 victories in other Panhellenic festivals. He is said to have consumed each day 20 lb of bread, 20 lb of meat, and 18 pints of wine. There is a well-known report of him that he once carried a 4-year-old bull around the stadium at Olympia on his shoulders, killed it with a single blow of his fist, and then ate the whole animal in 1 day.

According to Xenophon, athletes did not eat bread, presumably because they felt that the starch, although they did not recognize it as such, would make them fat; Epictetus said that athletes should observe restraint in their eating and that they should avoid rich confectionery. Philostratus wrote a book, apparently the only one which has survived to this day, devoted entirely to athletics. He regarded the professional athletic performers as effeminate and claimed that they were fed on soft cakes sprinkled with poppy seeds. They apparently ate considerable amounts of fish, however, although there is a great controversy as to which fish were the best types to be used. They also ate pork, and there were restrictions on the pasturing of the pigs which provided meat.

It would be very interesting to know what the performances of ancient Greeks were like in terms of times for various events, but there seems to be little information about this subject. There was, unfortunately, no way of measuring time for the Greeks except over 24-hr periods; the interest in athletics was simply to acclaim a particular winner each year irrespective of what the measure of his performance was compared with previous years. The type of information we could get about the excellence of athletes would be, for instance, a record of a runner who could run fast enough to catch a hare. Another beat a horse in a race from Coronea to Thebes. As far as endurance records are concerned, Herodotus claims that Pheidippides ran a distance of 150 mi, that is from Athens to Sparta, in a period of 2 days. Pheidippides is also said to have been the Greek who ran to Athens with the news of the victory of Marathon, an event which inspired the modern marathon race. However, it is obviously impossible to compare the excellence of the Greeks with the present-day records.

II. Protein in Athletics

Since the time of the Greeks, organized sports seem to have lapsed until approximately 100 years ago. For instance, the first annual Oxford and

Cambridge boat race was held in 1856, and the first modern Olympic games were held in Athens in 1896. Captain Webb swam the Channel in the year 1875.

Eggleton (1948) has drawn attention to the fact that in the early days athletes and sportsmen came from a very picked population. It was only the wealthy that had the time and energy to be able to indulge in athletics. In England, for instance, probably only 5% of the population had such an opportunity, which meant that all the athletes were drawn from a population of about a half-million people, excluding children and females. In the last 70 years, however, more of the lower income groups, particularly women, have been able to take to sports. There are probably now at least 3- to 4-million people in Britain who indulge in some form of athletics. This applies, of course, not only to England but to America and other countries of the world. Possibly this is the reason why we are seeing continuous breaking of records.

It was during this period that there developed the popular belief that any form of violent or sustained muscular exercise required a large quantity of meat foods. Until very recently there were many athletes who were firm believers that the best type of diet for an athlete was one which consisted primarily of underdone meat. In the latter part of the nineteenth century the person probably responsible for this view was Liebig. Liebig postulated that during exercise the substance of the muscle is consumed, and therefore hard work would remove a considerable portion of the actual material of muscle and could only be replaced by eating animal protein in its place. He actually said "All experience proves that this conversion of living muscular substance into compounds destitute of vitality is accelerated or retarded according to the amount of force employed to produce motion." He was such an important man scientifically that no one dared to challenge his opinion, although one Englishman, Dr. Edward Smith (Eggleton, 1948), did so, but little attention was paid to his findings. Dr. Smith made a careful investigation in one of the English penitentiaries of the food eaten by the prisoners, paying special attention to the amount of nitrogen that they excreted, which, of course, was an index of the degree of breakdown of muscle substance. He found that the amount of nitrogen excreted bore no relation at all to the amount of muscular work carried out by the men and that the amount of nitrogen excreted was related exclusively to the amount of nitrogen in the food. It is extraordinary that this critical experiment was completely ignored. Later on, two scientists in Zurich, Fick and Wislicenus (Eggleton, 1948), climbed one of the peaks of the Bernese Oberland and lived on a diet which contained no nitrogenous foods at all. They found that both during the climb and immediately after it when they were resting quietly the amount of nitrogen that was excreted was not increased by their physical effort. This really served as the basis for the modern outlook on the relationship of muscular performance to nutrients, which is that the muscle oxidizes the sugar and fat for the production of its energy and does not use up its own substance. Therefore, it is only in starvation or, in fact, in inactivation of muscles that the muscle substance is actually used up, and that the best way to preserve muscle substance is actually to use the muscles. It is of interest that the Medical Tribune of September 7, 1966, reports a rise in plasma protein excretion in urine after exercise (Poortmans and Jeanloz, 1966). In some cases the level was found to be 100 times normal and the quality of protein changed. In normal urine the proteins were mainly globulins, but the postexercise urine contained albumin and an appreciable amount of transferrin and γ-globulin. This phenomenon is related to the mechanisms of excretion and reabsorption in the kidneys themselves and not to any breakdown of muscle as a result of the exercise. The types of exercise used in this study were a 5-mi cross-country run and a high school football game.

III. Food and Energy

A. Energy Requirements for Various Tasks

There is no doubt that the energy output of an individual depends primarily on the type of work the person is called upon to do. It is also modified by other factors. Generally speaking, a woman is regarded as requiring only four-fifths of the calories needed by a man, although this figure cannot be rigidly adhered to because there are obviously many women whose calorie requirements are equal to, or greater than, those of many men. The energy requirements also vary considerably with age; a newborn baby requires less total energy than either a man or woman. Individuals themselves, even in health, vary to a certain extent in their calorie requirements; and in certain diseases the requirement will vary even more. In a cold climate or season there will be a greater loss of heat to the surrounding air, consequently, more food will be required to make good this heat loss. In a hot climate or season the air temperature may be hotter than that of the body, and there will be less food required because there will be no heat loss for which to compensate. The actual body temperature in a hot climate or temperature cannot be appreciably reduced by reducing the amount of food eaten, but it can be reduced to a certain extent by reducing the amount of protein eaten and by eating foods containing more water in order to cause greater sweating.

The energy requirement of a man lying in bed and kept at an equable temperature has been calculated. If he does nothing but this for 24 hr, he will require 1700 to 2000 cal; and every movement he makes will require additional energy for its performance. If he sits for 6 hr, he will require an additional 170 cal. If he does 6 hr slow walking, he will require a further 400 cal; and if he does 6 hr moderate exercise, he will need another 600 cal. Most of the nutritional books carry lists of calorie requirements for the performance of various tasks, but we will note a few of them. Mottram and Graham (1941) recorded a monk in a cloister as requiring 2304 cal, and a teacher or an office clerk requiring 2600. On the other hand, each member of a university boat crew required 4085 cal; a blacksmith, 4117; a woodcutter, 5500; and a brick-maker (which is presumably an American estimate), 8848 cal/day.

The difference between the calorie requirements for carrying out various types of physical activity were originally published by Mary Schwartz Rose in the United States, and noted here are 2 or 3 items of interest. Sleeping requires 65 cal/hr; standing relaxed, 105 cal; light exercise, 170; walking slowly, 200; walking moderately fast, 300; severe exercise, 450; running slowly, 570; very severe exercise, 600; and very fast walking, 650 cal/hr.

This relationship of calories to work output and exercise in general has been very well realized in times of war. For example, during the last war, the Germans had a very complex rationing system which classified the population into normal workers, light workers, medium workers, heavy workers, very heavy workers, and miners; each category receiving a different ration. The relationship of calories to work was also recognized in the rationing system in England but not to such a detailed degree. The usual procedure was that heavy industrial workers and miners were given extra rations of particular items of foodstuff. Eggleton (1948) has indicated that a robust man can metabolize 4000 cal of food in a working day, and he raised the question as to whether one variety of food is better than another in making up the calories consumed by those engaged in strong exercise. He says a good deal of evidence from the work on muscles and muscle extracts indicates that carbohydrate is the main fuel of exercise (although it has been shown since that a proportion of muscle fibers metabolize fat for energy). He also points out that there is evidence that manual laborers do not choose to eat carbohydrates if they can avoid it, but show a decided preference for fat and protein. He points out the firm belief, which until recently has been fixed in the minds of athletes as well as laborers, that meat is of very great value in the performance of muscular work. He feels that this belief may possibly have a justification in that meat is a good source of some of the vitamin B group and that the creatine content might possibly have some physiological value.

Another justification of belief in the value of meat consumption by heavy workers is the large number of calories needed for the performance of their work. A very large amount of carbohydrate would be required to provide the necessary calories if this were to be the main source of their calories. Pure carbohydrate provides 1860 cal/lb and so does pure protein; but pure fat provides 4200 cal/lb. Every time meat is eaten a certain amount of fat is eaten with it, therefore, the total amount of food required to provide the same amount of calories is less. It may be that it is almost impossible, eating carbohydrate foods, for people engaged in heavy laboring work to obtain enough calories without discomfort.

B. Oxygen Consumption in Exercise

A laborer uses about 5 or 6 cal/min during periods of working. Professor Hill (1925) showed that men running for a few minutes at a time at a pace which they could sustain without any serious respiratory problems used oxygen at the rate of 4 liters/min, with a caloric equivalent of about 20, or 4 times that used by the laborers. Four liters of oxygen is a large amount of oxygen to be pumped into the body every minute, and it cannot be maintained forever. Exercise which has to go on for some hours at a time must be scaled down to a level of about 1 liter/min. An athlete, however, is capable of working for short periods at a rate which would provide a combustion rate of something like 100 times that of a resting individual. He does this, of course, simply by using up the energy store maintained in the muscle which can be used immediately, whereas food taken into the body would have to go through a slow process of digestion and transport to the muscles before it could be oxidized.

However, the energy used up by the muscles has to be repaid, hence the well-known oxygen debt which athletes are able to build up. An athlete is able to build up an oxygen debt of about 16 liters of oxygen, in other words, the amount of oxygen that could be pumped by the heart over a period of about 4 min at the normal rate. Thus, it is only possible to build up a significant oxygen debt in events that have a maximum duration of less than 4 min; in actual practice it is in events of less than 1 min that the oxygen debt really becomes a significant factor. The 100-yd sprint, for example, is run almost entirely on oxygen debt. The runner produces (Eggleton, 1948) from 10 to 13 hp in this process, which is equivalent to an oxygen intake rate of about 23 liters/min, or about 6 times more than the heart could achieve if the muscle had to get its oxygen from the pumping of the heart. The chemistry of the oxygen debt and the production of lactic acid and its subsequent oxidation is a well-known biochemical story and, in any case, does not have a place in this chapter and will be left to be dealt with by other authors in this volume.

C. Calories Required for Athletic Performance

The actual number of calories used in the performance of a particular athletic event is not, in actual fact, very large. Even in the marathon race of about 26 mi, it is probable that the total calorie consumption during this time is only about 2500 cal. In the Oxford and Cambridge or Harvard and Yale boat races the oarsmen probably do not use more than about 600 cal for the actual event itself. It is obvious, therefore, that the calorie requirement is not a significant factor in most of these events. The same is true of the calorie requirement of the athlete in training. Although some athletes (e.g., some of those before the Rome Olympic games) were known to run as much as 100 mi a week in training, the majority of them in a training day probably do not use more than 300 or 400 cal for the extra work involved in the training. Therefore, the evidence now is probably that a high caloric intake is not an important factor in the training of athletes. This is a break with the figures claimed by some authors, e.g., Schenk, who in 1936 claimed that an Olympic athlete in training required around 7300 cal. He based his figure on what he claimed to be an inquiry into the diets of 4700 competitors from 42 nations at the 1936 Berlin Olympics. Abrahams (1948) pointed out that it is difficult to understand how he arrived at these figures, and it is now generally believed by most experts in athletic diets that these figures are way beyond what is required. In most cases, probably 300 or 400 cal above the normal calorie requirements of the individual athlete would be adequate.

IV. Protein, Fat, or Carbohydrate for Athletic Performance?

More controversial is the composition of the diet, particularly from the point of view of the ratio of protein, fat, and carbohydrates in the diet in relation to athletic performance. In discussing the quality of the diet for athletes with regard to protein, fat, and carbohydrates, we have to consider two points of view: (1) whether an excess of any one of these 3 nutrients is more important than any of the others during the training period, and (2) whether the administration of one or the other of them on the day of the event or immediately before the event is likely to be of much significance.

As far as the latter problem is concerned, the only nutrient which is likely to have any significant effect taken before an event is obviously sugar. Four ounces of sucrose, for example, are absorbed from the gut in a 2-hr period; whereas a pint of raw milk will take 6 hr to be absorbed. On the other hand, glucose is absorbed much more rapidly even than sucrose and might possibly have an effect since it would be more readily available for raising the blood sugar immediately before an event. Abrahams (1948) points out that he does not believe that any compound such as this can produce the kind of explosive result which would be advantageous in a particular athletic event. He further states that he himself had given sugar to athletes and that the men who have consumed it have performed well enough to attribute some credit to the sugar. But Abrahams is not convinced that it necessarily did have this effect, and that the effect may have been psychological. Abrahams says that he has seen this psychological element function with some substances simpler than sugar and sometimes with quite inert substances.

Haldi and Wynn (1946) studied carbohydrate intake of swimmers, using the 100-yd swim for that purpose. This was part of a study of the relationship of breakfast to performance. The composition of the meal, as far as carbohydrates are concerned, did not affect either the blood sugar level at the end of the swim or the performance. They concluded that the energy reserves of the body were more important than the composition of a preswim meal.

Von Dobeln (1963) has recently reviewed the subject of diet and work metabolism. He refers to the work of Drabkin (1959) who discussed in some detail the proportion of energy in exercise obtained from carbohydrate. However, Andres *et al.* (1956) have drawn attention to the importance of the plasma nonesterified fatty acids in this role and have, in fact, claimed that only 7% of the oxygen uptake of the muscles of the human forearm at rest could be attributed to oxidation of glucose. Jokl (1964), however, doubts if skeletal muscle can extract free fatty acids from the plasma. The studies of Issekutz *et al.* (1963) demonstrated that athletes on high carbohydrate diets used a higher proportion of carbohydrate with exercise, while those on a low carbohydrate diet used fat for this purpose. Subjects consuming diets low in both carbohydrate and fat tended to use an increased proportion of fat for energy production in exercise, i.e., they behaved as would an individual on a high fat diet. Karpovich (1941) also showed that the amount of carbohydrate metabolized in exercise was dependent upon the amount of carbohydrate in the diet, and the lower the carbohydrate in the diet the higher the amount of fat metabolized.

Lewis *et al.* (1959) have demonstrated in animal experiments that glucose decreases the oxidation of fatty acids such as palmitic acid but that fat does not cause a decrease of carbohydrate oxidation. The physiological mechanism producing these results is not known.

Karpovich also claims that when energy is derived from fats the work performed is actually 10% less economical than when the energy is derived from carbohydrates. Thus, to do the same amount of work using fat as the main energy source would require more oxygen than if carbohydrate were used.

There is little doubt that protein and fat, since they need a long digestion period, will produce little benefit by being administered immediately before a race or even some hours before. As far as the training diet is concerned, the situation is perhaps a little more complex. It has been claimed that sugar is the main fuel of muscle, but there is evidence now that most muscles actually contain a significant proportion of fibers for which fat is the principal fuel. The muscles which contain most of these fat oxidizing fibers are those which are involved in more sustained work. Such fibers, for instance, are much more common in postural muscles which are operating against gravity.

The old conception of the intake of large quantities of protein is now disregarded; but it is of interest that Yamaji (1951) found that in rigorous training, protein actually accumulated in muscles with a corresponding decrease of blood proteins. He feels that as a result, training program diets, particularly those where heavy muscular work is involved, should contain an excess of protein. This does not, of course, necessarily mean large quantities of meat. Van Itallie *et al.* (1960) point out also that in many cases an athlete is still in the growing phase and will need extra protein to meet his growth requirements in addition to the extra protein he will require while training. Dr. Reed S. Clegg, Medical Director of the University of Utah Athletic Department, has, according to the Medical Tribune of August 17th, 1966, been feeding high protein diets together with anabolic hormones to basketball players. The object of this was to add muscular bulk to the thin and more fragile members of the University's basketball teams without impairing their speed and strength. The results of the experiment are not yet available.

There seems to be no particular requirement for fat in the diet. Recent evidence, however, suggests that unsaturated fatty acids have a role in nutrition, but there is no reason to believe at this time that they have any specific importance in athletic performance. It is of interest that heart and skeletal muscle are said to use free fatty acids during exercise (see above). That fat is of value as a conveyor of some vitamins is, of course, of significance. The presence of fat in the diet reduces the total quantity of food that needs to be taken, and this may or may not be of significance to a particular individual.

The advantage of a meal shortly before an athletic event, which has been advocated by some, has been discussed by Dr. G. M. Asprey of the Department of Physical Education for Men, University of Iowa. At an A.C.S.M. Regional Meeting in Iowa City, he described the results of giving a 500-cal meal to subjects before they indulged in a 440-yd, half mi, 1-mi, and 2-mi runs, and in free-style swimming of 200 and 400 yd. The meal was 500 cal and contained cereal, toast, sugar, butter, and whole milk. It was given half an hour before the event. He found that there was no particular advantage nor any disadvantage in giving such a meal so close to the event. The possibility that such a meal would interfere with a performance, however, seems fairly likely. The present author had some success in the field of mile running in Australia many years ago and found that he obtained his best performance if his last meal was consumed 4 hr before the event took place; it consisted of an extremely light meal, probably around 200 or 300 cal. However, there is little doubt that the matter of time of food consumption before events is very much a personal matter which has to be worked out for each individual, and it seems undesirable to lay down general rules and regulations.

V. Vitamins and Athletic Performance

It has been suggested by Bourne (1948) that the desire for meat by some athletes may be related to the fact that there is an increased demand for riboflavin and nicotinic acid, and that by eating large amounts of meat in the training period these additional vitamins were obtained. There has been some controversy as to the possible increased requirements by athletes for vitamins. Many vitamins, particularly those of the vitamin B complex, form part of the reaction chains which are concerned with carbohydrate and fat metabolism. Vitamin B_1, for instance, is concerned with the decarboxylation and carboxylation of pyruvic acid, one of the intermediary degradation products of carbohydrate breakdown. It also incidentally appears to prolong the activity of acetylcholine at nerve endings by the process of inhibition of the formation of cholinesterase which hydrolyzes and inactivates the neuromuscular chemical transmitter of acetylcholine. As a matter of interest, it has been reported that cholinesterase is actually increased in vitamin B_1 deficiency (Glick and Antopol, 1939). Vitamin B_6, pantothenic acid, riboflavin, and nicotinic acid all form parts of the reaction chains associated with metabolism, and in muscular exercise it is reasonable to assume that the requirement for them will be increased. The important thing, however, is to what extent it is increased and to what extent the increased demand and requirement may be met by normal diets.

It has been stated (Bicknell and Prescott, 1945) that the vitamin B_1 requirements of an individual may be increased 15 times in severe exercise. This means that if the daily requirement of 1.5 mg for a sedentary man weighing 70 kg (which is the U.S. National Research Council's recommended dose in 1945) is increased by this amount, he would require in severe exercise 22.5 mg of vitamin B_1. To do this he would require 12.5 kg of lean meat, 90 gm of dried brewers yeast, or 750 gm of commercial wheat germ. It seems, therefore, rather unlikely that he could eat enough of these materials to obtain the amount of vitamin B_1 that would be required, and it seems more likely that this figure is in error.

There is very little evidence that large doses of vitamins of the B complex or any other vitamins will have very significant effect on the ability to perform in athletic events. The literature is very confusing in this area. Gounelle (1940) claimed that the supplementation of the diet of cyclists with vitamin B_1 improved their performance. McCormick (1940) made a similar claim for swimmers; but Karpovich and Millman (1942) obtained results contrary to these. Simonson et al. (1942) found that supplements of aneurine, nicotinamide, and riboflavin did not improve the performance in simple muscular work but did delay the onset of fatigue in neuromuscular work, a result which was also supported by the work of Hills (1942) who found that extra vitamin

B_1 reduced proneness to accidents in a group of workers. Keys and Henschel (1942) added mixed vitamins to normal army rations but found that they did not retard the development of fatigue nor did they hasten recovery from it. On the other hand, Harper *et al.* (1943) found in a series of carefully controlled experiments that mixed vitamin supplementation increased the vital capacity of a group of students. The present author (Bourne, 1943) found that rats injected with aneurine or aneurine ascorbate ran longer on a treadmill before becoming fatigued than did untreated rats. However, this difference was not of a high statistical significance.

There is no evidence that vitamin C is concerned with the carbohydrate cycle, but Giroud and Ratsimamanga (1939) pointed out that vitamin C is concerned with the elimination of lactic acid after exercise. Various authors have tried large quantities of vitamin C and claimed that it had a beneficial effect on muscular exercise. These include Rugg Gunn (1938), Sobecki (1939), and Brunner (1941), but Jetzler and Haffter (1939) were not able to support this effect.

It is of interest that more recently a number of investigators, mostly Russians, have claimed a beneficial effect of vitamin C on work performance, particularly on athletes in training and in sports contests. According to Van Huss (1966), Dr. Ludwig Prokop, Chief of the Sports Physiology Department of the Institute of Physical Education at the University of Vienna, claimed that he had observed a considerably improved physical performance following the administration of doses of 100 mg of vitamin C to athletes who already had normal ascorbic acid levels in their serum. Russian workers have claimed that there is a direct relationship between the intensity of the work which has to be carried out and the amount of vitamin C required. One of these is N. N. Yakovlev, corresponding member of the Academy of Sciences of the U.S.S.R., who has published a table in which he claims that requirements of vitamin C vary from 75 mg daily during the recovery period from athletic events or muscular exercise up to 300 mg daily during a competitive period. Similarly, V. V. Efremova claims that vitamin C requirements range from 100 mg per day for those engaged in light physical exercise to 200 mg per day for those engaged in heavy exercise. A. Desmarais, from the Faculty of Sciences, University of Ottawa, Canada, claims from his studies that rats running in a revolving drum required a larger quantity of vitamin C than controls. They were able to continue work for a longer period of time than the controls when they were given supplemental doses of 50 mg per day of sodium ascorbate.

All these results seem to lead to the conclusion that vitamin C permits greater physical endurance for longer periods of time. Van Huss then quoted A. W. Hoitink of the University of Vrije, Amsterdam, Holland, who tested a number of individuals on a bicycle ergometer before and after 1 or 2 weeks on a daily dose of 300 mg of vitamin C. One to 2 weeks after the second test was made the measurements were repeated with no supplement of vitamin C in between, and blood samples were also taken prior to and after the period of exercise. According to Hoitink, the vitamin C increased the total amount of work performed. He also said that it increased the serum ascorbic acid which is not surprising, but also that it reduced recovery pulse rate, respiration rate, and systolic blood pressure. He concluded that saturation with vitamin C improves performance.

Van Huss himself carried out a series of studies on the effects of vitamin C on athletes at Michigan State University, comparing vitamin C obtained from orange juice and from synthetic vitamin C. He used 10 male subjects, all active, well trained and all graduate students between 20 and 30 years of age. His procedure was as follows:

"Part one involved the effect on the economy of medium intensity, near steady state work, and associated measures. Part two was concerned with the effects on maximal oxygen intake and on high-intensity, all-out work, and associated measures." In the first part of this study, the students ran on a motor driven treadmill at a speed of 6 mi/hr with no grade; they also ran at 10 mi/hr up an 8% grade. All the subjects were found to have a normal range of serum ascorbic acid before tests began. In other words, they were all above 1.20 mg%. They were all able to tolerate relatively large doses of vitamin C, and they were all tested 1, 2, and 3 hr following the ingestion of three experimental drinks: (a) orange juice in which all but 15 mg of the vitamin C had been destroyed, (b) reconstituted frozen orange juice which provided 2.98 mg of vitamin C per kilo of body weight, and (c) beverage containing no vitamin C. They found that for single performances the vitamin C did not improve the work performance. However, they found that it did improve recovery following the performance of the work, a finding which is in keeping with Giroud and Ratsimamanga's statement that vitamin C helps in the removal of lactic acid. Van Huss did not believe that the one day tests which he carried out were adequate to distinguish between any possible differences in value of synthetic ascorbic acid and orange juice. The author emphasized at the conclusion of his recorded interview and research reports that this study was on a short term basis only and should be extended over a much longer period.

During World War II, Frankau (1943) carried out a series of studies on the acceleration of coordinated muscular effort by nicotinamide. The author points out that there have been reports in the literature of the addition of certain vitamins to the diet, especially vitamin B_1, improving resistance to fatigue and increasing muscular ability. Others, however, have failed to show, either in brief extreme exercise or even in prolonged severe exercise and also in semistarvation, any effect of vitamin supplementation of U.S. Army rations on muscular ability, endurance, resistance to fatigue, or recovery from exhaustion. However, Frankau indicated that the addition of certain vitamins to the normal diet of healthy young men did result in some increased efficiency in carrying out a fairly severe test which required both physical efficiency and coordination. His studies were carried out on Royal Air Force personnel who were in excellent physical training. The test chosen was one which involved "running rapidly, bending and turning quickly, and dropping discs accurately on a closely fitting shaft." Experiments were carried out on 20 subjects, 10 receiving vitamin tablets containing: vitamin A, 8000 IU; vitamin D, 1200 IU; thiamine, 2 mg; riboflavin, 4 mg; ascorbic acid, 100 mg; and nicotinamide, 40 mg. The remaining ten received placebos.

These experiments were carefully controlled. They seem to have been largely ignored in recent years and are rarely referred to in the literature. They demonstrated clearly that the addition of nicotinamide alone or nicotinamide and other vitamins to the diet of young men who could be described as physically fit resulted in increased efficiency in carrying out severe tests involving both physical effort and coordination; and furthermore, not only were they able to perform the tests statistically more rapidly, but they appeared to be less exhausted if they were taking the vitamins. The conclusion was that continued heavy or enduring physical work would benefit by increasing the dose of nicotinamide. It is probable that the action of this particular vitamin is a pharmacodynamic effect; in other words, it acts as a drug rather than as a vitamin, and by dilating the capillaries permits greater flow of blood through the muscular system.

More recently, vitamin E has come into the picture of muscular activity. Several papers have been published claiming its value in postponing fatigue. However, recent studies have suggested that wheat germ oil, in addition to vitamin E, may contain a factor that is important in the production of physical effort. Some of this work was carried out by Cureton (1955) who used a bicycle ergometer and timed treadmill runs at a standardized pace and slope accompanied by a study of the "T" wave of the electrocardiogram. He also studied all-out exercise with oxygen intake determinations. The amount of wheat germ oil used was one teaspoonful (60 minims) a day, although some much larger doses were given. Wheat germ oil was found to be more effective than corn oil with synthetic vitamin E or cottonseed oil. Wheat germ itself provided changes as good in reaction time but did not give the same improvement in endurance or in the circulatory measurements which correlate rather highly with endurance. Cureton recommends the administration of the wheat germ oil just after periods of progressive exercise. It seems to have a very beneficial effect during the training and permits the improvements in performance which have been mentioned. Wheat germ oil supplied alone, however, produced negligible gains unless it was also combined with physical training; training alone without the wheat germ oil was not as effective. Experiments carried out on older subjects gave more striking results even than with younger subjects. Studies by Ershoff and Levine (1955) had also demonstrated that there was an unidentified factor in wheat germ oil which beneficially affected the swimming performance of guinea pigs. The conclusions concerning Cureton's work were that wheat germ oil improved the endurance of middle-aged men running all out on a treadmill, and produced results significantly better than a matched group which took the same course in conditioning exercises for 8 weeks without the wheat germ oil. The gains in endurance were paralleled by improvements in the brachial pulse wave of the upper arm, the heartograph area and systolic amplitude, the "T" wave of the ECG, the systolic blood pressure and the Schneider Index.

Although these workers had claimed that their researches had shown that a beneficial effect was obtained using wheat germ oil and not using vitamin E itself, Percival (1951) had reported that vitamin E produced a decrease in the recovery pulses of men following a step test to exhaustion and a 440-yd run. This was obviously beneficial, but Ershoff and Levine (1955) found that α-tocopherol (vitamin E) did not affect the swimming of their guinea pigs. Consolazio et al. (1964) found that neither wheat germ oil, vitamin E, nor octocosinal improved the swimming performance of rats. So the value of vitamin E and the unknown factor in wheat germ oil in physical exercise is still controversial. Dr. Jyunichi Aoki, one of a group of doctors at Juvtendo University, Japan, recently (October, 1967) told a meeting of the Japan Society for Sports Medicine that vitamin E facilitates the utilization of oxygen by athletes and reduces the accumulation of lactic acid in the blood.

VI. Milk and Athletic Performance

There have also been some claims that milk taken before physical performance or even included in the diet can have a deleterious effect for various reasons. The studies by Nelson (1960), Van Huss (1962), and Asprey et al. (1965), did not show any agreement with this; in fact, they all showed that the drinking of milk or the eating of cereal and milk prior to various physical exercise did not affect the performance. Van Huss (1962) found no difference in training, response, or performance whether milk was included or excluded from the diet.

VII. Conclusions

The role of diet in athletic performance still remains controversial. However, it now appears that the old-fashioned massive meat diet is not only unnecessary but could even be disadvantageous. Nor does it appear that excessive calorie consumption is necessary or desirable. The evidence that specific substances or vitamins, e.g., sugar, vitamin C, vitamin B1, vitamin E, or an unknown factor in wheat germ oil, are of special value in physical exercise or athletic performance is still equivocal. The possible beneficial effect of nicotinamide may be related to its pharmacodynamic effect in causing capillary dilation.

It seems that the best diet for an athlete is one based on fresh fruit and fruit juices, vegetables, milk, first-class protein (such as that found in meat, fish, cheese, and eggs), and whole wheat bread, in other words, the type of diet that is recommended for good health for the rest of the population. An athlete who bases his diet on such a nutritional basis will probably find that extra vitamins will have no effect on his performance or his recovery from it; and it seems likely that only in those athletes whose diet is already defective is a special vitamin supplement likely to be beneficial.

REFERENCES

Abrahams, A. (1948). *Brit. J. Nutr.* **2**, 266.
Andres, R., Cader, G., and Zierler, K. L. (1956). *J. Clin. Invest.* **35**, 671.
Asprey, L. E. (1965). *Res. Quart.* **36**, 233.
Asprey, L. E., Alley, W., and Tuttle, W. (1965). *J. Am. Dietet. Assoc.* **47**, 198.
Bicknell, F., and Prescott, F. (1945). "The Vitamins in Medicine." Heineman, London.
Bourne, G. H. (1943). Unpublished work.
Bourne, G. H. (1948). *Brit. J. Nutr.* **2**, 261.
Brunner, H. (1941). *Schweiz. Med. Wochschr.* **71**, 715.
Consolazio, C. F., Matoush, L. O., Nelson, R. A., Isaac, G. J., and Hursh, L. M. (1964). *J. Appl. Physiol.* **19**, 265.
Cureton, T. K. (1955). *Scholastic Coach* **24**, 36 and 67.
Drabkin, D. L. (1959). *Perspectives Biol. Med.* **2**, 473.
Drummond, J. C., and Wilbraham, A. (1939). "The Englishman's Food." Jonathan Cape, London.
Eggleton, P. (1948). *Brit. J. Nutr.* **2**, 249.
Ershoff, B. H., and Levine, E. (1955). *Federation Proc.* **14**, 431.
Frankau, I. M. (1943). *Brit. Med. J.* **II**, 601.
Giroud, A., and Ratsimamanga, A. R. (1939). *Arch. Hosp.* **II**, 891.
Glick, D., and Antopol, W. (1939). *J. Pharmacol. Exptl. Therap.* **65**, 389.
Gounelle, H. (1940). *Bull. Soc. Med. Hop. Paris* **56**, 225.
Haldi, J., and Wynn, W. J. (1946). *J. Nutr.* **31**, 525.
Harper, A. A., MacKay, I. F. S., Raper, H. S., and Camm, G. L. (1943). *Brit. Med. J.* **I**, 243.
Harris, H. A. (1966). *Proc. Natl. Soc.* **25**, 87.
Henschel, A. (1943). *Res. Quart.* **8**, 230.
Hill, A. V. (1925). *Lancet* **II**, 481.
Hills, H. W. (1942). *Brit. Med. J.* **II**, 587.
Issekutz, B., Birkhead, N. C., and Rodahl, K. (1963). *J. Nutr.* **79**, 109.
Jetzler, A., and Haffter, C. (1939). *Wien. Med. Wochschr.* **89**, 332.

Jokl, E. (1964). "Nutrition, Exercise and Body Composition." Thomas, Springfield, Illinois.

Karpovich, P. V. (1941). *Res. Quart.* **12**, Suppl., 432.

Karpovich, P. V., and Millman, N. (1942). *New Engl. J. Med.* **226**, 88.

Keys, A. (1943). *Federation Proc.* **2**, 164.

Keys, A., and Henschel, A. F. (1942). *J. Nutr.* **23**, 259.

Lewis, K. F., Allen, A., and Weinhouse, S. (1959). *Arch. Biochem. Biophys.* **85**, 499.

McCormick, W. J. (1940). *Med. Record* **152**, 439.

Mottram, V. H., and Graham, G. (1941). "Hutchinson's Food and the Principles of Dietetics," 9th ed. Arnold, London.

Nelson, D. O. (1960). *Res. Quart.* **31**, 181.

Percival, L. (1951). *Shute Foundation J. Med. Res.* **3**, No. 2.

Poortmans, J. R., and Jeanloz, R. W. (1966). *13th Ann. Meeting Am. Gll. Sports Med.* p. 301.

Rugg Gunn, M. A. (1938). *J. Roy. Naval Med. Serv.* **3**, 199.

Simonson, E., Enzer, N., Baer, A., and Braun, R. (1942). *J. Ind. Hyg.* **24**, 83.

Sobecki, G. (1939). *Med. Prakt.* **13**, 299.

Stromgren, G. (1960). *The Athletic Journal* Oct., p. 32.

Van Huss, W. D. (1962). *Res. Quart.* **33**, 120.

Van Huss, W. D. (1966). *Nutrition Today* March, p. 20.

Van Itallie, T. B., Sinisterra, L., and Stare, F. J. (1960). *In* "Science and Medicine of Exercise and Sports" (W. R. Johnson, ed.), p. 203. Harper, New York.

von Dobeln, W. (1963). *Nutr. Rev.* **21**, 211.

Yamaji, R. (1951). *J. Physiol. Soc. Japan* **13**, 476a and 483b.

6

TEMPERATURE REGULATION

I. The Achievement of Thermal Balance

Thomas Adams and P. F. Iampietro

The discussion that follows cannot aspire to be a complete analysis of the environmental or physiological factors involved in temperature regulation; it attempts only to be an introduction in this field and to offer a critical appraisal of selected interests. If it can afford the beginning student an understanding and appreciation of the general area, and give the advanced student and professional reader an outline of current concepts, it will have fulfilled its responsibilities. More detailed information and extended bibliographies are available in several reviews (Adams, 1960a, b; Burton and Edholm, 1955; Day, 1943; Fry, 1958; Hardy, 1960; Robinson, 1952; Winslow and Herrington, 1949).

A. The Homeotherm and His Environment

In defending its acquired thermal balance, the homeotherm is presented with a dual thermostatic responsibility. Whereas it must appropriately adjust its own physiology to meet environmental thermal demands (during heat and cold exposures), it must also be prepared to rebalance biothermal heat exchange mechanisms to dissipate metabolic heat loads during exercise, regardless of the environmental thermal imposition. Both internal and external thermal threats generally marshal the same physiological defenses against hyperthermia, as discussed below.

Metabolic processes, like the rates of most chemical reactions, are catalyzed by heat. Metabolic independence from the influence of environmental temperature, within the limits of successfully achieved homeostasis, gives the warm-blooded animal a considerable advantage over the poikilotherm. Thermally affected metabolic processes depend upon the regulated, relatively constant internal temperature for the homeotherm, but for the cold-blooded animal, upon the more capricious and extreme environmental thermal changes. This freedom from other than extreme environmental thermal exposure has been identified as having had evolutionary importance (Bogert, 1959; Burton and Edholm, 1955). The observation that all homeotherms thermoregulate within a relatively narrow temperature range (36°C for the elephant to 41°C for the birds) supports the suggestion that at least one other homeothermic advantage is internal thermal stability at a metabolically efficient level; ca. 37°C has been suggested to be an optimum temperature for many metabolic reactions (Burton and Edholm, 1955).

Although a reasonably sharp distinction can be made between homeotherms and poikilotherms on the basis of body temperature stability through physiological, reflexly mediated action, it has been demonstrated that poikilotherms can limit internal temperature fluctuations through behavioral adjustments. It is the degree of precision and the type of body temperature control that separates the so-called cold- and warm-blooded animals. Whereas most homeotherms can control mean body temperature within a fraction of a degree by reflex adjustments of metabolism, blood flow, etc., poikilotherms are restricted to providing a less discrete body temperature set only by behavior and selection within the environment.

The homeotherm's ability to isolate metabolic processes from the influence of the environment does not come without cost. Total energy dissipation is usually greater than for the poikilotherm even at moderate exposure temperatures due to the steeper gradient between the homeotherm's skin surface temperature and environmental temperature. In winter, the warm-blooded animal is faced not only with a greater heat loss due to lower ambient and environmental temperatures but also with reduced metabolic energy sources (food supplies). Besides improving, extending, and supplementing its thermal protection by additional fur growth and cold acclimatization processes, the warm-blooded animal so stressed may augment these protections by physically removing itself from the stressing environment (e.g., burrowing or migrating), or surrender its homeothermic status and retreat into a temporary state of modified poikilothermy (hibernation or pseudohibernation). In either event, the obligated high energy flux is avoided. Humans adapt further by using the "psychosociological" (Burton and Edholm, 1955) tools of shelter, clothing, heating and air conditioning systems, etc., and thereby establish for themselves greater thermal freedom than any other warm-blooded animal.

B. THE PHYSICAL BASIS FOR HOMEOSTASIS

A constant temperature for any object is achieved [Eq. (1), Fig. 1] when sources of heat gain are equally matched by avenues of heat loss, with such a balance represented by an unchanging heat content ($\Delta H = 0$). For animals [Eq. (2), Fig. 1], the thermal steady state is reached when metabolism (always a source of heat production) is coupled with, or balanced against, effective avenues of heat exchange, and no net heat gain or loss takes place. A constant internal temperature is the direct result of the algebraic sum of these influences, and nothing else. Such a thermal situation exists for the homeotherm after enough heat has been stored to elevate its temperature above that of the environment and within the thermal control zone ($37°$–$39°C$ for most mammals).

EQUATION

1. $\Delta H = (\text{HEAT GAIN}) - (\text{HEAT LOSS})$
2. $\Delta H = \text{METABOLISM} \pm \text{HEAT EXCHANGE}$
3. $\Delta H = \text{METABOLISM} \pm C_d \pm C_v \pm R_d - E_v$

WHERE:

$\Delta H = $ NET HEAT FLUX; IF EQUAL TO ZERO, A THERMAL STEADY STATE IS ACHIEVED.

$C_d = $ CONDUCTION
$C_v = $ CONVECTION
$R_d = $ RADIATION
$E_v = $ EVAPORATION

Fig. 1. Basic heat exchange equations.

Specifically, the avenues of heat exchange are [Eq. (3), Fig. 1] conduction (Cd), convection (Cv), radiation (Rd), and evaporation (Ev), each of which (except evaporation) can be a source of heat gain or loss, depending on environmental and physiological circumstances. Heat flow along any of these routes requires an energy potential gradient. For conduction, convection, and radiation, a thermal gradient is required; heat loss by evaporation requires a difference in water vapor pressures. Detailed examination of the physical variables associated with each of these energy exchange avenues is available elsewhere (Adams, 1960b; Brengelmann and Brown, 1965; Burton and Edholm, 1955; Newburgh, 1949; Winslow and Herrington, 1949); the present discussion will be limited to evaluating each of these forces as they supply the physical framework for homeostasis.

Heat transfer by conduction is defined as thermal energy exchange through a medium, between objects in physical contact, or by the transfer of kinetic intramolecular energy, without involving the physical transfer of material. With an existing temperature difference, heat can be exchanged (gained or lost) between the bottoms of the feet and the floor, between the skin and contact clothing, between and through adjacent body tissues, etc. Since homeotherms normally have only a small body area in contact with other objects in the environment (except for clothing), conduction is usually not a major avenue of environmental heat exchange for the warm-blooded animal.

Convection, a special case of conduction, is most often considered as a separate avenue of heat exchange. It is distinguished as a route of thermal energy flow depending upon the movement of a fluid over a surface which is at a different temperature. Two types of convection are usually identified. In natural (or passive) convection, the fluid (liquid or gas) flow is a function of differences in density within the fluid produced by differences in temperature (e.g., warm air rising from a flame or over a warm surface). Forced convection, which increases the rate of heat exchange, requires an additional energy source external to the heat exchanging system itself to move the fluid (e.g., an electric fan or a stirring motor). In addition to the physical considerations for conduction, heat exchange by convection also varies with the fluid characteristics (viscosity, density, etc.) and the surface features of the object which affect surrounding fluid movement (surface texture, irregularities, shape, etc.). Most important and effective convective heat exchange within the body occurs by tissue blood flow. Since the movement of blood through the circulatory system depends ultimately on the expenditure of myocardial metabolic energy, tissue perfusion is an example of forced convection. The free movement of blood through the vasodilated body serves not only to minimize intracorporeal temperature differences, but also is an important mechanism for exchange of body heat with the environment.

Heat exchange by convection between the body surface and the surrounding air (or water) can be reduced by the interposal of any material which would inhibit free fluid flow. Trapping air within or beneath clothing or within fur provides a still fluid layer in contact with the skin which reduces heat exchange by convection and establishes an important protective microenvironment immediately surrounding the animal. Any factor which damages the integrity of this still fluid layer facilitates increased convective heat exchange. For example, exercise in the cold air can increase heat loss markedly from the skin surface due to limb and body movements (Carlson *et al.*, 1954; Hart, 1952). Less heat would be lost were the same amount of exercise performed isometrically.

Heat transfer by the exchange of electromagnetic energies between facing surfaces is called radiation. This heat exchange route is unique in that it does not depend upon contact between heat exchanging masses, but can take place through low density environments (e.g., as solar radiation does through "space"). All objects above a temperature of absolute zero ($-273°C$) exchange radiative energy with every other facing object (or with its own facing surfaces), with the net gain or loss of heat depending upon differences in temperature and other surface characteristics (e.g., emissivity: whether an object is a good "reflector" or "emitter" of radiant energy) (Brengelmann and Brown, 1965; Newburgh, 1949).

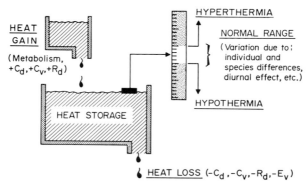

Fig. 2. Body temperature is maintained within a normal range as the amount of stored heat is balanced by rates of net heat gain and loss.

Heat loss by evaporation depends upon thermal transfer in the conversion of a material from a liquid to a gas phase. Evaporation is always a heat-dissipating phenomenon; the energy stored by gas molecules can be released during the process of condensation. The dissipation of heat by evaporation can occur from any wetted body surface exposed to a less than saturated gaseous environment (e.g., from the respiratory tract surfaces, from the skin with or without sweat gland activity, or from the wetted fur). Homeotherms exposed to environmental temperatures higher than skin temperature depend solely upon heat loss by evaporation to retain a thermal steady state [Eq. (3), Fig. 1]. If exposed under such a condition in air that is saturated with water vapor (i.e., at 100% relative humidity, no vapor pressure gradient can be established), progressive hyperthermia develops at the accumulated rates of metabolic heat production and heat gains from the environment through conduction, convection, and radiation. Even if sweat gland activity (or panting) were maximal under these conditions, no effective cooling could occur since evaporative processes would be precluded.

An analogy expressing the interaction of these factors is presented in Fig. 2.

In conceptualizing a specific thermal exposure, it is important to recognize that seldom do any of the four avenues of heat exchange operate alone in effective biothermal responses; the thermal threat to the homeotherm and the countering physiological defense is effected rather in terms of the algebraic sum of these interacting forces.

C. THE PHYSIOLOGICAL BASIS FOR BIOTHERMAL CONTROL

Figure 3 shows how the avenues of heat exchange operate together to transfer thermal energy (during an air exposure) from the clothed- or bare-skin surface. This body cross section shows the three major temperatures to be considered, air (T_a), skin (T_s), and "core" (T_r) or deep body temperature, usually evaluated as rectal temperature. Modifying heat exchange rates along this axis are the summing insulations of the outer body area ("shell") [I_t], the clothing [I_{c1}] and the air [I_a]. Tissue insulation [I_t] can vary due to rates of local blood flow [C_{cv}], i.e., internal body convection, to make the "shell" (that portion of the body mass in which there are temperature gradients and which will change its temperature during thermal stress) occupy approximately one half of the total body mass (during massive peripheral vasoconstriction and extended cold exposure), or bring the "core" (that portion of the body which is at a near constant temperature)* close to the skin surface (during cutaneous vasodilation and heat exposure). Heat exchange (double headed arrows) can occur by conduction (C_d) both within the body between adjacent tissues at different temperatures, or with objects touching the skin surface (including clothing). Heat loss (single headed arrows) by evaporation can occur directly from deep body masses (within the "core") by evaporation from nasopharyngeal, buccal, lingual, palatine, and respiratory-tract surfaces (E_{va}) or from the skin and clothing surfaces (E_{vb}). Heat exchange by radiation (R_d) and convection (C_v) to the surrounding environment can take place from any exposed surface. The terms "core" and "shell" are, of course, functionally defined in terms of the heat content and thermal gradients within different body masses; they do not have fixed anatomical counterparts.

* Small temperature differences exist both between organs and structures deep in the body and within the ventricular cavities during different phases of the cardiac cycle (due to heat released during myocardial contraction). Although these differences in temperature should be considered in evaluating the rationale for selecting a single temperature measurement to reflect accurate internal mean temperature, it should not be confusing in the general, but conceptually valuable, identification of the "core."

Partitional calorimetric testing has shown that during a whole body exposure (human) with air and wall temperatures at 24°C and with low relative humidity and little forced air movement, evaporation accounts for approximately 21%, radiation 37%, and conduction and convection together 42% of the total dissipated heat (Winslow and Herrington, 1949). These proportions can be drastically different for exposures in environments with other characteristics.

A situation analogous to that presented in Fig. 3 can be envisioned for a water rather than an air exposure. Additional appreciation of the physical factors involved in the avenues of heat exchange may also be gained by speculating how the equations in Fig. 1 would have to be rebalanced, or the avenues of heat exchange shown in Fig. 3 re-evaluated for a water exposure or during exposure to environments of low density ("space").

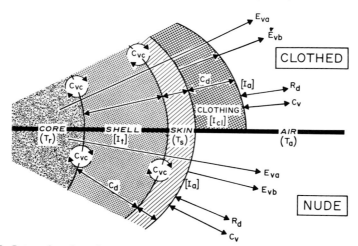

Fig. 3. Internal and environmental physical heat exchange routes are indicated for both clothed (upper) and nude (lower) air exposures.

At least 3 separate thermal functions can be attributed to that portion of the body near the skin surface, the shell, which is not (as defined) at deep body temperature. In addition to serving as a site for convective heat exchange by perfusing blood, decreased heat loss during cold exposure results as the uniformly warm body mass (core) withdraws from the skin surface to deeper body areas, interposing a vasconstricted tissue mass between itself and the environment (Wood et al., 1958). This shell, so established, offers some degree of thermal insulation ($[I_t]$, Fig. 3) which can be calculated (Adams, 1963b, Burton and Edholm, 1955). These circulatory adjustments can bring about a change in tissue insulation from approximately 25 to 10 kcal/hr·m²·°C with a change in ambient temperature from 35° to 10°C (Day, 1943). Deposition of subcutaneous fat layers can increase tissue insulation over that achieved by vasoconstriction alone in the human (Buskirk *et al.*, 1963; Carlson *et al.*, 1958), as it can in arctic animals (Irving, 1966). Since the shell can transiently change its heat content, it can serve an additional role of thermal capacitance which acts as a buffer to internal temperature changes by means of its ability to affect either positive or negative heat storage. This effect has been shown to be of functional importance at least to desert mammals (Schmidt-Nielsen, 1959).

Besides the physiological adjustment of the avenues of heat exchange (physical temperature regulation), most homeotherms can provide large amounts of thermal energy during an acute cold exposure by involuntary muscular activity, shivering (Iampietro *et al.*, 1960) (chemical temperature regulation), or by voluntary activity (Table I). For the human, both metabolic heat production and skin surface evaporation of secreted sweat are critically important in extending the environmental thermal limits provided only by circulatory adjustments in which a thermal steady state can be enjoyed, as shown in Fig. 4. Although the ambient temperature at which chemical temperature regulation begins (so-called critical temperature) (Scholander *et al.*, 1950) is only a degree or so below normal room temperature for the human, some furred animals are able to maintain a constant internal temperature

TABLE I

DIFFERENT LEVELS OF PHYSICAL ACTIVITY
WITH CORRESPONDING VALUE OF HEAT
PRODUCTION[a]

Activity	Metabolic rate[b]	Met[c]
Sleeping	36	0.7
Basal	40	0.8
Sitting (resting)	50	1.0
Standing	60	1.2
Walking (level)		
1.5 mph	90	1.8
3.0 mph	130	2.6
4.0 mph	180	3.6
Running (level)		
10 mph	500	10.0
Heavy work	860	17.2

[a] Adams (1960a).
[b] In kcal/hr·m².
[c] One met = 50 kcal/hr·m².

without augmenting physical defenses by shivering in air temperatures as low as −40°C (Scholander *et al.*, 1950). Increases in heat production by shivering are effective in maintaining thermal balance only in acute cold stress; protection during chronic cold exposure must rest upon mechanisms for retaining rather than generating heat (Irving, 1966).

A very general estimate of the flexibility of the interacting influences of clothing and physical activity during exposure to cold is shown in Fig. 5. More accurate relations for "comfort" and behavioral integrity are available elsewhere (Burton and Edholm, 1955; Kaufman, 1963; Kaufman and Pittman, 1964; Winslow and Herrington, 1949). Predictions of homeothermal status are made available for extreme exposures through the use of computor analogues of operating thermoregulatory systems (Brown, 1963; Crosbie *et al.*, 1963), as well as through human testing.

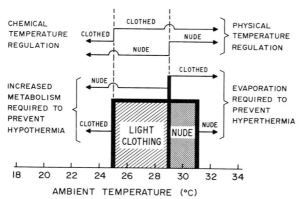

Fig. 4. The temperature ranges of effective vasomotor regulation are shown for the human nude and with light clothing. Exposure to temperatures above each upper limit requires sweat gland activity to maintain normothermia; normal temperature stability during an exposure to temperatures below each lower limit requires metabolic heat production.

Internal body temperature can be protected during a cold exposure not only by appropriate and effective physiological reflexes which reduce heat loss at the body surface and increase metabolic heat production, but also by critically redistributing stored calories. Analogous to the conservation of body fluids by renal countercurrent mechanisms, decreased heat loss has been described to take place in the extremities of many animals (including humans) by a circulatory, countercurrent heat exchange system (Schmidt-Nielsen, 1963). Figure 6 shows how this effect occurs. During a cold exposure, venous blood normally returning through cutaneous channels is shunted by vasomotor adjustments to veins deeper in the axis of the extremity. Through the anatomical juxtaposition of these arteries and veins (vena comites), warm

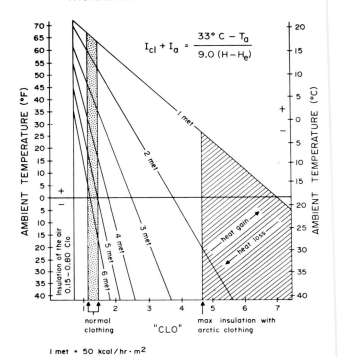

I met = 50 kcal / hr · m²

I met = 0.18 °C / kcal · m² · hr

= the amount of insulative clothing required to maintain a resting-sitting man with a metab. of I met indefinitely comfortable at an envir. temp. of 21 °C (70 °F)

Fig. 5. This chart shows the approximate relationship between ambient temperature and the units of insulation (expressed as "clo") required to maintain thermal comfort. It will in addition indicate the varying degrees of heat loss (or gain) and levels of thermal equilibrium under varying degrees of heat production and exercise. No estimates can be made with this diagram to include the effects of wind velocity greater than 20 ft/min. From Adams (1960b).

EXAMPLE: 72°F with normal clothing at rest (1 met) is thermally equal to 54°F with 3 clo, is equal to 41°F with 4 clo, is equal to 27°F with 5 clo, etc.

EXAMPLE: 0°F with 7.2 clo at rest is equal to 3.7 clo at 0°F at 2 met, is equal to 2.5 clo at 0°F at 3 met, etc.

EXAMPLE: −40°F with 2.5 clo at 4 met is an isothermal condition equal to 57°F with normal clothing at 2 met, is equal to 54°F with 3 clo at rest, etc.

EXAMPLE: The heat loss (degree of thermal stress) at rest with normal clothing at 40°F is equal to the thermal stress encountered at 45°F with no clothing at rest, is equal to 20°F with 3 clo at rest, etc.

EXAMPLE: The thermal stress at −35°F with 3 clo at 3 met is equal to 46°F with no clothing at 3 met, is equal to 0°F with 2.1 clo at 3 met, is equal to 30°F with normal clothing at 3 met, etc.

EXAMPLE: The heat loss at 15°F with 4.5 clo at 1 met is equal to the heat loss at 10°F with 2.7 clo at 2 met, is equal to the heat loss at 5°F with 2 clo at 3 met, etc.

arterial blood, coursing peripherally, can lose heat by conduction (C_d) to the corresponding vein carrying cooler blood centrally. The temperature difference between the warm arterial blood and the cooler venous blood is due, of course, to some heat loss to the environment at the skin surface. The end effect is to establish an additional site for this exchange of heat within the body (by heat transfer to the returning venous blood) which keeps the thermal energy within the body and reduces heat loss to the environment (extremity temperature is reduced since the arterial blood entering the peripheral portions of the limb is cooler). This type of thermal response, in conjunction with skin vasoconstriction reflexes, establishes a temperature gradient longitudinally as well as transversely in the extremity (Bruck and Hensel, 1953).

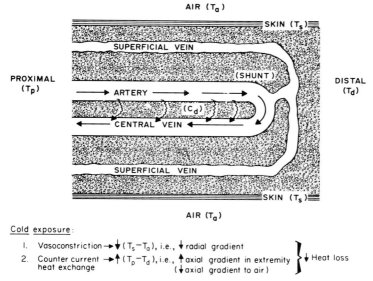

AIR (T_a)

SKIN (T_s)

SUPERFICIAL VEIN

PROXIMAL (T_p)

(SHUNT)

DISTAL (T_d)

ARTERY

(C_d)

CENTRAL VEIN

SUPERFICIAL VEIN

SKIN (T_s)

AIR (T_a)

Cold exposure:

1. Vasoconstriction → ↓ ($T_s - T_a$), i.e., ↓ radial gradient
2. Counter current → ↑ ($T_p - T_d$), i.e., ↑ axial gradient in extremity
   heat exchange   (↓ axial gradient to air)

} ↓ Heat loss

Fig. 6. Section through an extremity showing the circulatory basis for countercurrent heat exchange.

Figure 7 illustrates how the alternate superficial venous return pathways can also have thermoregulatory importance. During exposure to air warmer than skin temperature, venous blood shunted to the skin surface decreases the gradient along which (and the rate at which) heat is gained from the environment (skin temperature approaches environmental temperature). Similarly, during exercise at ambient temperatures lower than skin temperature, the increased heat loss required to maintain thermal balance in the face of increased metabolic heat production is facilitated by increasing (even more) the skin-ambient temperature gradient.

Both in the case of heat exposure and of exercise at lower air temperatures, required heat loss from the skin surface by evaporation is increased due to the increase in water vapor pressure accompanying the rise in skin temperature; sweat gland activity consequently becomes a more efficient mechanism for losing heat as long as the environment is not saturated with water vapor.

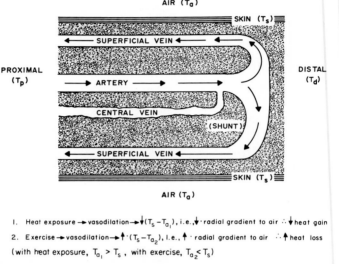

1. Heat exposure → vasodilation → ↓($T_s - T_{a_1}$), i.e., ↓ radial gradient to air ∴ ↓ heat gain

2. Exercise → vasodilation → ↑($T_s - T_{a_2}$), I.e., ↑ radial gradient to air ∴ ↑ heat loss

(with heat exposure, $T_{a_1} > T_s$, with exercise, $T_{a_2} < T_s$)

Fig. 7. Section through an extremity showing the circulatory adjustment for environmental heat exchange at the skin surface.

In addition to satisfying skin metabolic requirements, the cutaneous circulation can vary considerably in performing its role in thermoregulation. Skin blood flow in a nude resting man at 82°F ambient temperature is estimated to be 400 ml/min (Greenfield, 1963). This flow can be increased by a factor of 3 with work at 70°F (Brouha and Radford, 1960), or during rest at 100°F; working at 100°F will raise cutaneous circulation to approximately 9000 ml/min (Brouha and Radford, 1960).

Succinctly, an acute human response to cold is characterized by: (1) peripheral cutaneous vasoconstriction (which results in an increase in tissue insulation), expansion of the shell, and withdrawal of the core; (2) increased heat production by shivering; and (3) shunting of venous blood in the extremities to deep vessels for countercurrent heat exchange.* An acute human response to heat stress is characterized by (1) peripheral cutaneous vasodilation (decrease in peripheral tissue insulation), expansion of the core, re-

---

* In furred animals, this series of responses would be supplemented by piloerection which would trap air near the skin and reduce the rate of skin surface convective heat loss.

duction of the shell; (2) increased sweat gland activity; and (3) the superficial return of venous blood.†

In spite of the cursory presentation here, it should be clearly recognized that the physiological responses to heat and cold stress and the consequent re-adjustment of heat within the body is far from simple and their details are not completely understood. More detailed descriptions of the characteristics of heat, cold, hibernation, etc., are available elsewhere (Burton and Edholm, 1955; Hardy, 1963).

D. The Neurophysiological Control of Body Temperature

As might be expected for any unit which remains as stable as homeothermic deep body temperature (although not necessarily total body heat content due to thermal transients within the shell) under the buffeting of internal and external thermal loads, the subserving control system is complex. As with any control system, however, it retains the basic components of input (internal and skin temperature) and output (metabolism, shivering, sweating, vasomotor control, etc.) operating through an integrational level (hypothalamic central nervous system areas). Figure 8 presents an outline of these operational levels for responses to cold.

The general response pattern for cold elicited reflexes shown in Fig. 8 is that temperature receptors within the skin (Hensel, 1963) provide information (via the lateral spinothalamic tract) afferently into neurointegrational levels within the diencephalon (hypothalamus) which reflexly relays appropriate effector responses through the sympathetic and somatic motor pathways and into metabolic channels. A similar, grossly oversimplified circuit can be described for defenses against hyperthermia.

Just before the turn of this century, it became apparent that internal body temperature, in addition to the more obvious influence of local skin temperature, was influential in triggering thermal responses (Ott, 1887; Richet, 1885). It became clear later that the neurons and synaptic activity in regions of the anterior hypothalamus were especially susceptible to local temperature effects (Hasama, 1930; Magoun *et al.*, 1938), and that the temperature of this area serves functionally as an additional thermal input into the biothermal control system. Since there are no anatomically identifiable temperature receptors in the anterior hypothalamus, as there are in the skin, it should be emphasized that the effect of temperature within the central nervous system is a direct, thermal modification of activity rather than one in which information (in the form of action potentials) is fed into a central integrational area; the

† In furred animals, in the absence of effective sweat gland activity, increased evaporative cooling would occur through panting, and in extreme body heating, by copious salivation and licking of the fur.

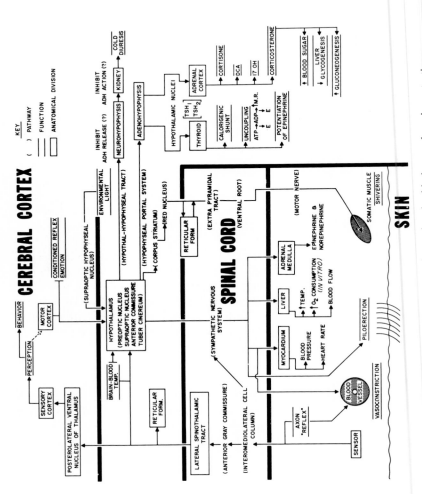

Fig. 8. A general outline of the reflex pathways involved in homeothermic protections against hypothermia.

terms "thermal sensibility" (to denote the action of temperature directly on central nervous system cells) and "thermal sensitivity" [to identify peripheral (skin) temperature receptor function] seem appropriate (Adams, 1963a).

Local anterior hypothalamic heating and cooling in unanesthetized animals (Adams, 1963a; Freeman and Davis, 1959; Fusco, 1963) has emphasized the earlier suggestion that local central temperature as well as skin temperature must be considered as a functional temperature regulation control system input. Local diencephalic heating produces many of the characteristic heat responses as does (to a more limited extent) local hypothalamic cooling initiate predictable cold defenses. Questions related to the preferential influence of either of these factors in cold and heat exposure and acclimatization largely remain open. The identification of the neural characteristics of anterior hypothalamic neurons, in contrast to others within the central nervous system, is not complete (Hardy, 1960). The basic features of control system regulation which are most likely involved in body temperature control have been presented (Hardy and Hammel, 1963).

It should not be forgotten that thermal control effectors serve other functions for the organism and may operate effectively outside of hypothesized biothermal control. For example, it has been shown recently that sweat gland activity is triggered almost immediately upon initiation of voluntary activity (Van Beaumont and Bullard, 1963; Meyer *et al.*, 1962), before there are any measurable changes in skin or central temperature; the total response, however, can (under some circumstances) be greatly influenced by skin temperature (Van Beaumont and Bullard, 1963; Benzinger *et al.*, 1963). Although it can be argued teleologically that this response is involved in the preparatory phases of thermal control and is effected in anticipation of the increased heat production associated with exercise, details of its action are missing. The control of sweating during exercise is discussed in greater detail in Section II.

Sweating, panting, shivering, peripheral vasomotor responses and other thermoregulatory effector actions serve the same biothermal ends, to offset net heat fluxes impinging through environmental and exercise induced heat stress, and to retain a constant internal temperature. Matching of appropriate responses to the thermal situation is the role of central neural reflexes subserving temperature regulation. Research leading to the detailed elucidation of these controls has only begun.

II. Thermal Balance during Exercise and Environmental Stress

P. F. Iampietro and Thomas Adams

When man exercises, he must dissipate the heat produced by the muscles or increase body temperature. If heat generated during exercise can be lost to the environment, a new thermal steady state can be achieved; voluntary activity is then limited by factors other than elevated body temperature. If humidity is high, or if clothing inhibits heat loss by radiation, convection, conduction and the evaporation of sweat, body temperature increases as a function of the exercise rate with voluntary activity terminating as hyperthermia ensues.

A. EXERCISE IN HEAT AND HUMIDITY

Seminude man resting at 82°F (a "neutral" temperature) produces heat at the rate of 80 kcal/hr. Approximately 20 kcal/hr are dissipated as water evaporates from respiratory and skin surfaces (without sweating, so-called "insensible water loss"); 60 kcal/hr are lost by radiation, convection and conduction. During heavy exercise, heat production may rise as high as 960 kcal/hr (12 times resting). The major portion of this heat is brought to the body surface by increased skin blood flow (400 ml/min at rest compared to 1200 ml/min during exercise) (Brouha and Radford, 1960); skin surface heat loss is further increased by the evaporation of sweat. Since each milliliter of water evaporated requires 0.58 kcal, a sweating rate of 3000 ml/hr can dissipate heat at a rate of 1740 kcal/hr.

In addition to attempting heat dissipation during exercise, an advantage may be taken of the thermal capacitance of the shell with some heat being stored (increasing body temperature; see page 180). This effect is valuable in heavy exercise for short periods (e.g., track events of a mile or less). No satisfactory explanation is available to indicate why body heat storage is tolerated better during exercise than by resting man during heat exposure.

The neurophysiological control system through which heat is dissipated by increased skin surface evaporative water loss is particularly important in extending the upper limit of physical temperature regulation (see Fig. 4) during whole body heat exposure, and especially during prolonged exercise. There appears to be a thermoregulatory response to exercise in which internal body temperature is controlled at a new, higher level. The elevation over resting internal temperatures depends upon the rates of work (Nielsen and Nielsen, 1965) and is generally uninfluenced by ambient temperature (within the limits of biothermal ability). Further, during different steady state workloads at a uniform ambient temperature, sweat rates and internal temperatures are linearly related and skin temperature remains constant. Conversely, when the same level of work is performed at different ambient temperatures, internal body temperature remains constant and sweat rates rise as a linear function of average skin temperature (Nielsen and Nielsen, 1965). These data provide a valuable extension of the relationship between sweat rate and internal temperature reported earlier (Benzinger *et al.*, 1963).

Resting man (nonheat acclimatized) exposed to a hot environment (as high as 120°F) can maintain a normal body temperature by increasing cardiac output and skin blood flow, and evaporating sweat. Superimposition of requirements to dissipate metabolic heat during exercise increases circulatory strain (the requirement to provide blood flow to the exercising muscles and to the skin for heat dissipation) leading to increased internal body and skin surface temperatures, nausea, dizziness and syncope (Robinson, 1963). Heat production approximately 8 times resting at 100°F increases skin blood flow about 4 times over resting levels at the same temperature (Brouha and Radford, 1960). Heat dissipation at ambient temperatures greater than skin temperature depends solely on the evaporation of secreted sweat. The less clothing which may form a vapor barrier and the drier the surrounding air, the greater ease with which exercise can be performed in the heat. Human heat acclimatization involves changes in blood volume and peripheral circulation which reduces cardiovascular strain during exercise in the heat, and improves sweating efficiency (Ladell, 1964).

The comfort and ease of physiological adjustment to a heat stress, either at rest or during exercise, is a combined function of ambient temperature and humidity (Goldman *et al.*, 1965; Iampietro and Goldman, 1965). Those geographical areas which typically have high ambient temperatures in the summer (100°F or more), usually have low relative humidity. This allows for the rapid and complete evaporation of sweat on the skin and clothing and a relatively effortless thermal adjustment. Those areas, however, with high water vapor pressures (although lower ambient temperatures) have a much

TABLE II

SWEAT RATES FOR TWO LEVELS OF ACTIVITY AT TWO DRY BULB TEMPERATURES AND AT VARIOUS HUMIDITIES

	Reference	Dry bulb (°F)	Wet bulb (°F)	Relative humidity (%)	Sweat rate (liter/hr)
Rest (80 kcal/hr)	Goldman *et al.* (1965)	80	66	47	0.05
	Goldman *et al.* (1965)	110	82	30	0.42
	Goldman *et al.* (1965)	110	95	57	0.84
	Goldman *et al.* (1965)	110	105	84	1.38
Work (350 kcal/hr)	Adolph *et al.* (1947)	80	—	Low	0.45
	Adolph *et al.* (1947)	110	—	Low	1.05
	Iampietro and Goldman (1965)	110	90	46	1.60
	Iampietro and Goldman (1965)	110	95	57	1.90

less tolerable summer climate. Since the ready evaporation of sweat is not possible with high relative humidity, exercise thermal tolerances are thereby limited (Wyndham *et al.*, 1965). The same, or greater, amount of water and salt may be lost in secreted sweat in the wet-hot climate, in contrast to the dry-hot environment; the thermal balance question is more related to its evaporation than simply its production. Table II illustrates how sweat secretion increases when humidity is increased. Resting man at 110°F ambient temperature more than triples sweat secretion when relative humidity increases from 30% to 84%. Working man at the same dry bulb temperature almost doubles sweat secretion when relative humidity increases from "low" (about 30%) to 57%. The excellent chapter by Ladell (Ladell, 1964) should be consulted for a comprehensive treatment of the physiological effects of humid heat in man.

B. WATER AND WORK

Sweating removes from the body both water and salts. The loss of water leads to dehydration, and eventually decreased performance. As blood volume decreases with the progressive loss of body water, metabolic as well as heat exchanging circulatory functions become impaired. Further dehydration (3.0% of body weight) reduces sweat gland activity (Pearcy *et al.*, 1956). Sweat gland function during exercise in either hot or cold environments brings about the same general effects. After exercise, rehydration by voluntary water intake does not replace the total amount of water lost until several days (Adolph *et al.*, 1947; Iampietro *et al.*, 1956); the physiological mechanism for this latency is not clear.

Inattention to body hydration levels during competitive sports can result directly in reduced performance, or more seriously, set the stage for heat exhaustion. A decrease in body water by 5% reduces maximum oxygen consumption (the highest rate at which aerobic work can be performed) (Buskirk *et al.*, 1958) and performance (the skill required for a particular task) (Adolph *et al.*, 1947). Whereas particular attention should be paid to drinking adequate amounts of water during and after exercise (Ladell, 1955), the requirement to replace lost Na, K, and Cl can be normally met during meals (Fregly and Iampietro, 1958; Johnson *et al.*, 1942). Since both water and inorganic salt are lost in the sweat, excessive water intake alone can result in below normal levels of tonicity and consequent discomfort and/or heat cramps. The periodic replacement of body water and salts during work in hot environments, or at any time when sweating is maintained, is essential to insure performance standards and general well being (Johnson *et al.*, 1942). Figure 9 illustrates the importance of water replacement when men work in a hot environment. Rectal temperature of the "no water" group exceeds 102°F after 4 hr of work while rectal temperature of the "water ad lib" group remains below 102°F for more than 5 hr.

C. THERMAL ACCLIMATIZATION

Chronic exposure to hot or cold environments results in a progressive change in the way an animal defends internal thermal stability. These adjustments have been characterized (Fry, 1958) as:

1. Acclimation: systemic or cellular changes in an individual on a daily basis in direct response to an identified stress
2. Acclimatization: long term responses or adjustments of an individual to an identified stress
3. Adaptation: phylogenetic adjustment or compensation to any environmental condition

Physiological heat acclimatization processes for humans are well defined (Bass *et al.*, 1955; Bass, 1963), although for cold acclimatization they remain somewhat equivocal. Heat acclimatized individuals demonstrate an increased ability to work in the heat and respond to an acute heat stress with a more rapidly elicited sudomotor reflex and the production of a more dilute sweat. Although the total potential for sweat secretion is enhanced, less sweat is produced for mildly stressing heat exposures (at rest) compared to matching responses of nonheat acclimatized humans. Heat acclimatization has also been reported to be accompanied by a decrease in "cardiovascular stress" (Bass, 1963) during acute heat exposures and an increase in total blood volume. This latter claim may have to be identified by the measurement method and the experimental condition (Bazett *et al.*, 1940; Robinson, 1963). The most striking component of human heat acclimatization is the increased ability and ease with which the superimposed stresses of exercise and acute heat exposure are met during the first 5–7 days of chronic heat exposure. It is thought that acclimatization to heat is not complete unless work is performed in the heat; exposure to heat alone confers but little acclimatization. Recent work, however, indicates that acclimatization may be accomplished by controlled hyperthermia alone (Fox, 1965).

This evidence may have practical importance in competitive events involving teams with different thermal histories. Men normally exercising in warm or hot environments may well be expected to perform better in competition at high ambient temperatures than others usually exercising at comfortable or cool temperatures. Individuals from climates cooler than that in which exercise is to be performed may improve competitive potential by thermal "preconditioning." Moderate exercise (about 350 kcal/hr) for 2–3 hr daily at an ambient temperature a few degrees warmer than that anticipated for an impending event, 10–14 days before competition, could conceivably extend thermal exercise limits, improve performance, and reduce physiological strain.

The experimental identification of human, whole body cold acclimatization has stirred a controversy for many years which at present is far from resolved. Although regional skin cold acclimatization for the human is well documented (Adams and Smith, 1962; Elsner et al., 1960; LeBlanc et al., 1960; Miller and Irving, 1962; Nelms and Soper, 1962), the precise character of whole body changes with chronic cold stress remains elusive. Experimental programs reporting physiological changes in "indoor" men who (for the purposes of the experiment) live in a cold environment must face the question of possible artifacts introduced by physical fitness changes (Adams and Heberling, 1958; Heberling and Adams, 1961; Keatinge, 1961). These programs must also identify how thermal stress occurs when, in many studies, the subjects are provided with thermally insulating clothing; it would seem that exposure to the microclimate established by such clothing would preclude the required experimental condition of cold exposure (except perhaps for the hands, feet, and face). Attempts to demonstrate cold acclimatization in human populations indigenous to arctic or subarctic regions leaves unresolved problems of (at least) racial, ethnic, and dietary involvements (Adams and Covino, 1958). Although a large number of reports have been published in this area, equivocation on the basis of subject selection, use, training and maintenance, the nature of the chronic and acute cold exposures used in the tests, adequacy, appropriateness and precision of employed physiological tests and, of course, individual data interpretation in view of these variables, serve to cloud the issue.

Nonetheless, some experiments in which subjects have been chronically exposed to cold (unprotected by microenvironments generated by thermally insulating clothing) strongly suggest that increased heat production without shivering (so-called "nonshivering thermogenesis") can be developed in humans (Carlson and Thursh, 1959; Davis, 1963) as it can in other species (Cottle and Carlson, 1956; Hannon, 1963). Although much more data must be available before these questions are answered, the general pattern of human cold acclimatization is hinted to be related to increased heat production through shivering (Iampietro et al., 1958) and endocrine or intracellular adjustments, a greater heat flux with increased shell and decreased core partitioning of the main body mass (i.e., increased tissue insulation) (Carlson et al., 1951), but reduced peripheral vasoconstriction (Wood et al., 1958) leading to warmer hands and feet. Although obligating a source of increased heat loss, the warmer extremities may play the protective role of reducing peripheral cold injury and maintaining manual dexterity. There is little evidence to support the suggestion that a reduced thermoregulatory "set-point" accompanies these changes (LeBlanc, 1956). Paralleling tests of heat acclimatization and exercise, some effort has been directed toward defining in man cold acclimatization in terms of metabolic responses to exercise in the cold (Andersen *et al.*, 1952).

In spite of difficulty in identifying the whole body cold acclimatization indexes, local cold acclimatization for the human has been well documented both by "field" and laboratory testing (Adams and Smith, 1962; Elsner *et al.*, 1960; Miller and Irving, 1962; Nelms and Soper, 1962). Humans who chronically expose their extremities to cold air or water show an alteration in local circulation during acute cold stress (extremity immersion in well-stirred ice water) which can be interpreted as a protective adjustment. Their extremities do not cool as deeply and remain generally warmer than those of persons not having experienced long term local cold exposure. Increased protection against local cold injury and maintained manual dexterity may well be achieved prior to *de facto* cold stress by repeated, local cold exposures.

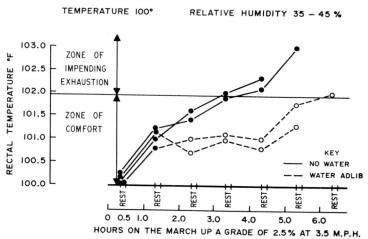

Fig. 9. The effect of water intake on rectal temperature during work in the heat (after Johnson *et al.*, 1942).

The physiology of exercise cannot be separated from the homeothermic demands of the environment. Performance capability can be easily sacrificed by a lack of understanding or respect for thermoregulatory requirements. The cost is, of course, the termination of voluntary exercise by hyperthermia before cardiovascular, muscular, and pulmonary limits are met. The recognition of only a few thermoregulatory concepts can pay a multifold return in improved individual and group performances.

REFERENCES

Adams, T. (1960a). "The Control of Body Temperatures," Tech. Rep. 59–21. AAC, Arc. Aeromed. Lab., Alaska.

Adams, T. (1960b). "Environmental Factors Influencing Thermal Exchange," Tech. Rep. 59–22. AAC, Arc. Aeromed. Lab., Alaska.

Adams, T. (1963a). *J. Appl. Physiol.* **18**, 772.

Adams, T. (1963b). *J. Appl. Physiol.* **18**, 778.

Adams, T., and Covino, B. G. (1958). *J. Appl. Physiol.* **12**, 9.

Adams, T., and Herberling, E. J. (1958). *J. Appl. Physiol.* **13**, 226.

Adams, T., and Smith, R. E. (1962). *J. Appl. Physiol.* **17**, 312.

Adolph, E. F., and associates (1947). "Physiology of Man in the Desert." Wiley (Interscience), New York.

Andersen, K. L., Strommie, S., and Elsner, R. W. (1952). "Metabolic and Thermal Responses to Muscular Exercise in the Cold," TD Rept. No. AAC-TDR-61-52. Fort Wainwright, Alaska.

Bass, D. E. (1963). *In* "Temperature, Its Measurement and Control in Science and Industry" (J. D. Hardy, ed.), Vol. 3, Part 3, Chapter 28. Reinhold, New York.

Bass, D. E., Kleeman, C. R., Quinn, M., Henschel, A., and Hegnauer, A. H. (1955). *Medicine* **34**, 323.

Bazett, H. C., Sunderman, F. W., Doupe, J., and Scott, J. C. (1940). *Am. J. Physiol.* **129**, 69.

Benzinger, T. H., Kitzinger, C., and Pratt, A. W. (1963). *In* "Temperature, Its Measurement and Control in Science and Industry" (J. D. Hardy, ed.), Vol. 3, Part 3, Chapter 56. Reinhold, New York.

Bogert, C. M. (1959). *Sci. Am.* **200**, 105.

Brengelmann, G., and Brown, A. C. (1965). *In* "Physiology and Biophysics" (T. C. Ruch and H. D. Patton, eds.), Chapter 54, p. 1050, Saunders, Philadelphia, Pennsylvania.

Brouha, W. L., and Radford, E. P., Jr. (1960). *In* "Science and Medicine of Exercise and Sports" (W. R. Johnson, ed.), Chapter 10, pp. 190, 193. Harper, New York.

Brown, A. C. (1963). "Analog. Computer Simulation of Temperature Regulation in Man," TD Rept. No. AMRL-TDR-63-116. Wright-Patterson AFB, Ohio.

Bruck, K., and Hensel, H. (1953). *Arch. Ges. physiol.* **257**, 70.

Burton, A. C., and Edholm, O. G. (1955). "Man in Cold Environment." Arnold, London.

Buskirk, E. R., Iampietro, P. F., and Bass, D. E. (1958). *J. Appl. Physiol.* **12**, 189.

Buskirk, E. R., Thompson, R. H., and Whedon, G. D. (1963). *In* "Temperature, Its Measurement and Control in Science and Industry" (J. D. Hardy, ed.), Vol. 3, Part 3, Chapter 37. Reinhold, New York.

Carlson, L. D., and Thursh, H. L. (1959). "Human Acclimatization to Cold," Contract No. AF41(657)-212. Wright-Patterson AFB.

Carlson, L. D., Young, A. C., Burns, H. L., and Quinton, W. F. (1951). "Acclimatization to Cold Environment," USAF Tech. Rept. No. 6247. Wright-Patterson AFB.

Carlson, L. D., Pearl, D., and Scheyer, W. (1954). *Am. J. Physiol.* **179**, 625.

Carlson, L. D., Hsieh, A. C. L., Fullerton, F., and Elsner, R. W. (1958). *J. Aviation Med.* **29**, 145.

Cottle, W. H., and Carlson, L. D. (1956). *Proc. Soc. Exptl. Biol. Med.* **92**, 845.

Crosbie, R. J., Hardy, J. D., and Fessenden, E. (1963). *In* "Temperature, Its Measurement and Control in Science and Industry" (J. D. Hardy, ed.), Vol. 3, Part 3, Chapter 55. Reinhold, New York.

Davis, T. R. A. (1963). *In* "Temperature, Its Measurement and Control in Science and Industry" (J. D. Hardy, ed.), Vol. 3, Part 3, Chapter 38. Reinhold, New York.

Day, R. (1943). "The Effect of Cold on Man," Rev. Ser. 1(2)L1-64. Josiah Macy, Jr. Found., New York.

Elsner, R. W., Nelms, J. D., and Irving, L. (1960). *J. Appl. Physiol.* **15**, 662.

Fox, R. H. (1965). *In* "The Physiology of Human Survival" (O. G. Edholm and A. L. Bacharach, eds.), Chapter 3, p. 71. Academic Press, New York.

Freeman, W. J., and Davis, D. D. (1959). *Am. J. Physiol.* **197**, 145.

Fregly, M. J., and Iampietro, P. F. (1958). *Metab., Clin. Exptl.* **7**, 624.

Fry, F. E. J. (1958). *Ann. Rev. Physiol.* **20**, 207.

Fusco, M. (1963). *In* "Temperature, Its Measurement and Control in Science and Industry" (J. D. Hardy, ed.), Vol. 3, Part 3, Chapter 51. Reinhold, New York.

Goldman, R. F., Green, E. B., and Iampietro, P. F. (1965). J. Appl. Physiol. **20**, 271.

Greenfield, A. D. M. (1963). *In* "Handbook of Physiology" (Am. Physiol. Soc., J. Field, ed.), Sect. 2, Vol. 2, p. 1328. Williams & Wilkins, Baltimore, Maryland.

Hannon, J. P. (1963). *In* "Temperature, Its Measurement and Control in Science and Industry" (J. D. Hardy, ed.), Vol. 3, Part 3, Chapter 41. Reinhold, New York.

Hardy, J. D. (1960). "The Physiology of Temperature Regulation," Rept. No. 22, NADC-MA-6015. U.S. Naval Air Develop. Center, Johnsville, Pennsylvania.

Hardy, J. D., ed. (1963). "Temperature, Its Measurement and Control in Science and Industry," Vol. 3, Part 3. Reinhold, New York.

Hardy, J. D., and Hammel, H. T. (1963). *In* "Temperature, Its Measurement and Control in Science and Industry" (J. D. Hardy, ed.), Vol. 3, Part 3, Chapter 54. Reinhold, New York.

Hart, J. S. (1952). *Can. J. Zool.* **30**, 90.

Hasama, B. (1930). *Arch. Exptl. Pathol. Pharmakol.* **153**, 257.

Heberling, E. W., and Adams, T. (1961). *J. Appl. Physiol.* **16**, 226.

Hensel, H. (1963). *In* "Temperature, Its Measurement and Control in Science and Industry" (J. D. Hardy, ed.), Vol. 3, Part 3, Chapter 19. Reinhold, New York.

Iampietro, P. F., Vaughan, J. A., MacLeod, A. R., Welch, B. E., Marcinek, J. G., Mann, J. B., Grotheer, M. P., and Friedemann, T. E. (1956). "Caloric Intake and Energy Expenditure of Eleven Men in a Desert Environment" Tech. Rept. EP-40. Quarter Master, Research and Development Center, U.S. Army, Natick, Massachusetts.

Iampietro, P. F., Bass, D. E., and Buskirk, E. R. (1958). *Metab., Clin. Exptl.* **7**, 149.

Iampietro, P. F., Vaughan, J. A., Goldman, R. F., Kreider, M. B., Masucci, F., and Bass, D. E. (1960). *J. Appl. Physiol.* **15**, 632.

Iampietro, P. F., and Goldman, R. F. (1965). *J. Appl. Physiol.* **20**, 73.

Irving, L. (1966). *Sci. Am.* **214**, 94.

Johnson, R. E., Belding, H. S., Consolazio, C. F., and Pitts, G. C. (1942). "The Requirements of Water and of Sodium Chloride for the Best Performance of Men Working in Hot Climates," Harvard Fatigue Lab. Rept. No. 13.

Kaufman, W. C. (1963). *Aerospace Med.* **34**, 889.

Kaufman, W. C., and Pittman, J. C. (1964). *Aerospace Med.* **35**, 1167.

Keatinge, W. R. (1961). *J. Physiol.* (*London*) **157**, 209.

Ladell, W. S. S. (1955). *J. Physiol.* (*London*) **52**, 11.

Ladell, W. S. S. (1964). *In* "Handbook on Physiology" (Am. Physiol. Soc., J. Field, ed.), Sect. 4, Chapter 39. Williams & Wilkins, Baltimore, Maryland.

LeBlanc, J. (1956). *J. Appl. Physiol.* **9**, 395.

LeBlanc, J., Hildes, J. A., and Heroux, O. (1960). *J. Appl. Physiol.* **15**, 1031.

Magoun, H. W., Harrison, F., Brobeck, J. R., and Ranson, S. W. (1938). *J. Neurophysiol.* **1**, 101.

Meyer, F. R., Robinson, S., Newton, J. L., Ts'ao, C. H., and Holgersen, L. O. (1962). *Physiologist* **5**, 182.

Miller, L. K., and Irving, L. (1962). *J. Appl. Physiol.* **17**, 449.

Nelms, J. D., and Soper, D. J. G. (1962). *J. Appl. Physiol.* **17**, 444.

Newburgh, L. H., ed. (1949). "Physiology of Heat Regulation and the Science of Clothing." Saunders, Philadelphia, Pennsylvania.

Nielsen, B., and Nielsen, M. (1965). *Acta Physiol. Scand.* **64**, 314.

Ott, I. (1887). *J. Nervous Mental Disease* **14**, 152.

Pearcy, M., Robinson, S., Miller, D. I., Thomas, J. T., and Debrota, J. (1956). *J. Appl. Physiol.* **8**, 621.

Richet, C. (1885). *Arch. Ges. Physiol.* **37**, 624.

Robinson, S. (1952). *Ann. Rev. Physiol.* **14**, 73.

Robinson, S. (1963). *In* "Temperature, Its Measurement and Control in Science and Industry" (J. D. Hardy, ed.), Vol. 3, Part 3, Chapter 27. Reinhold, New York.

Schmidt-Nielsen, K. (1959). *Sci. Am.* **201**, 140.

Schmidt-Nielsen, K. (1963). *In* "Temperature, Its Measurement and Control in Science and Industry" (J. D. Hardy, ed.), Vol. 3, Part 3, Chapter 14. Reinhold, New York.

Scholander, P.F., Hock, R., and Walters, V. (1950). *Biol. Bull.* **99**, 237.

Van Beaumont, W., and Bullard, R. W. (1963). *Science* **141**, 643.

Winslow, C. E. A., and Herrington, L. P. (1949). "Temperature and Human Life." Princeton Univ. Press, Princeton, New Jersey.

Wood, J. E., Bass, D. E., and Iampietro, P. F. (1958). *J. Appl. Physiol.* **12**, 357.

Wyndham, C. H., Strydom, N. B., Morrison, J. F., Williams, C. G., Bredell, G. A. G., Maritz, J. S., and Munro, A. (1965). *J. Appl. Physiol.* **20**, 37.

7

DOPING AND ATHLETIC PERFORMANCE

Richard V. Ganslen

I. History

Five thousand years ago Chinese physicians used extracts of the Ma huang plant to strengthen heart action and raise blood pressure; they had discovered ephedrine, not chemically identified until 1924. For millennia, according to Huxley (1957), man has sought self-transcendence by experimenting with nature's products in their natural or altered state.

Man has sought magic elixirs in every fruit, berry, root, and flower to enhance his feelings of well-being or to help him cope with his afflictions. Early, perhaps before written history, man accidentally discovered the by-product of fermentation, alcohol, which has served as a wonderful soporific through the centuries. One will never know whether the soldiers of Ghengis Khan used wine to reduce the tensions of the chase or to allay fatigue.

Perhaps the greatest feat in athletic history should be credited to the Greek Olympic runner Pheidippides, whose performance we honor with the modern Marathon. In the year 490 BC the bronze-clad Athenians marched into battle against the Persians and among these foot soldiers was Pheidippides. During the fighting Pheidippides was sent to Sparta for reinforcements, a 2-day journey. At the end of the battle he discarded his armor and ran to Athens where he fell dead with the words of victory on his lips. We ask ourselves, how much motivation does it take to make a man run himself to death in defiance of all the inhibitory functions of his central nervous system?

II. Nature of the Problem (Definition)

We define "doping" as orally or parenterally medicating a competitive athlete with the sole intention of artificially and unnaturally increasing his competitive performance.

One must discriminate very carefully between the therapeutic application of drugs or chemical agents to save life or protect man from unusual stress and the use of chemical agents to produce extraordinary performance by inducing a "hyperactive state."

Many drug substances are available that will produce a biological state of hyperactivity, in man, without necessarily improving performance efficiency. It is imperative to point out that some of these substances are natural constituents of the body. The fact that the body produces excessive amounts of stimulating substances under stress complicates the legislative control of drug administration in competitive sports where these identical substances could be used.

Man, exposed to severe environmental stress, such as cold, may respond by a marked decrease in energy output to preserve life (decreased reactivity). The hyperreactive state associated with intensive athletic competition, involving great emotional stress, lies at the other end of the scale of physiological reactivity.

III. Philosophical Considerations

When one considers the administration of a drug or a chemical agent to enhance a performance, he must face the dilemma of equating philosophical, ethical, and biological questions which, in the past, have been oversimplified. Many questions must be satisfied.

Bøje (1939) reviewed the early work on doping and recommended that the practice be absolutely forbidden. Karpovich (1965) has reviewed some of the more recent literature in this area. The wealth of material on this subject in many satellite fields of physiology is easily overlooked. One gains considerable insight into the wealth of literature available by examining, at first hand, the newer pharmacological textbooks such as one by Goodman and Gilman (1965). Many discussions of drugs pertinent to this review have been incorporated into the general textbooks in physiology where they are less liable to attract attention. Charlier's book (1961) on coronary agents is a classic in the field. Recent papers by La Cava (1961), Porritt (1965), and Prokop (1965) are also of interest.

Exercise physiologists are interested in the broad problems of muscle energetics, hypoxia, fatigue, and recuperation. Incidents related to this are specific studies of the by-products of biochemical transformation which sometimes can be correlated with the magnitude of energy transformation. Enhancement of energy production with drugs, without deteriorating the physiological reserves, is a challenge which has intrigued man for centuries.

The supreme efforts of man have been accomplished in times of travail, turmoil, and stress without the necessity for psychic energizing substances. The progressive improvement of athletic records does not suggest that man has, as yet, exhausted his natural resources. Yet, need for knowledge of substances to bring man to a level of normal functional efficiency after hurtful stress and to preserve life is of paramount importance.

IV. Methods of Study

Physiology is largely the science of unravelling the mysteries associated with the remarkable properties of the autonomic nervous system. That this system is subservient to the central nervous system does much to complicate the inquiry.

The remarkable coordinative properties of an autonomic response to a stressor, provoking physiological disequilibrium, has been the foundation stone for thousands of investigations of mammalian organisms. From the study of peripheral responses, science has tediously progressed to the study of individual cells and the alteration of their properties in the presence of substance found within or alien to their structure. Pharmacological science, therefore, proceeds at a rate consistent with the inroads of biochemistry into the study of cellular physiology.

Despite tremendous advances in cellular physiology and chemistry, pharmacodynamics is still a jungle, barring comprehensive explanations of how drugs work. The selection of criteria unsuited to the complex nature of the problem is a dilemma of major proportions which confronts pharmacodynamic investigators in all of the biological disciplines.

Enthusiasm for the double-blind or placebo approach is misleading. Investigators frequently take a hostile defensive attitude toward a design weakness with demonstrable deficiencies. Even the most naive subjects and supposedly ignorant investigators note differences in experimental subjects a short interval after an agent has been ingested.

If one could equate personalities, then the testing of pharmacological agents would be more fruitful. Paradoxically, it has frequently been observed that subjects on placebos show statistically significant improvement, as great as 40%, upon which the test substance does not substantially improve, Agersborg and Shaw (1962). The objective testing of drugs on human subjects is a dream, perhaps not realizable in our lifetime.

PHYSIOLOGICAL DYNAMICS

Pharmacological agents act by disturbing cell enzymes, cell membranes, or specialized functional components of a cell. To have some effect on man, the agent must arrive at the site of action in adequate concentration and the receptor must demonstrate an altered biological energy state as long as the agent is present.

For convenience, one must accept the concept of drug reception at an effector cell. The receptor must demonstrate sensitivity to a certain concentration of the neurotransmitter trigger which initiates somatic or motor disturbances. Receptor selectivity may be demonstrable.

A drug, acting at a site, may act as an antimetabolite to prevent normal neurotransmitter response, or it may exaggerate response or trigger the release of inhibitor substances. The positive or negative triggering action may be localized or take place in some remote corner of the CNS, e.g., digitalis, used to strengthen the heart function, acts on contractile muscle proteins, electrolyte, fluxes, and heart muscle energy utilization. Which is the most important? Which is primary? Are these all one mechanism in disguise? We do not know.

Aspirin and morphine are efficacious in controlling pain. However, morphine works at all levels of pain intensity, while aspirin is only useful at lower pain thresholds. Drugs often, if not always, produce side effects that are worthy of concern but are obscured by the primary effects, which are usually emphasized. Morphine may suppress cough, cause histamine release, act as an antidiuretic, and precipitate a respiratory crisis; all are secondary effects of genuine concern.

V. Research Methods and Pitfalls

One may measure changes in the electrical conductivity of a cell, cell assembly, or organ isolated from the body, and arrive at some very definite conclusions, but subsequent observations of the same organs in the intact body refute the prior investigation. One can, more conveniently, study the blood pressure, pulse rate, circulatory, respiratory, or neuromuscular response in the intact organism with great success without ever knowing what really happened within the organism.

The persistent effects of drugs are quite easily studied; however, the transient effects are often of tremendous significance and offer the greatest challenge to the investigator; e.g., Dave Sime, one of the world's greatest sprinters, was observed to have a heart rate of 28 beats per minute in the blocks; by the time he had made his sixth step, his pulse rate was over 120. Was his heart rate acceleration due to simple mechanical venous pumping mechanisms or was it triggered by sympathetic adrenal factors?

A study of cumulative heart rates in exercise may be worthless in a pharmacological investigation because it may obscure vital transitory effects on the heart only detectable by an EKG, where the individual beats are evaluated. If the ventricular force from pulse waves or via strain gauges is measured, in some manner, the results are distorted or completely nullified by changes in heart volume without any loss of cardiac efficiency. One can only conclude that the ingested substance affected the ventricular force, but by what mechanism one can only hazard a guess.

In studies of circulation, one may be interested in the pharmacodynamics of a certain blood pressure (vasopressor substance). The investigator must now contend with all the vascular deflections which are smoothly integrated for maximum biological adaptability. The vascular beds, acting as blood pools, may be mediated by nerve stimuli, local metabolites such as oxygen or carbon dioxide, the heart rate changes, or local pressure heads. Thus, unless steady state conditions can be achieved in the course of experiment, one often obtains interesting but meaningless data.

Any stress changes reactivity and may aggravate the effects of pharmacological agents designed to evaluate the stress situation. This may or may not impair future reactivity. Exposure to altitude is a stress, the stressor mechanisms of carbon dioxide and oxygen lack react to improve resistance to subsequent exposures to altitude.

VI. Drug Dosages

One cannot give physiologically identical doses of drug substances to people, only quantitatively identical doses. Individuals receive the drug substances in different states of physiological receptivity which thus alters the quality of the response. As the drugs' doses are repeated, the physiological re-activity becomes depressed; we label this "tolerance." Tolerance to drugs, especially the sympathomimetics, tranquilizers, barbiturates, and CNS depressants, increases with drug dose frequency, yet the causal factors for the increased tolerability (hyporeactivity) remain obscure.

In animal experimentation, too little or too much of a given agent degrades an improvement observed with the optimal drug dose (Parin *et al.*, 1964). It is also true, in animal experimentation, that the end point may be "survival." There is often a tendency to ignore disturbances in reactivity prior to expira-tion or recovery, which do not seem to degrade performance; e.g., an endurance swimming test in a rat must assess cardiodynamics, hemodynamics, hypo-thermia, muscle chemistry, and central nervous system excitability (motiva-tion) to explain survival. We may be interested in the postactivity effects of the drug on an EKG, but this may not tell us whether or not myocardium is functionally normal, only that the EKG is normal.

The logical approach to pharmacological experimentation, therefore, is to give the subject an agent with known properties and then administer a similar, but not identical, substance, not a blank cartridge. Discrimination between two sympathomimetic agents is more meaningful in normal subjects than the use of a stimulant preceded by or followed by a placebo, especially when the subjects' reactions must be solicited. The investigator must be extremely conscious of the limitations of his data in any pharmacological in-vestigations where extrapolation is hazardous.

A. Sympathomimetic Drugs

The sympathomimetic drugs are substances whose effect is similar to a stimulation of the adrenergic nerves. Effects include: excitatory or inhibitory functions, stimulation of metabolic functions in the liver and muscles (glycogenolysis), cardiac excitement, and, last but not least, central nervous system excitatory action.

Although there are approximately 30 drugs in this category, only three have special CNS effects, nine are known to have pressor activity (blood pressure elevation) and four have known influence on cardiac function.

The CNS drugs are: hydroxamphetamine, amphetamine, and metham-phetamine. These drugs are sold under a variety of trade names such as Benzedrine, Dexedrine, Pervitan, Elastonon, Isophan, Desamin, etc.

The specific cardiac stimulators are: epinephrine, norepinephrine (lev-arterenol), hydroxamphetamine, and ephedrine.

Charlier's book (1961) on the coronary vasodilators listed more than 900 references and discussed hundreds of drugs which have been used in connection with heart and circulatory function.

It is imperative to point out that a complete listing of pharmacological agents which influence the CNS, listed by trade name, would include over 100 titles.

B. Adrenaline-Noradrenaline and Performance

The catecholamines, adrenaline (A) (epinephrine), and noradrenaline (NA) [levarterenol (norepinephrine)] play a significant role in maintaining circulatory function at high levels of efficiency during work. These natural constituents of the body exert their effects by strengthening cardiac contraction or altering the resistance of blood vessels.

The early work of Dill *et al.* (1930) emphasized the role of the corticoadrenal secretion in assisting the body in mobilizing fuel by direct effects on the liver. Experimentally, it was demonstrated that dogs responded as well during treadmill work to glucose as they did to adrenaline injections. In one case, an adequately fed dog jogged for 17 hr continuously (82 mi).

Since, at an early date, it was suspected that adrenaline and noradrenaline were secreted by sympathetic nerves as well as the adrenal gland, Campos *et al.* (1928), sympathectimized dogs. No performance decrement was observed. When adrenaline (0.02 mg/kg) was injected, the dogs' work performance was normal, but if too much adrenaline was used, the dogs became excited and could not perform.

Vendsalu (1960) has completed one of the most comprehensive studies of A and NA to date. Blood samples were collected during bicycle ergometer work equivalent to 200 kgm/min.

At rest, the A and NA levels for the subjects ranged from 0.06–0.08 μg and 0.30–0.42 μg/liter, respectively. At the heaviest work load the adrenaline concentration reached 0.30 mg/liter while noradrenaline peaked at 1.3 mg/liter. Within 5 min of the completion of work the A and NA levels were back to normal.

Drastic alteration in energy output and maintenance of reasonable tonus in the blood vessels is closely correlated with reflex secretion of adrenaline and noradrenaline from the adrenal gland and adrenergic nerves. Assays reveal that 90% of the body's adrenaline is stored in the adrenal gland proper. In animal studies where the animals have been stressed by surgery, work, or hypothermia, the adrenal gland is found to be completely devoid of these hormones immediately after the stress.

The increasing popularity of the orthostatic tolerance test (tilt-table) led Vendsalu to examine the effects of this fitness test on A and NA secretions. This work raises some questions with respect to the validity of tilt-table tests to appraise fitness.

Persons who do not adapt well to tilting experience syncope which is evidenced by increases in noradrenaline secretion 5 to 10 times normal. Normal persons who may evidence some hypotension do not demonstrate this response. The reflex secretion of A and NA is therefore a positive reflex response to an excessive gravitational stressor effect. Figure 1 illustrates this response.

Tilt-table tests tend to discriminate between simple postural hypotension and arterial orthostatic anemia where excessive blood pooling may occur.

Ganslen *et al.* (1964) also used the tilt-table test to assess the effects of tranquilizer and vasodilator drugs. However, the mechanisms involved in orthostatic syncope under a central nervous system depressant may be very dissimilar.

The fact that adrenaline and noradrenaline may undergo four- to tenfold increases under various stressor conditions, with or without hard muscular work, make the evaluation of blood or urine samples of these substances extremely difficult, Elmadjian (1961).

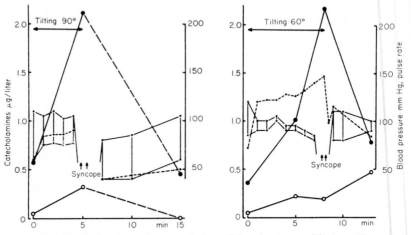

Fig. 1. The catecholamine response during tilting in two subjects with syncope. Solid line, noradrenaline; open circles, adrenaline; dashed line, pulse; crosses, blood pressure.

C. TRANQUILIZER AND VASODILATOR DRUGS

Ganslen *et al.* (1964) experimented with the effects of caffeine-Metrazol, Equanil (meprobamate), and a potent vasodilator Recordil (7-flavonoxyacetic acid ethyl ester). Subjects were subjected to tilt-table tests as well as an all-out treadmill walk at 3.4 mph up a progressively increasing grade (1% per minute). See Fig. 2.

Caffeine and Metrazol taken separately had no influence on performance. However, a combination of caffeine-Metrazol (0.2 gm caffeine plus 0.4 gm Metrazol) increased the maximal O_2 intake 3.3 ml/kg/min and resulted in a decreased pulse rate during work. The systolic and diastolic blood pressure was 6 to 10 mm Hg higher.

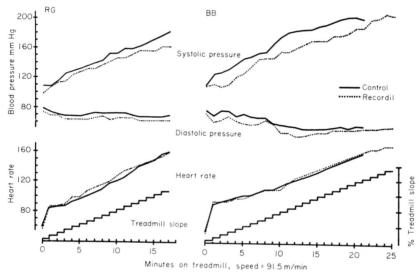

Fig. 2. Effects of Recordil 7-flavonoxyacetic acid ethyl ester on cardiovascular response to the standard treadmill test.

Recordil proved to be a potent vasodilator. Subjects ingested 200 mg 4 hr prior to the tilt-table and treadmill tests. Both experienced subjects exceeded all previous performances on the treadmill. In contrast to the caffeine-Metrazol mixture, the pulse rate was increased while both the systolic and diastolic blood pressures were lower.

Equanil (400 mg) was ingested every 4 hr over periods as long as 24 hr. Work performances were unchanged although there was marked disinclination to work and some ataxia. Single doses of 400 mg were ineffective. In larger doses, there was evidence of a decrease in cardiac output.

Asmussen and Bøje (1948) experimented with nitroglycerin as a coronary vasodilator in bicycle ergometer work of short duration. Subjects were always conscious of having taken the drug. No performance improvements were demonstrated.

D. AMPHETAMINES AND CAFFEINE IN WORK PERFORMANCE

Weiss and Laties (1962) have completed the most comprehensive review of performance enhancement with caffeine and the amphetamines.

Studies on energizing compounds date back to the work of Rivers and Webber (1907), who fed 500 mg of caffeine citrate to subjects doing ergographic work and produced consistent increases in performance. Foltz et al. (1942) worked 4 subjects to exhaustion on a bicycle ergometer and in the retest increased their work capacity with caffeine sodium benzoate. They then experimented with amphetamine (10–15 mg), methamphetamine (5 mg), caffeine sodium benzoate, and a placebo. Amphetamine administered 30 min before the task was ineffective, methamphetamine produced a significant effect, and caffeine fell somewhere in between. Using 23 subjects, Foltz et al. worked subjects to exhaustion on a step test. With 10 mg caffeine or amphetamine no improvements were noted, but the subjects improved with the training. These subjects, who carried knapsacks weighing 33% of their body weight, may have been handicapped by their lack of leg strength for this specific exercise. Alles and Feigen (1942), using the Mosso ergograph, obtained performance improvements with 20 mg amphetamine. Ten mg had no influence. The response with 400 mg of caffeine was much less marked. Knoefel (1943), using the bicycle ergometer, compared amphetamine, metamphetamine, and dextro-isomers of both. He reported increased work output, greatest with the dextro-isomer. Lehmann et al. (1939) used 3 subjects repeatedly on the bicycle ergometer and noted that the time to exhaustion was prolonged by doses of 5, 10, and 15 mg of metamphetamine when compared to placebo.

Graf (1950) conducted a number of studies in Germany during World War II using various agents to prevent fatigue and improve work performance. He tested Cardiazol and caffeine separately, and then tested them when mixed. Many of the tasks were tedious arithmetic calculations; hand steadiness and fine-motor-coordination effects were also investigated. He also experimented with Isophen (methamphetamine). Graf concluded that there were always optimal doses a drug has of which no improvement could be obtained. In long, monotonous tasks, subjects improved substantially under the influence of the drugs. The drugs seemed to produce fatigue delay at the expense of fine-motor-coordination steadiness. Graf emphasized that stimulants may act at different levels in the cerebral cortex, and one should not expect identical excitatory effects from two different substances. It may be pertinent to point out that European Benzedrine compounds are not chemically identical to their American counterpart.

As a result of the German activity with drug substances (stimulants), Seashore and Ivy (1953) launched an extensive series of experiments in which they tried to mimic military conditions insofar as possible. Four substances were investigated: caffeine sodium benzoate (450 mg); amphetamine sulfate (10 mg); methamphetamine hydrochloride (5 mg); and lactose placebo. The subjects hiked 18–20 mi and then performed guard duty until 4:30 AM. This was followed by $1\frac{1}{2}$ hr of testing. Other test periods included up to 20 hr of truck driving and marches with full packs in hot moist and hot dry air. The drugs were definitely superior to the placebo in improving performance.

Somerville (1946) tested 100 subjects divided into two groups. One group received 15 mg amphetamine 1 hr before the end of a march lasting 17 hr. After the hike, the men were taken to the obstacle course and rifle range. No significant performance differences were noted. In a second military exercise lasting 56 hr and including some hiking, two of three groups were fed 30 and 35 mg of amphetamine 22 hr before the termination of the problem. No significant difference was noted in these two groups when compared to the controls on a lactose palcebo. Cuthbertson and Knox (1947) tested the effect of 15 mg methamphetamine on performance of an 18-mi march after 24 hr of sleeplessness. The "drop-out" number was lower with the drug group.

VII. Athletic Performance

G. M. Smith and Beecher (1959, 1960) conducted comprehensive studies of swimmers using secobarbital and amphetamine sulfate. This study was severely criticized by Pierson and an adequate rebuttal to his statements was written by Cochran et al. (1961).

Fifteen college swimmers each swam his preferred event twice on 12 consecutive days. The second swim was started 15 min after the end of the first swim. On the fourth and twelfth days each subject received a dose of amphetamine equal to 14 mg/70 kg body weight; on 4 other days he received control medication, and on 4 other days he received secobarbitual equal to 100 mg/70 kg body weight. The amphetamine was fed 2–3 hr before the swimming tests, and the secobarbital 55 min in advance of the tests. Events included 100–200 yd swimming all styles against the clock. Fourteen of the fifteen subjects were significantly improved on amphetamine. Although the improvement was only 1.16% in swim time, it would take tremendous training in a trained athlete to expect such a performance gain. In the second test series, only the 100-yd events were improved while the secobarbital impaired all performances. In another series of tests using track runners, three ran 600-yd, three ran 1000-yd, and three ran 1-mi tests. Eight out of nine men improved on amphetamine. In another experiment, college weight throwers averaged 4.39% improvement on amphetamine. In the final test series 16 swimmers were challenged to earn a steak dinner by improving their last 3 competitive meets. Each swimmer swam 6 times, three with amphetamine and three with the placebo. Where the times for the 100- and 200-yd swims were combined, 11 of the 16 men improved on amphetamine.

In the latest study by G. M. Smith *et al.* (1963) 15 inexpert and 15 expert swimmers were compared as to the effects of amphetamine and secobarbital on performance. Each subject swam 24 times: 8 times after taking amphetamine, 8 times after taking secobarbital, and 8 times after taking a placebo. Amphetamine improved the performance of both groups of swimmers to a similar degree. The results of the experiment were very carefully examined statistically, demonstrating clearly that the variability in performance with the inexpert swimmers was 5 times greater than with the experts.

Karpovich (1959) gave 10–20 mg of amphetamine to subjects 30 min before running to exhaustion on the treadmill two successive times with 10 min rest between tests, and reported no beneficial effects. It is possible that this short interval between drug ingestion and the treadmill run did not permit maximum absorption of the drug.

Golding and Barnard (1963) used 15 mg of amphetamine administered 2–3 hr before an all-out treadmill run at 10 mph up an 8.5% grade. No significant performance improvements were noted, although the resting pulse rate and blood pressures were significantly higher. Eysenck and Easterbrook (1960) and Haldi and Wynn (1946) failed to detect any effect of amphetamine on performance. They used only a 5 mg dose with 12 inexpert swimmers. One should not expect much in the way of results from any ineffective therapeutic dose.

A. CAFFEINE

Caffeine, cola, and tea are classified as xanthines often containing theobromine and several other alkaloids of little practical interest.

The average cup of coffee contains about 150 mg caffeine. Although the caffeine of tea leaves exceeds that of the coffee bean, much more dilution is usually noted in a cup of tea. A cola drink may contain as much as 55 mg caffeine and some theobromine.

The appeal of these beverages lies primarily in their central stimulating effect eulogized in the literature since the discovery of coffee (850 AD) by the Arabian goat herder, who, according to legend, noted his goats frisking around after a meal of coffee beans. The ready availability of coffee and the habituation of Navy men to the coffee pot in open messes has recently been a matter of concern (Paul, 1963). Men surveyed drank from 2 to 25 cups of coffee per day and reported with headaches, cardiac arrhythmias, and distressing digestive symptoms.

German citizens, deprived of coffee for long periods, found caution necessary when it later became available, confirming the tolerance build-up with habitual use. Caffeine is useful in coronary patients because it increases diuresis and promotes coronary vasodilation. Some subjects have a more severe reaction to caffeine doses at low concentrations than they experience with the amphetamine compound.

Cola seems to stimulate the individual in a different manner with respect to the central nervous system when compared with Cardiazol, caffeine, or amphetamine, e.g., without the side effects occasionally noted with caffeine but this mechanism is not understood.

The action of caffeine on muscle metabolism was first noted by Hartree and Hill (1924) who demonstrated that caffeine produces a sustained spontaneous liberation of heat from the muscles, persisting even after the muscle becomes inexcitable. This suggests that caffeine acts on the skeletal muscles chemically. Larger than normal amounts of lactic acid appear from muscles exposed to caffeine and muscle metabolism (O_2 consumption) is elevated.

There is a marked influx and efflux of calcium ions in the muscles in the presence of caffeine (Bianchi, 1961; Feinstein, 1963).

B. Nikethamide (Coramine)

Nikethamide (Coramine) is a derivative of nicotinic acid with a moderate CNS stimulating effect. It is primarily used as a respiratory stimulant and was once thought to be of value as a heart stimulant. It produces inconsistent blood pressure responses. It is occasionally used as a respiratory stimulant in cases of extreme obesity and treatment of pellagra (Dulfano and Segal, 1963).

C. Cardiazol (Metrazol)

Cardiazol (Metrazol) pentylenetetrazol experiments to date by Graf (1950) and Ganslen *et al.* (1964) discount Cardiazol as a worthwhile cardiovascular stimulant in exercise. Slight increases in oxygen intake and systolic blood pressure with caffeine-Cardiazol mixtures were demonstrated with no increase in working capacity. See Fig. 3. Cardiazol has little popularity therapeutically except in the diagnosis of latent epilepsy. Cardiazol is very useful in reversing the depressant effects of an overdose of barbiturates.

D. Cocaine

Cocaine is obtained from the leaves of the erythroxylon cocoa tree found in Peru, Bolivia, and Java. The cocoa leaves have been chewed by Indian natives for centuries to allay fatigue and stimulate the CNS.

Cocaine stimulates the CNS from above downward, producing excitement, garrulousness, and extreme restlessness. Increased muscular performance of

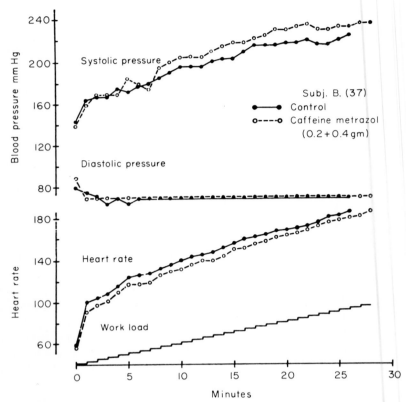

Fig. 3. Effects of caffeine-Metrazol on cardiovascular response to gradually increased energy expenditure.

natives under the influence of cocaine is attributed to the absence of fatigue sensations.

The addiction to cocaine has so powerful a hold on an animal that a monkey fitted with an indwelling catheter will, after a few injections, press the injection button in excess of 6000 times to get another shot.

Physiologically, cocaine first stimulates and then depresses the CNS. In small doses it may slow the heart, but larger doses step up the heart rate. The toxic action of the drug on the heart muscle is thought to be a cause of cardiac failure. Cocaine (a) elevates body temperature by its direct effect on the skeletal muscle; (b) induces vasoconstriction, which reduces blood flow to the skin's surface; and (c) disturbs the heat control center. Cocaine exaggerates the action of epinephrine and norepinephrine. Severe toxic reactions may appear with doses as little as 20 mg.

E. Sulfa Drugs

Sulfanilimide inhibits the action of carbon anhydrase at rest and during exercise in concentrations as low as 10^{-5}–10^{-9} M. Thus there is direct interference with the mechanism involved in the release of carbon dioxide in the lungs.

F. Alcohol

Alcohol has been used since the dawn of history, and the Arabs are supposed to have introduced the art of distillation into Europe in the Middle Ages.

Alcohol is often thought of as a stimulant, when in reality it is a powerful anesthetic and depressant in large doses. Moderate amounts of alcohol stimulate respiration, slow the electroencephalogram, and impair muscular performance. The blood pressure, pulse rate, and cardiac output may not be significantly altered, but the subject feels warm because of pronounced peripheral vasodilation. Asmussen and Bøje (1948) were unable to demonstrate performance improvements on the bicycle ergometer with 25–75 gm of pure alcohol given 30–45 min before bicycle ergometer rides. In the same test series, caffeine seemed to produce some benefit. The ingestion of alcohol causes a rise in both blood and urine lactate due to oxidative disturbances, but the carbohydrate content of alcohol cannot be utilized effectively for strenuous work. Despite the 7 cal of energy per gram of alcohol, body heat adjustments under the influence of alcohol are poor and there is marked depression of the heat control centers in the brain. The use of alcohol in a cold environment for work improvement is contraindicated, although its therapeutic value, in small amounts, should not be underestimated.

G. Ultraviolet

Lehmann and Szakall (1932), Ronge (1948), and Allen and Cureton (1954) have reported improvements in fitness with exposure to artificial ultraviolet light. Ronge's definitive work in this area is of special interest.

In studies of Swedish school children, the amount of work of a submaximal nature the children could perform, assessed in terms of cardiovascular stress, was found to improve significantly when the children were regularly exposed to artificial light. Fluctuation in blood calcium, vitamin D, and conversion of organic phosphate were considered as the principal causal factors influencing these improvements. Phosphate compounds and balanced calcium levels play a vital role in muscle and nerve energetics. The vitamin D mobilization and its effect on energy production can be dramatically demonstrated by ingesting rachitic dogs with concentrated vitamin D and observing the remarkable recovery of the animals. Muscle energy liberation depends upon adequate calcium and phosphorus levels mobilized in the presence of vitamin D. Vitamin D alone may be effective in the absence of ultraviolet light exposure.

H. GELATIN

Gelatin as a potent source of energy was unduly advertised in the late 1930's. Remarkable influences of this protein on the muscle tissue were part of the advertising campaign.

Karpovich and Pestrecov (1941), using jail inmates, concluded that the improvements of subjects on gelatin with farina as a placebo were attributable to training.

Gelatin contains a number of amino acids, most prominent of which is glycine (25.5%), plus alanine, phenylalanine, tyrosine, methiamine, and fractional amounts of serine and cystine. In nutritional studies of rats, gelatin proved to be an inadequate amino acid source and had to be supplemented with cystine, isoleucine, choline, and tryptophan for minimal health.

Early studies with gelatin (Karpovich and Pestrecov, 1941) were misleading, and critical examination of these investigations reveals the lack of controls in the design of the experiments. No one denies the necessity for glycine or other essential amino acids in the diet, but to extrapolate and attribute improved performance to these substances alone is not justifiable.

I. VITAMINS AS DRUGS

Vitamins exert their action when present in very minute amounts. This implies that they are very potent substances. A daily intake of one gram of vitamin B_{12} is sufficient to reverse severe cases of pernicious anemia.

Under normal circumstances the danger of toxic reactions to high vitamin intakes is low and with the exception of parenteral injections of thiamin, deaths have not been attributed to excess vitamin intake.

Prolonged ingestion of excessive amounts of vitamins A and D are capable of potentiating serious bone and liver disturbances. The toxicity of panthothenic acid, riboflavin, p-aminobenzoic acid, or ascorbic acid has never been determined. In scurvy, 1000 mg of ascorbic acid can be assimilated daily without harm.

A great deal of interest in ascorbic acid levels of the body has been centered on its presence in the adrenal cortex where it may play a vital role in the enzyme systems related to hormone production in this gland. Elsewhere in the body the coenzyme function of ascorbic acid has always been of significance in the health of the capillaries. Many clinical studies have demonstrated a need for increased vitamin C intake in the treatment of colds, tuberculosis, rheumatic fever, and pregnancy.

The excessive intake of vitamins is not justified. Studies of performance improvement as a consequence of increased vitamin intake, alone, are very difficult to control.

J. Oxygen and Oxygen Toxicity

Asmussen and Nielsen (1958) demonstrated that by increasing the partial pressure of oxygen to an athlete on a bicycle ergometer it would substantially increase his oxygen intake. However, the blood is normally 97% saturated with oxygen at sea level. The inability to maintain maximum saturation of the blood with oxygen in exercise is a circulatory rather than a simple respiratory phenomenon. At altitude, the athlete with maximum circulatory efficiency and maximal efficiency as a running machine is best able to survive. Efficiency may be independent of age, as Balke (1960) has demonstrated.

The tremendous popularity of SCUBA diving and the development of hyperbaric chambers for surgery and the treatment of certain respiratory ailments has called attention to the toxic effects of oxygen under pressure. Lambertsen (1964, 1968) and Roth (1963) have reviewed this problem in detail.

Men exposed to above normal atmospheric pressure of 100% O_2 or at partial pressure of O_2 equivalent to 2 atm of pressure, develop central nervous system disturbances and convulsions. The onset of the convulsions may be very rapid with little forewarning. The dynamics of this situation are not fully understood, but two suggestions have been offered: (a) the PO_2 in the red cells is so tightly bound that reduction in hemoglobin is not sufficient to release base to transport CO_2 which, therefore, accumulates in the brain and a true acidosis condition results; (b) Zirkel et al. (1965) have recently demonstrated the clinical features of oxygen toxicity in the central nervous system. Sports divers must be extremely wary of long exposure to hyperbaric oxygen mixtures which may result in drowning as a consequence of seizure of unknown cause with zero warning time. Sports divers, returned promptly to the surface and normal atmosphere pressure, respond quickly without apparent ill effects.

VIII. Drug Tolerance and Toxicity

It is of vital importance to recognize that pharmacological substances can be stored in fat, tissue proteins, and the liver. So significant is this storage that a single dose of Suramin, an effective treatment for trypanosomiasis, confers protection for 3 months or more.

The mobilization of the body's reserves, or their exploitation, is always accomplished at some cost to the individual. Even the almost reciprocal action of the parasympathetic and sympathetic nervous system in the presence of an environmental stress *involves sacrifice of efficiency for expediency*. Thus, overfatigue, excessive demands for output efficiency, disturbed rest, emotional tension, or nutritional deficiencies help to popularize pharmacological dependence (habituation) to the borderline of addiction in weak willed individuals.

The recent deaths of three prominent public figures were traced directly to the free mixing of barbiturates, energy pills, and alcohol. Drug synergism haunts the shadow of every physician who chances to simultaneously treat a patient with two different drugs. Drug toxicity may only reflect enzyme disturbance, but many enzymes at the neuromuscle junction and in the brain are essential to life. *No drug is free of toxic effects*. However, some effects are trivial in nature compared to the benefits derived from their use. Extension of a drug's effect may trigger serious problems. Vasodilation may be desirable, but excessive vasodilation may trigger syncope, blood dyscrasias, or drug allergies.

The central excitatory effects of the antifatigue drugs, psychic energizers, is largely, if not entirely, due to the release of norepinephrine in the brain potentiating excitatory effects elsewhere in the body. According to Eddy *et al.* (1965) and Seevers (1966) more than $9\frac{1}{2}$ billion amphetamine tablets are manufactured in the U.S. each year, of which number only 50% are sold through legitimate drug channels. At the recent First National Institute on Amphetamine Abuse, it was reported that some addicts could consume as much as 1700 mg of amphetamine daily. A normal therapeutic dose seldom exceeds 15 mg.

In work experiments the psychic energizers make the subject oblivious to fatigue symptoms and impending disaster. This pharmacological approach bypasses the individual's "will" at the possible expense of physiological disaster.

IX. Legislative Controls

The thought of routine saliva, blood, and urine analysis to detect the presence of stimulants in athletic competition is, in itself, repugnant to all sportsmen. The technical difficulties involved in such postcompetitive analysis are enormous, but not impossible.

From a biological viewpoint, the effects of sympathomimetic drugs (energizers) are mediated through the nervous system. The chemical by-products of this stimulation are *natural constituents of the body*. It can be demonstrated that identical levels of noradrenaline or adrenocortitropic hormones can be reached by hard muscular exercise or excitement which can be achieved by intravenous or muscular infusion of the neurohumoral agent. The work of Vendsalu (1960) emphasizes how rapidly these substances disappear from the blood stream. The state of reactivity of the individual, his blood pressure, and/or pulse in work may be significant in determining urine accumulation of hormones and correlate little, or not at all, with the amount of a given substance ingested or injected. Thus, the psychological as well as physiological state of the individual influencing the level of vital neurohumoral transmitters, would tend to nullify most scientific attempts at biochemically policing athletic competition.

X. Sportsmanship

Sportsmanship is a code of conduct evolved by gentlemen which is evidenced when a man engaged in competition *can take an unfair advantage of his opponent, but does not take advantage.*

The use of drugs to improve performance is a violation of this code. When the athlete steps on the athletic field, he faces an encounter with himself; he *encounters* his opponent and the skill to be mastered. This is his moment of truth. Athletics, along with the arts, constitute the ultimate form of human expression. The real satisfaction in athletics is in overcoming and surviving all of the demoralizing situations with which one must contend, often in the absence of biological perfection.

The evil in drugs lies not in their existence, but in the willingness of men trained in the highest ideals of a profession, i.e., coaches and team physicians, to prostitute their ideals to the transitory satisfaction of winning a contest.

There often exists a very thin line of demarcation between doping and the therapeutic use of drugs in sports training rooms. Only knowledgeable team physicians should have access to pharmacological stores.

XI. Conclusion

Fatigue is the expected consequence of sports competition. Fatigue is a part of the body's built-in biological warning system. Drugs make men ignore danger signs which are a threat to man's physiological and psychological reserves. Bartley and Chute (1947), Bartley (1965), and Ganslen (1958) have discussed these phenomena in detail.

The team physician who enters the training room with stimulating drugs in his medical kit exposes himself to temptation and censure. The star athlete may feel tired. The injection of novacaine in the presence of serious trauma violates the principles of good medicine, but in the case of a minor strain constitutes therapy.

Can we censure the coach who permits his athletes to drink strong coffee and tea when we know that caffeine has potential for performance enhancement? Does the administration of a tranquilizer drug, to relieve pregame tension, constitute the same violation of medical and sports ethics that exists with the use of psychic energizing substances to produce alertness? Should a team physician administer barbiturates to promote sleep the night before competition? Will the use of 100% O_2 between competitions in Mexico City adhere to the principles of good sportsmanship?

The fact remains, despite damning criticism of the use of drugs, that drugs can improve strength and circulation; they can allay fatigue and enhance certain types of athletic performance.

XII. Epilogue

We do not know of a pharmaceutic substance which will improve the athlete's biological reserves for competition more than adequate nutrition and sleep and hard physical training.

REFERENCES

Agersborg, H. P. K., and Shaw, D. L. (1962). *J. Sports Med.* **2**, 217.
Allen, R. M., and Cureton, T. K. (1945). *Arch. Phys. Med.* **26**, 641.
Alles, G. A., and Feigen, G. A. (1942). *Am. J. Physiol.* **136**, 392.
Asmussen, E., and Bøje, O. (1948). *Acta Physiol. Scand.* **15**, 109.
Asmussen, E., and Nielsen, M. (1958). *Acta Physiol. Scand.* **43**, 365.
Balke, B. (1960). *In* "Science and Medicine of Exercise and Sports" (W. R. Johnson, ed.), p. 343. Harper, New York.
Bartley, S. H. (1964). *J. Sports Med.* **4**, 153.
Bartley, S. H. (1965). "Fatigue (Mechanism and Management)." Thomas, Springfield, Illinois.
Bartley, S. H., and Chute, E. (1947). "Fatigue and Impairment in Man." McGraw-Hill, New York.
Bianchi, C. P. (1961). *J. Gen. Physiol* **44**, 845.
Bøje, O. (1939). *Saertryk Nord.* **2**, 24.
Campos, F. A. de M., Cannon, W. B., Lundin, H., and Walker, T. T. (1928). *Am. J. Physiol.* **87**, 680.
Charlier, R. (1961). "Coronary Vagodilators." Pergamon Press, Oxford.
Cochran, W. G., Smith, G. M., and Beecher, H. K. (1961). *J. Am. Med. Assoc.* **177**, 347.
Cureton, T. K., and Pohndorf, R. H. (1955). *Res. Quart.* **26**, 391.
Cuthbertson, D. P., and Knox, J. A. C. (1947). *J. Physiol. (London)* **106**, 42.
Dejours, P. (1964). *In* "Handbook of Physiology" (Am. Physiol. Soc., J. Field, ed.). Sect. 3, Vol. I, pp. 631–648. Williams & Wilkins, Baltimore, Maryland.
Dill, D. B., Edwards, H. T., and Talbott, J. H. (1930). *J. Physiol. (London)* **69**, 61.
Dulfano, M. J., and Segal, M. S. (1963). *J. Am. Med. Assoc.* **185**, 69.
Eddy, N. B., Nalbach, H., Isbell, H., and Seevers, M. H. (1965). *Bull. World Health Organ.* **32**, 721.

Elmadjian, F. (1961). *In* "Performance Capacity" (H. Spector, J. Brozek, and M. S. Peterson, eds.), pp. 22–50. Natl. Acad. Sci., Washington, D.C.

Eysenck, H. J., and Easterbrook, J. A. (1960). *J. Mental Sci.* **106**, 831.

Feinstein, M. B. (1963). *J. Gen. Physiol.* **47**, 151.

Foltz, E. E., Ivy, A. C., and Barborka, C. J. (1942). *Am. J. Physiol.* **136**, 79.

Foltz, E. E., Ivy, A. C., and Barborka, C. J. (1943). *J. Lab. Clin. Med.* **28**, 603.

Ganslen, R. V. (1958). *Arkansas Alumnus* **12**, 2.

Ganslen, R. V., Balke, B., Nagle, F. J., and Phillips, E. E. (1964). *Aerospace Med.* **35**, 630.

Golding, L. A., and Barnard, J. R. (1963). *J. Sports Med.* **3**, 221.

Goodman, L. S., and Gilman, A. (1965). "The Pharmacological Basis of Therapeutics." Macmillan, New York.

Graf, O. (1950). *In* "German Aviation Medicine," Vol. II, Chap. XI. U.S. Dept. of Air Force, Washington, D.C.

Grob, D. (1961). *Ann. Rev. Pharmacol.* **1**, 239.

Haldi, J., and Wynn, W. (1946). *Res. Quart.* **17**, 96.

Hartree, W., and Hill, A. V. (1924). *J. Physiol. (London)* **58**, 441.

Hauty, G. T., Payne, R. B., and Bauer, R. O. (1957). *J. Pharmacol. Exptl. Therap.* **119**, 385.

Huxley, A. (1957). *Ann. N.Y. Acad. Sci.* **67**, 673.

Juvrup, A., and Muido, L. (1946). *Acta Physiol. Scand.* **11**, 60.

Karpovich, P. V. (1959). *J. Am. Med. Assoc.* **170**, 558.

Karpovich, P. V. (1965). "Physiology of Muscular Activity." Saunders, Philadelphia, Pennsylvania.

Karpovich, P. V., and Pestrecov, K. (1941). *Am. J. Physiol.* **134**, 300.

Knoefel, P. K. (1943). *Federation Proc.* **2**, 83.

La Cava, G. (1961). *J. Sports Med.* **1**, 49.

Lambertsen, C. J. (1964). *In* "Handbook of Physiology" (Am. Physiol. Soc., J. Field, ed.), Sect. 3, Vol. I, pp. 545–555. Williams & Wilkins, Baltimore, Maryland.

Lambertsen, C. J. (1968). *Ann. Rev. Pharmacol.* (in press).

Lehmann, G., and Szakall, A. (1932). *Arbeitsphysiol.* **5**, 278.

Lehmann, G., Straub, H., and Szakall, A. (1939). *Arbeitsphysiol.* **10**, 690.

McKenzie, R. E., and Elliott, L. L. (1965). *Aerospace Med.* **36**, 774.

Mommerts, W. F. H. M. (1961). *Ann. Rev. Physiol.* **23**, 529.

Parin, V. V., Vasilyev. P. V., and Belay, V. Ye. (1964). *NASA, Tech. Transl.* **F277**.

Paul, O. (1963). *Circulation* **28**, 20.

Porritt, A. (1965). *J. Sports Med.* **5**, 166.

Prokop, L. (1965). *J. Sports Med.* **5**, 88.

Rivers. W. H. R., and Webber, H. N. (1907). *J. Physiol. (London)* **37**, 33.

Ronge, H. E. (1948). *Acta Physiol. Scand.* **15**, Suppl. 49, p. 145.

Roth, E. M. (1963). *NASA, Tech. Note* **TN D-2008**.

Roughton, F. J. W., Dill, D. B., Darling, R. C., Graybiel, A., Knehr, C., and Talbott, J. H. (1941). *Am. J. Physiol.* **135**, 77.

Seashore, R. H., and Ivy, A. C. (1953). *Psycho. Monographs* **67**, No. 15, 1.

Seevers, M. H. (1966), *Proc. 1st Natl. Inst. Amphetamine Abuse, Grafton, Illinois, 1966* (sponsored by Southern Illinois University, Grafton, Illinois) not published.

Smith, C. K. (1963). *Ann. Rev. Pharmacol.* **3**, 223.

Smith, G. M., and Beecher, H. K. (1959). *J. Am. Med. Assoc.* **170**, 542.

Smith, G. M., and Beecher, H. K. (1960). *J. Am. Med. Assoc.* **172**, 1502.

Smith, G. M., Weitzner, M., and Beecher, G. F. (1963). *J. Pharmacol. Exptl. Therap.* **139**, 119.

Somerville, W. (1946). *Can. Med. Assoc. J.* **55**, 470.
Vendsalu, A. (1960). *Acta Physiol. Scand.* **49**, Suppl. 173, p. 75.
Weiss, B., and Laties, V. G. (1962). *Pharmacol. Rev.* **14**, 1.
Zirkel, L. G., Mengel, C. E., Horton, D. D., and Duffy, E. J. (1965). *Aerospace Med.* **36**, 1030.

8

LONGEVITY, GENERAL HEALTH, and EXERCISE

James S. Skinner

I. Introduction

There have been many statements in the scientific literature, popular press, and in the classroom concerning the relationship between exercise and health. Unfortunately, many of these have been unqualified statements based on uncontrolled observations and popular beliefs. Their proponents have attempted to draw many firm conclusions in a research area where few are as yet justified. Many persons believe that exercise is a panacea for innumerable ailments and problems. Their statements have confused the issues and have driven people to extreme positions on the relative merits of exercise for health.

It is the purpose of this chapter to review and outline important research findings, allowing the reader to decide for himself whether increased activity is of any value in each particular study.

II. Problems in Research on Exercise

Before reviewing the scientific literature, it is necessary to point out some of the many problems inherent in studying the effects of exercise on topics as complex as longevity and general health.

First of all, it is difficult, if not impossible, to isolate the exercise factor and its effects. An example of this is shown by the study of Kasanen *et al.* (1963), in which the mode of living of 100 subjects who had recently had a myocardial infarction was compared with that of 100 control patients of the same age. Although the infarction patients were less active, they also consumed more fat, had a higher serum cholesterol, smoked more, took more analgesics and soporifics, were under more stress in their work, were psychologically more labile, and had a greater family history of cardiovascular disease. With this number of differences, it becomes difficult indeed to dissect out whether activity was a major factor in the etiology of coronary disease. The important thing to remember is that one would have to prove that the two groups were alike in all other significant respects to support the probability that exercise contributed significantly to their difference in coronary disease rates.

Many studies which have claimed differences due to one factor or another are retrospective, i.e., they measure characteristics and relate them to a past episode. The investigators assume that the environment has not changed from the time of the event or that the individual was not changed by the event. A major obstacle in these studies is determining whether the differences found are "merely coincidental, the cause of, or the result of" the process being studied (Bronte-Stewart and Krut, 1962). A correlation between two variables does not necessarily mean that a "cause and effect" relationship is present.

Transfer of workers from one occupation to another has been a problem in studies which classify people according to the amount of activity involved in their present or last occupation. Due to changes in health, a man doing strenuous work for 40 years may elect or be advised to take a less active job. If he has a clinical episode in the next few years, he may be classified with other sedentary workers and this fact used as evidence that sedentary living is associated with a greater incidence of that particular health problem.

One of the biggest problems in studies comparing active and inactive groups is personal selection. People may select or tend to belong to an occupational group as a result of underlying socioeconomic, physical, or psychological reasons which, though not apparent, may also influence or reflect their health or longevity. Bassett (1962) found a significant difference in the amount of deliberate activity engaged in by healthy medical students with and without a family history of heart disease, i.e., those with a positive history had a decreased tendency to exercise. This may represent a behavior pattern acquired at home and may account for their higher lipid values and greater relative weight. However, one might speculate that the coronary prone individual is under continual pressure from within to succeed (Friedman and Rosenman, 1959) and is, therefore, faced with the choice of leaving his work (usually sedentary) to exercise or of continuing to work toward his goals.

Athletes are a poor group to compare with the general public as they may be different for many reasons. People seldom continue with active sports until "old age" and those few who do become an even more select group.

The range and amount of energy expenditure among most occupations is so small that it is difficult to obtain adequate numbers of very active men to be compared with the large group of sedentary men found in the United States today. These few, whose occupation involves strenuous labor, are usually poorly educated and from the lower socioeconomic strata of the population. Therefore, there may be differences in racial, ethnic, and dietary backgrounds which make the control necessary for meaningful comparisons even more difficult.

Information on the physical activity of occupational groups being compared has not been well documented. Investigators have classified men as active or sedentary or engaged in heavy, moderate, or light activity based on subjective evaluations of the present or last occupation. They have presumed that one group was more active without measuring whether this was so. This has been done in spite of the fact that many occupations do not require caloric expenditures over two to three times the resting metabolic rate. Likewise, these investigators have not measured nonvocational, leisure activities, assuming that this was negligible or constant for both groups. Although the measurement of energy expenditure may be inconvenient for both subject and investigator, too subjective, inexact, and may require a good deal of time, effort, and resources for validation, it is still necessary for a definitive study.

One problem in the interpretation of results in some studies has been the secondary changes that may occur when physical activity is increased. Some men become more "health conscious" when they begin to exercise and may change their diet, lose weight, stop smoking, etc. While this does not detract from the possible benefits of an exercise program, it may change certain factors of risk to general health or longevity and makes interpretation more difficult.

In view of the numerous problems just outlined, the reader may question the need for a review of studies which have related exercise, as a single factor, to the etiology or sequelae of complex health problems. However, if a thread of consistency can be found in the results of many investigations using different approaches, then insight may be gained.

III. General Health Related to Chronic Diseases

A. CARDIOVASCULAR DISEASES

Much has been written on the causes and associated phenomena of cardiovascular disease; it is generally accepted that multiple risk factors are involved. Comprehensive reviews of studies relating physical activity to cardiovascular health have been made by Fox and Skinner (1964), Montoye (1962), and Holloszy (1963). This review summarizes only the more important results and their implications.

1. Coronary Heart Disease (CHD)

Morris and his associates (1953) found that the incidence of CHD was less in conductors than in drivers of the London Transport Company. On the other hand, the incidence of angina pectoris was greater in the conductors. They presumed, but did not establish, that the conductors were more active because they walked up and down the stairs of the double-decker buses during their occupational hours. The same results were found among postal workers (Morris et al., 1953), i.e., the presumably more active postmen had a lower incidence of CHD and a higher incidence of angina.

Realizing that constitutional factors could have affected these differences, Morris and his coworkers (1956) studied characteristics of the transport employees. Drivers were found to be taller and heavier than conductors when they were initially employed; a difference in waist girth remained after a correction was made for differences in height. It was also discovered that those conductors who later became drivers had larger waists than conductors who remained conductors. The association between overweight and CHD and the personal selection factor which may have affected the occupational choice of these men raises doubts about the total value of the original study.

Zukel et al. (1959) found that farmers, who were presumably more active, had less CHD over a 1-year period than other men in North Dakota. On the other hand, they also had a higher rate of angina. When the data on "hours of heavy physical activity at usual occupation" were examined more closely (Fox and Skinner, 1964), the highest CHD incidence appeared in persons who performed no heavy work.

Brunner and Manelis (1960) studied the 10-year CHD incidence and mortality rates of workers living in 58 collective settlements in Israel. Although the groups were not age-matched, the incidence rates were markedly lower in the nonsedentary workers. Most environmental conditions were similar but although all workers ate from the same table it is possible that the more active workers ate varying quantities of the same foods and in reality had a different dietary intake. It would be of interest to know how homogeneous the groups were since marked differences in CHD and its risk factors were found among recent and early Yemenite, Iraqi, and European immigrants to Israel (Toor et al., 1960).

Kahn (1963) studied postal workers who remained clerks or carriers for five years or more. Among workers with service of 20 years or more in one category, clerks were found to have a higher mortality from CHD; this difference was greater when compensation was made for those carriers who switched to other categories. There was a suggestion that recent activity was more important than that done 5, 10, or 15 years previously.

In a study of civil service employees, Chapman et al. (1957) found no significant differences in actual and expected rates for CHD among active and sedentary workers. Re-examination in 1962–1963 revealed the same conclusions (Fox and Skinner, 1964).

Data from a study by Stamler et al. (1960) suggest that slightly less CHD was found in utility corporation workers whose occupation generally involved more activity. However, no jobs could be classified as involving heavy labor and there were other factors (hypertension, diabetes, obesity, and angina) which obscured the differences.

Taylor et al. (1962) studied railroad workers and reported that switchmen and section men had lower death rates from all causes, particularly arteriosclerotic heart disease, compared with more sedentary clerks. However, more clerks lived in urban communities where, for some reason, death rates are generally higher. Further studies revealed that clerks were also fatter (Brožek et al., 1963) and smoked more cigarettes (Blackburn et al., 1965).

In 89 confirmed cases of CHD among 1062 men aged 60–69 years, Brown et al. (1957a) reported a consistent increase in the frequency of CHD among sedentary patients. These men were placed in different activity categories by their own evaluation, which may or may not have been valid. The authors admit that certain highly prone individuals may have been eliminated by CHD before the age of 60. Nevertheless, differences in CHD prevalence were inversely associated with the physical activity and not with the mental stress of the occupation.

McDonough et al. (1965) found a significant difference in CHD prevalence between white and Negro males in Georgia. Rates for high social class white males (HSC-WM) were significantly greater than for low social class white males (LSC-WM) and Negro males (NM), with no difference between LSC-WM and NM. Dietary fat intake, cigarette smoking, or emotional stress could not explain these differences. On the other hand, there appeared to be marked differences in occupational physical activity, which was inversely associated with CHD prevalence rates.

These findings were confirmed by Skinner et al. (1966), who studied the physical working capacity (PWC) and physical activity patterns of representative samples of healthy men from the original group. While there were no mean differences in the response of blood pressures and pulse rates to exercise or in PWC measured by a treadmill test, there were significant differences in the amount of occupational activity engaged in, as determined by an objective questionnaire. HSC-WM were significantly less active than either LSC-WM or NM; there was little difference between NM and LSC-WM. A partial explanation for this apparent discrepancy is that the different activity levels may have been insufficient to cause a training effect reflected by differences in PWC. This raises some questions about the usefulness of measuring PWC and equating it with levels of activity.

Questionnaires from 355 Harvard football players were studied by Pomeroy and White (1958). Of the 87 men who had died 25 to 50 years after leaving the university, 25 infarcts occurred among those who decreased their activity; there were none among 38 players who continued to exercise heavily. There were many problems in this retrospective study on a select group, e.g., the less active group gained more weight, had a greater family history of CHD, smoked more, and had more divorces.

While single case studies reveal nothing about CHD epidemiology, they may provide some insight. An autopsy was performed after embalmment on Clarence DeMar, a famous endurance runner who died with rectal cancer at the age of 70 years (Currens and White, 1961). It revealed no obstruction, with moderate coronary sclerosis and atherosclerosis of the aorta. While the lumen of his coronary arteries was larger than normal, the variation among normals is too great for any definite conclusions.

Two autopsy studies have been reported by Spain and Bradess (1957, 1960). In the first of these, data from CHD mortality rates over a 7-year period in Westchester County, New York, were examined. It appeared that more men in sedentary occupations died from CHD before the age of 55 years than did men in moderately active or strenuous work. In the second study, there was no difference in the degree of atherosclerosis between 100 men whose last occupation was classified as sedentary and 107 men who had active occupations. All these men had died suddenly and unexpectedly from accident, homicide, or suicide.

Pathologists from 206 hospitals collaborated on a study reported by Morris and Crawford (1958) in which each examined about 25 consecutive, unselected autopsies of men aged 45 to 70 years. Analysis revealed that the prevalence of large fibrous patches (among hypertensive cases only), small multiple scars, large healed infarcts, and coronary occlusions was inversely associated with the amount of activity involved in the last occupation; the degree of atherosclerosis was not significantly different.

Some information on exercise and CHD can also be found in studies on animals. Although these studies provide data not usually obtainable in humans, it is not always possible to extrapolate from the results.

Eckstein (1957) surgically constricted the circumflex coronary arteries in dogs and found that increased collateralization was proportional to the degree of constriction in dogs who served as controls; no increase was found with mild constriction. In the dogs trained for 6 to 8 weeks, there was even greater collateral vascularization at mild, moderate, and severe constriction.

Using a corrosion-cast technique, Tepperman and Pearlman (1961) studied the effects of exercise on the coronary arteries of rats. In four experiments, exercised rats had a significantly greater cast weight (i.e., supposedly greater vascularization) and in two experiments the ratio of coronary-cast weight to heart weight was significantly increased. In one experiment on guinea pigs, however, there was no increase in cardiac hypertrophy due to training.

Using the same technique, Stevenson et al. (1964) found that rats forced to exercise had an increase in apparent coronary tree size, provided the exercise was "not too severely or frequently done." While they admit that the size of the coronary cast does not necessarily correlate with blood flow in vivo, they conclude that moderate exercise with adequate rest may be more beneficial than heavy, frequent exercise.

In summary, there is an inference that an inverse association exists between the level of occupational activity and the incidence of CHD. Recent activity may be more important than that done many years before. On the other hand, angina pectoris is reportedly more prevalent among those men in active occupations; the significance of this finding is unclear at the present time.

Autopsy studies reveal evidence of fewer previous infarcts among persons whose last occupation involved more activity but no difference in the degree of atherosclerosis. While these two statements appear contradictory, there are studies suggesting that exercise can increase the collateral circulation and the size of the coronary arteries in experimental animals. This, in turn, may affect the incidence of infarction but not the degree of coronary involvement.

2. Hypertension

There have been no well-controlled studies on the effects of exercise on hypertension. Andersen and Elvik (1955) found lower resting blood pressures in young athletes compared with nonathletes. Miall and Oldham (1958) and Kapeller-She (1963) noted a lower incidence of hypertension in active groups. Several Finnish army recruits in a study by Frick et al. (1963) had lower pressures after training; this might have been due to decreased anxiety during the second testing period.

These brief findings were confirmed somewhat by the autopsy study of Morris and Crawford (1958), in which manifestations of hypertension were found less frequently and at later ages in more active persons. Morris (1960) also reported that fewer conductors had diastolic blood pressures over 105 mm Hg than did drivers in the same age range.

On the other hand, Brown et al. (1957b) found no evidence that blood pressure levels were related to physical or mental demands of employment in 1045 men in the seventh decade. Many criticisms of their earlier study (Brown et al., 1957a) are also applicable here (see Section III, A, 1).

In summary, there seems to be insufficient evidence that exercise is related to the incidence of hypertension or that training will reduce its severity. This is an area, however, which has not been adequately studied and these conclusions can only be tentative.

3. Occlusive Arterial Disease

Few adequate studies have been done to determine the effects of exercise and especially training on the natural history of occlusive arterial disease; clinical impressions form the bulk of available information. One measure of disease severity is the time or distance walked before claudication forces an individual to stop. This criterion is subjective and there is usually little control over differences in pain sensitivity or factors which influence blood flow to the limb, such as environmental temperature, speed of walking, quality and grade of the walking surface, time since the last cigarette, etc. Zsotér et al. (1964) found that the time and composition of the last meal affected peripheral blood flow. With postprandial lipemia which usually follows a fatty meal, they noted a decrease in limb blood flow and a reduced claudication time in patients with arterial disease.

It is difficult to accurately measure blood flow at rest and during exercise. Wide variation in the normal resting flow raises questions about its significance when recorded.

An example of the poor quality of information available is a case study reported by Ebel (1958). A patient developing claudication after walking five blocks was given vasodilator drugs and told to walk to the point of tolerance several times daily. After 4 years, both posterior tibial pulses returned and he could walk unlimited distances at a slower pace. It is not known whether any other influencing factors were also altered during this period.

For many years, the main exercise for patients were passive movements developed by Buerger (1924), who theorized that blood vessels alternately emptied and distended would eventually accept an increased function in the transport of blood. However, a study by Wisham et al. (1953) does not support this concept. They studied 10 normals and 19 patients to determine the acute effects of active and passive exercises on blood flow to the gastrocnemius. Passive postural movements caused no change while increases in flow did occur during and shortly after active exercise. The effect of exercise appeared to increase in relation to its intensity.

Foley (1957) found that 21 of 22 patients with gangrenous feet healed faster when put on a walking program. This was mainly a clinical impression that would be difficult to quantify objectively.

Herron (1964) exercised 15 healthy middle-aged men with a walking and running program and found no effect on recovery blood flow in the calf muscle following 15 min of resisted planter flexion with free and occluded circulation. Total peripheral resistance was also unaffected.

Based on clinical impressions, Schoop (1964) theorized that the speed of blood flow, not ischemia, leads to dilatation and an increase in collateral circulation and that exercise is the simplest, most effective method for augmenting the circulation. Unfortunately, he presented little data on this theory and its effect on arterial disease.

Schlüssel (1965) had his patients walk until claudication pain first developed and used two-thirds of that time as the training load. The subjects did this three times, 10 to 20 min daily. They were retested at regular intervals, at which time a new training load was set. He reported substantial improvement in the claudication pain time (CPT) of his patients.

Larsen and Lassen (1966) measured the maximal walking time (MWT) of subjects with intermittent claudication by walking them at 3 mph up an elevation which gave rise to a CPT of 2–3 min. Seven subjects were then given a pedometer and urged to walk daily to MWT, rest, and walk again. After 1 hr the distance walked was recorded. After 6 months the 7 experimental and 7 control subjects were retested. There was little change in maximal blood flow or in the delay period (time from end of the ischemic period to the beginning of the maximal blood flow) for either group. The exercised group had significant increases in MWT from 2.9 to 8.2 min and in CPT from 1.7 to 3.5 min; there was little change in the control subjects.

Data from a study by Skinner and Strandness (1967a) suggest that acute progressive vasodilatation occurs with repeated exercise of sufficient intensity. This repeated stimulus for increased blood flow also appeared to have a training effect, since the four subjects increased their MWT and two increased their CPT. To investigate the possible training effect, five patients with arteriosclerosis obliterans were evaluated over a 3- to 8-month period of supervised, individualized treadmill exercise (Skinner and Strandness, 1967b). As a result of this training regimen there were significant increases in MWT and CPT in all five men (increases ranged from 1.4 to greater than 15 times the initial MWT). In all subjects there was also a significant increase in the systolic blood pressure recorded at the ankle after exercise; this would tend to indicate a reduction in the amount of ischemia and a greater capacity of the collateral vessels. These data signify that there was a significant increase in collateral circulation at rest, during exercise, and/or after exercise, improving the blood supply to the obstructed leg.

Although progress in this area of investigation has been hindered by the lack of accurate techniques for measuring (a) blood flow at rest and during exercise, and (b) the extent of vascularization, it appears that physical training may be of value in the treatment of occlusive arterial disease.

B. Metabolic Disorders

1. *Lipid Metabolism*

Although some investigators have reported reductions in serum cholesterol with increased activity, the metabolic pathway by which exercise can directly affect serum cholesterol remains unclear. According to Gould and Cook (1958), cholesterol is not broken down to fragments that can be oxidized to carbon dioxide and cannot, therefore, be considered a direct source of energy. Observations on the fate of radioactive cholesterol (cholesterol-4-^{14}C) reveal that no ^{14}C is detected in respiratory CO_2 (Chaikoff *et al.*, 1952) and that 95% of the intravenous dose is recovered in the feces within 15 days (Siperstein and Chaikoff, 1955).

One reason for confusion is the misinterpretation of results from animal experimentation. Since man's metabolism of cholesterol differs from that found in chickens, mice, and rabbits, it is inappropriate to extrapolate from data obtained in exercise studies on these animals.

Inadequate control over factors which can affect cholesterol levels has yielded inconclusive results in many exercise studies. Although diet has a major effect on the serum cholesterol concentration in normal persons, in some studies showing a reduction in cholesterol with exercise there has been no control or inadequate measurement of dietary intake during the training period (Chailley-Bert *et al.*, 1955; Golding, 1961).

Weight loss, by itself, may be accompanied by a decrease in cholesterol (Walker *et al.*, 1953) and it has been shown that the cholesterol level tends to fluctuate with changes in body weight (Anderson *et al.*, 1957; Montoye *et al.*, 1959). Thus, the interpretation of studies reporting reductions in body weight and in serum cholesterol as a result of training (Golding, 1961; Rochelle, 1961) are open to question and provide no definitive answers to this complex problem.

The need for adequate control is emphasized by the following results. Two subjects in a study by Holloszy *et al.* (1964a), who lost weight during the first few months of training, had concomitant reductions in their serum cholesterol. However, when their weights stabilized, their serum cholesterol returned to the initial values and remained constant during the next few months of even more strenuous training.

In studies where diet and body weight were unaltered, there was no change in the cholesterol level with increased activity (Mann *et al.*, 1955; Taylor *et al.*, 1961; Holloszy *et al.*, 1964a). Thus, when other factors are controlled, it appears that exercise has no effect on serum cholesterol. There is little doubt that exercise may cause a caloric imbalance which, in turn, may temporarily affect the cholesterol level but this does not mean that there is a direct or lasting effect.

Results obtained with studies on exercise and serum triglycerides (TG) are more consistent. Unlike cholesterol, there is a pathway by which exercise can affect this lipid fraction, i.e., the TG molecule can be broken down into glycerol and fatty acids, both of which can be metabolized for energy.

It appears well documented that exercise can inhibit the marked rise in TG normally seen after a fatty meal (Cohen and Goldberg, 1960; Nikkilä and Konttinen, 1963; Cantone, 1964). The fasting TG level has also been reduced for at least 44 hr after running 3 mi (Holloszy et al., 1964a). Prolonged, heavy exercise (competitive cross-country skiing for 8 to 9 hr) caused a significant, acute decrease in the serum TG (Carlson and Mossfeldt, 1964). No change was observed in the serum cholesterol.

Only the acute effect of exercise on TG has been substantiated. It is not known whether active people maintain lower TG levels than inactive people but there is a suggestion in the data of Holloszy et al. (1964a) that this is the case.

Changes in body weight can also affect the TG level. Albrink et al. (1962) and Albrink and Meigs (1965) have suggested that weight gain rather than obesity per se is associated with elevated TG.

In summary, it has been shown that weight gain can increase both the TG and cholesterol concentration and that weight loss can reduce the serum cholesterol. When diet and body weight are not altered, these lipids also tend to remain constant. Thus, if weight can be stabilized over a period of years through increased activity, this then might have a beneficial effect on lipid concentrations. This is especially important in our affluent society where the number of overweight persons is steadily increasing.

2. Diabetes Mellitus

Exercise was a main form of therapy for diabetes mellitus before insulin was discovered (Allen, 1915; Bürger, 1920) but since that time it has played a minor role. Although treatment of diabetes may include proper regulation of diet, drugs, and exercise (Joslin et al., 1959), only the first two are usually stressed by physicians. This may be partially due to the lack of knowledge about the acute and chronic effects of exercise on glucose metabolism and to the abundance of research on the nutritional and pharmacological aspects. However, a review of the evidence that increased activity may serve a useful role in the management of diabetes is warranted.

Knowles (1960) has shown that during periods of increased activity, a diabetic patient may decrease his insulin requirement. Conversely, it is known clinically that when he becomes less active he should increase his insulin dosage (Joslin et al., 1959). A change in insulin requirement, however, does not necessarily denote a change in the severity of diabetes but may only reflect a temporary alteration in metabolism.

Devlin (1963) found a significant decrease in plasma insulinlike activity (ILA) after exercise in 18 healthy volunteers. After a brief training period, there was a small decrease in ILA after exercise and no difference in the resting ILA. He theorized that some alteration of muscle metabolism occurred decreasing insulin requirement or that the postexercise blood glucose level was not as low after training.

A more controlled study by Sanders *et al.* (1964) on 4 nondiabetic and 2 juvenile diabetic subjects revealed evidence of increased glucose utilization during exercise. In normals, exercise reduced the arterial plasma glucose; glucose extraction decreased in the splanchnic bed and nonexercising muscles but increased in the exercising muscles. Glucose assimilation by the exercising muscles was increased in the diabetic subject. Regional glucose extraction was maximal immediately after exercise in both groups and was not contingent upon acute increases in the total amount of extrapancreatic insulin.

Larsson *et al.* (1962) noted a lower physical working capacity (PWC) in diabetic adolescent girls compared with normal girls of the same age. They also found a regular decrease in blood sugar of the diabetic girls during work; this effect was especially conspicuous in those girls with a high blood sugar level. After training, PWC increased in most subjects but there was no increase in the insulin requirement in spite of a 50% increase in caloric consumption.

Decreased PWC in diabetic girls was confirmed by Sterky (1963) and in diabetic boys by Larsson *et al.* (1964). In the former study, this reduction did not seem to be directly connected with the diabetic state but may have been the result of inadequate training since these diabetic girls were less active than normal girls. Conflicting results on diabetic girls and boys were reported by Elo *et al.* (1965), who also noted that duration of disease and insulin requirement had a low correlation with PWC.

There is evidence that weight control is an important factor in diabetes management, e.g., diabetes occurs more frequently in obese subjects and weight loss to normal levels may be followed by at least a temporary remission of overt diabetes (Smith and Levine, 1964). Yalow *et al.* (1965) state that "obesity can provide an additional stress in those who carry an inherited tendency to diabetes but does not in itself necessarily constitute a prediabetic state." It is possible, therefore, that exercise may have a beneficial effect on diabetes by helping to reduce or maintain body weight.

Albrink and Meigs (1965) summarize their earlier investigations by stating that (a) higher triglycerides (TG) were observed in men with a positive family history for diabetes, and (b) there is a low but significant relationship between fasting blood sugar and TG concentrations. In view of the effect of exercise on the serum TG (Section III, B, 1), this may represent another indirect means by which increased activity may affect the natural history of diabetes.

These studies suggest that exercise is a useful adjunct to other forms of diabetes management. Unfortunately, most have focused on only one segment of the diabetic population, those taking insulin. This reviewer has found no research on the effects of exercise on the larger number of adult-onset diabetics who are able to control their diabetes by oral hypoglycemic drugs and/or proper diet. Much more information is needed on the acute and long-term effects of regular exercise and training on the course and severity of the entire spectrum of diabetes mellitus. Again, many factors must be controlled before definitive information on exercise can be brought to the attention of the physician and his diabetic patient.

C. RESPIRATORY DISEASES

1. Asthma

Research in this area has been limited to studies on children. It was initially concerned with proper breathing exercises to strengthen respiratory muscles, to provide better ventilation, and to create more efficient breathing patterns.

Scherr and Frankel (1958) found that the frequency and severity of asthmatic attacks decreased after a program of respiratory exercises, gymnastics, and combative sports. A 30% decrease in attacks and drug therapy was noted by McElhenny and Peterson (1963) after 4 months of exercise. They also noted a significant increase in vital capacity (VC). These findings were confirmed in a later study of 8 months' duration (Peterson and McElhenny, 1965).

Itkin (1964) reported that 3 months of conditioning and athletics increased PWC and the ability to perform exercise. However, there was no significant change in bronchial obstruction as measured by the forced expiratory volume at one second (FEV_1) or in the amount of medication required.

Millman *et al.* (1965) studied the effects of a 4-month conditioning program. Maximal breathing capacity increased 55–89% but there was no difference in FEV_1 and a slight increase in VC. As a result of training, the children showed an improved cardiorespiratory adjustment to, and recovery from, a standard exercise test.

Some of the changes reported in these studies were probably psychological and reflected changes in attitude toward asthma by both the children and their parents. While this does not detract from the positive effects of exercise, it does not necessarily mean that the underlying disease is affected.

2. Emphysema

With the exception of a monograph by Haas and Luczak (1963), showing reduced oxygen consumption in emphysematous patients given proper breathing exercises, this reviewer has found only one article on training and emphysema. Pierce *et al.* (1964) found that a relatively modest amount of daily exercise resulted in decreased heart rates, respiratory rates, minute ventilation, oxygen consumption, and carbon dioxide production for any given level of exercise. There was an increase in the amount of exercise the patients could tolerate but no change in their pulmonary function tests.

It appears from this small amount of data that training may not alter the underlying pathology of asthma or emphysema but may affect the subject's ability to adapt to these diseases within the limits of his capacity.

3. Other Aspects of Heatlh

It has been suggested that the overabundance of food and the decrease in motor activity in affluent societies have created many new problems. Perhaps the most common "metabolic disorder" is the prevalence of obesity, which has been associated with a decreased life expectancy (Dublin and Marks, 1951) and an increased risk of CHD (Whyte, 1965; Bjurulf, 1959) and diabetes mellitus (Yalow *et al.*, 1965). Exercise can be of value in reducing obesity but it is not known whether this will also affect life expectancy or the risk of developing those diseases associated with it. As the problem of activity and weight control is a very complex one, the reader is referred to more adequate reviews by Mayer (1963) and Dabney (1964).

With the increasing number of older people, an area needing research is activity and its relation to physiological aging processes. An important geriatric problem is the prevalence of inactivity (Riccitelli, 1963), which may result in muscular atrophy, decreased appetite, bones becoming porous and fragile, and a slowing down of physiological processes. Skinner *et al.* (1964) showed that endurance training increased the body density and PWC of men 35–55 years old. In these same men, Holloszy *et al.* (1964b) found improvement in cardiovascular function measured by the ultralow frequency ballistocardiograph (BCG) and reflected by significant increases in wave amplitudes. Also, 4 of 5 men with abnormal BCG's had normal tracings after training. Normally, with aging there is a progressive decline in wave amplitudes (i.e., decreased contractile force of the heart) and an increased incidence of abnormality (Starr and Wood, 1961). Thus, it appears in a few instances that physical training may counteract some of the trends normally seen with aging. However, this does not necessarily denote that training is affecting the aging process.

This review has not dealt with the effects of training on "physical fitness" and its relationship to the total spectrum of "health" since both are complex, poorly defined terms which do not lend themselves to precise, objective investigation. Many aspects of health (e.g., psychological and social) could not be considered in this review. There are also many inadequate studies on disease and aging processes which have not been reviewed because their findings are too inconclusive and serve only to strengthen the need for objective, controlled research.

IV. Longevity

Longevity is associated with so many factors (disease, accidents, etc.) that it is difficult to assess how it may be affected by exercise. The effects of exercise on any of the disease or aging processes which have or have not been mentioned in this review can also influence mortality rates.

Hammond (1964a) asked 387,427 males with no history of stroke, heart disease, hypertension, or cancer to fill out a questionnaire on their personal habits and physical complaints. During the next 2 years 10,082 of the men died, 4468 in the first year and 5614 in the second. Death rates during both periods were much higher for men who said they did no exercise in their work or play than for men who said they did slight, moderate, or heavy exercise. Death rates decreased with increasing amounts of exercise.

A later report by Hammond (1964b) covering mortality over a 34-month period confirmed this relationship in 442,094 men aged 40 to 89 years. These men were categorized by 24 variables relating to family history, diet, occupation, religion, residence, height, exercise, etc., into 85 subgroups. Mortality rates of smokers and nonsmokers were then compared. The lowest rate in all 85 subgroups occurred in men who did not smoke and who said they exercised moderately or heavily. Even among smokers, the lowest rates were found in men who said they did moderate or heavy exercise.

The exact significance of these 2 studies by Hammond (1964a,b) is unclear since ill health may have reduced the ability or desire to indulge in exercise. It is not known whether the exercise was primarily done at work or during leisure time. There is also no information on how these arbitrary classifications of exercise were interpreted by each individual interviewed.

Studies of athletes, with all of the problems inherent in this type of investigation, form the bulk of information on longevity. Dublin (1932) and Rook (1954) found no difference in longevity after college between athletes and nonathletes. Likewise, Montoye *et al.* (1957) reported no difference between athletes and an age-matched group of students in cause of death, longevity, or cause of death of parents. After a period of 7 years, there was still no difference in results from 98% of the original study group (Montoye *et al.*, 1962).

Karvonen (1959) studied the longevity of 388 skiers from Finland. On the average, skiers lived 6 years longer than the general male population between the years 1931–1940 and 3 years longer than a similar population between the years 1951–1955. The significance of this trend was not clarified by the investigator and may be related to changes in the samples or the population studied.

There is insufficient evidence in these studies on athletes to say that activity in sports either increases life expectancy or that it has any adverse effects. Since most athletes train for only a short time during their youth, it seems unlikely that there would be any carry-over value 20 to 40 years later with regard to their health or longevity. Also, since each sport involves a different type of training, the athletes should not be grouped into one category to be compared with students who did not participate in varsity athletics but who may have been just as active in intramural sports or physical education classes.

V. Résumé

Attempting to make simple statements from such a vast amount of data may be as misleading as some of the individual studies reviewed. However, since one function of a review is to collate, distill, and generalize wherever possible, an attempt has been made to do just that.

It appears that the following statements are warranted or suggested from a review of the literature on exercise and health:

1. No unequivocal relationship between activity and general mortality has been proved.

2. Along with a decrease in activity in the general population, there has been an increase in the incidence of some chronic diseases (this does not necessarily denote a causal relationship).

3. Regular, moderate exercise may be of value in reducing the incidence and severity of coronary heart disease.

4. Persons with occlusive arterial disease, emphysema, and asthma may be benefited by regular activity.

5. There is little evidence to show whether physical training will affect the incidence or severity of hypertension.

6. Exercise may be a useful adjunct to other forms of management for diabetes mellitus.

7. Theoretically, an important benefit of regular exercise can be the control of body weight, which may indirectly affect general mortality, coronary heart disease, diabetes, and lipid metabolism.

8. Exercise may not directly affect some disease processes but may improve the adaptation of the organism to the restrictions resulting from them.

9. Changes in health and longevity may not be directly attributed to exercise patterns since many other factors (e.g., personal selection, health consciousness, habits, heredity) can operate simultaneously.

10. The vast spectrum of "health" has not been adequately studied.

VI. Implications

The implications of this review are clear: too little is known about the chronic and acute effects of exercise on health and longevity. Even though adequate control over the many interdependent factors is difficult, this is an area of research where such control is absolutely essential before definitive answers can be obtained.

There is a need for greater communication among those persons interested in the many aspects of health. In this way, physical educators, physiologists, physicians, psychologists, public health personnel, etc., can better comprehend the role and possible contributions of each field in solving the many questions in this complex area of investigation.

Since so many interdependent factors need to be understood and controlled and because research on human beings involves many scientific disciplines, a team approach to research may be an optimal method for obtaining definitive information. This crossfertilization of men and ideas through joint investigation should improve the quality of the research.

More information on the metabolic costs of various types, durations, intensities, and amounts of exercise is needed. A "pharmacopoeia of exercise" would be an invaluable tool for prescribing activity as well as for studying and understanding its acute and chronic effects on the human organism.

There are no easy solutions for the major problems outlined in this review. At the present time, we cannot fit exercise and its possible effects on health and longevity into Koch's postulates. Neither can we put the many interdependent factors into simple formulae and get definitive answers. However, by critically appraising the evidence and the trends that appear, we can hope to arrive at the proper conclusions. If this review has stimulated the reader to think critically about research in this field, then it has accomplished its purpose.

REFERENCES

Albrink, M., and Meigs, J. (1965). *Ann. N.Y. Acad. Sci.* **131**, 673.
Albrink, M., Meigs, J., and Granoff, M. (1962). *New Engl. J. Med.* **266**, 484.
Allen, F. (1915). *Boston Med. Surg. J.* **173**, 743.
Andersen, K. L., and Elvik, A. (1955). *Acta Med. Scand.* **153**, 367.
Anderson, J. T., Lawler, A., and Keys, A. (1957). *J. Clin. Invest.* **36**, 81.

Bassett, D. (1962). *Am. J. Med. Sci.* **243**, 741.

Bjurulf, P. (1959). *Acta Med. Scand.* **166**, Suppl. 349, 1.

Blackburn, H., Taylor, H. L., Parlin, W., Kihlberg, J., and Keys, A. (1965). *Arch. Environ. Health* **10**, 312.

Bronte-Stewart, B., and Krut, L. (1962). *J. Atherosclerosis Res.* **2**, 317.

Brown, R., Davidson, L., McKeown, T., and Whitfield, A. (1957a). *Lancet* **II**, 1073.

Brown, R., McKeown, T., and Whitfield, A. (1957b). *Can. J. Biochem. Physiol.* **35**, 897.

Brožek, J., Kihlberg, J., Taylor, H. L., and Keys, A. (1963). *Ann. N.Y. Acad. Sci.* **110**, 492.

Brunner, D., and Manelis, G. (1960). *Lancet* **II**, 1049.

Buerger, L. (1924). "The Circulatory Disturbances of the Extremities." Saunders, Philadelphia, Pennsylvania.

Bürger, M. (1920). *Arch. Exptl. Pathol. Pharmakol.* **87**, 233.

Cantone, A. (1964). *J. Sports Med. Phys. Fitness* **4**, 32.

Carlson, L. A., and Mossfeldt, F. (1964). *Acta Physiol. Scand.* **62**, 51.

Chaikoff, I., Siperstein, M., Dauben, W., Bradlow, H., Eastham, J., Tomkins, G., Meier, J., Chen, R., Hotta, S., and Srere, P. (1952). *J. Biol. Chem.* **194**, 413.

Chailley-Bert, Labignette, P., and Fabre-Chevalier. (1955). *Presse Med.* **63**, 415.

Chapman, J., Goerke, L., Dixon, W., Loveland, D., and Phillips, E. (1957). *Am. J. Public Health* **47**, 33.

Cohen, H., and Goldberg, C. (1960). *Brit. Med. J.* **II**, 509.

Currens, J., and White, P. D. (1961). *New Engl. J. Med.* **265**, 988.

Dabney, J. (1964). *Ann. Internal Med.* **60**, 689.

Devlin, J. (1963). *Irish J. Med. Sci.* **6**, 423.

Dublin, L. (1932). *Sta. Bull. Met. Life Insurance Co.* **13**, 5.

Dublin, L., and Marks, H. (1951). *Tr. A. Life Insurance M. Dir. Am.* **35**, 235.

Ebel, A. (1958). *In* "Therapeutic Exercise" (S. Licht, ed.), pp. 770–785. E. Licht, New Haven, Connecticut.

Eckstein, R. (1957). *Circulation Res.* **5**, 230.

Elo, O., Hirvonen, L., Peltonen, T., and Välimäki, I. (1965). *Ann. Paediat. Fenniae* **11**, 25.

Foley, W. (1957). *Circulation* **15**, 689.

Fox, S. M., and Skinner, J. S. (1964). *Am. J. Cardiol.* **14**, 731.

Frick, M., Konttinen, A., and Sarajas, H. (1963). *Am. J. Cardiol.* **12**, 142.

Friedman, M., and Rosenman, R. (1959). *J. Am. Med. Assoc.* **169**, 1286.

Golding, L. (1961). *Res. Quart.* **32**, 499.

Gould, G., and Cook, R. P. (1958). *In* "Cholesterol" (R. P. Cook, ed.), p. 273. Academic Press, New York.

Haas, A., and Luczak, A. (1963). "The Application of Physical Medicine and Rehabilitation to Emphysema Patients." Inst. Phys. Med. Rehabil., New York University, New York.

Hammond, E. C. (1964a). *Am. J. Public Health* **54**, 11.

Hammond, E. C. (1964b). *J. Natl. Cancer Inst.* **32**, 1161.

Herron, R. (1964). Unpublished Ph.D. Thesis, University of Illinois, Urbana, Illinois.

Holloszy, J. (1963). *J. Am. Geriat. Soc.* **11**, 718.

Holloszy, J., Skinner, J. S., Toro, G., and Cureton, T. K. (1964a). *Am. J. Cardiol.* **14**, 753.

Holloszy, J., Skinner, J. S., Barry, A., and Cureton, T. K. (1964b). *Am. J. Cardiol.* **14**, 761.

Itkin, I. (1964). *J. Am. Phys. Therapy Assoc.* **44**, 815.

Joslin, E. P., Root, H., White, P., and Marble, A. (1959). "Treatment of Diabetes Mellitus." Lea & Febiger, Philadelphia, Pennsylvania.

Kahn, H. (1963). *Am. J. Public Health* **53**, 1058.

Kapeller-She, A. (1963). *Federation Proc.* **22**, T-778.

Karvonen, M. (1959). *Ergonomics* **2**, 207.

Kasanen, A., Kallio, V., and Forsström, J. (1963). *Ann. Med. Internae Fenniae* **52**, Suppl. 43, 1.

Knowles, H. (1960). *A.D.A. Forecast* **13**, 1.

Larsen, O. A., and Lassen, N. A. (1966). *Lancet* **II**, 1093.

Larsson, Y., Sterky, G., Ekengren, K., and Moller, T. (1962). *Diabetes* **11**, 109.

Larsson, Y., Persson, B., Sterky, G., and Thoren, C. (1964). *J. Appl. Physiol.* **19**, 629.

McDonough, J., Hames, C., Stulb, S., and Garrison, G. (1965). *J. Chronic Diseases* **18**, 443.

McElhenny, T., and Peterson, K. (1963). *J. Am. Med. Assoc.* **195**, 142.

Mann, G., Teel, K., Hayes, O., McHailey, A., and Bruno, D. (1955). *New Engl. J. Med.* **253**, 349.

Mayer, J. (1963). *Ann. Rev. Med.* **14**, 111.

Miall, W., and Oldham, P. (1958). *Clin. Sci.* **17**, 409.

Millman, M., Grundon, W., Kasch, F., Wilkerson, B., and Headley, J. (1965). *Ann. Allergy* **23**, 220.

Montoye, H. (1962). *J. Sports Med. Phys. Fitness* **2**, 35.

Montoye, H., Van Huss, W., Olson, H., Pierson, W., and Hudec, A. (1957). "The Longevity and Morbidity of College Athletes." Phi Epsilon Kappa, Ann Arbor, Michigan.

Montoye, H., Van Huss, W., Brewer, W., Jones, E., Ohlson, M., Mahoney, E., and Olson, H. (1959). *Am. J. Clin. Nutr.* **7**, 139.

Montoye, H., Van Huss, W., and Nevai, J. (1962). *J. Sports Med. Phys. Fitness* **2**, 133.

Morris, J. (1960). *Mod. Concepts Cardiovascular Disease* **29**, 625.

Morris, J., and Crawford, M. (1958). *Brit. Med. J.* **II**, 1485.

Morris, J., Heady, J., Raffle, P., Roberts, C., and Parks, J. (1953). *Lancet* **II**, 1053 and 1111.

Morris, J., Heady, J., and Raffle, P. (1956). *Lancet* **II**, 569.

Nikkilä, E., and Konttinen, A. (1962). *Lancet* **I**, 1151.

Peterson, K., and McElhenny, T. (1965). *Pediatrics* **35**, 295.

Pierce, A., Taylor, H. F., Archer, R., and Miller, W. (1964). *Arch. Internal Med.* **113**, 28.

Pomeroy, W., and White, P. D. (1958). *J. Am. Med. Assoc.* **167**, 711.

Riccitelli, M. (1963). *J. Am. Geriat. Soc.* **11**, 299.

Rochelle, R. (1961). *Res. Quart.* **32**, 538.

Rook, A. (1954). *Brit. Med. J.* **I**, 1773.

Sanders, C., Levinson, G., Abelmann, W., and Freinkel, N. (1964). *New Engl. J. Med.* **271**, 220.

Scherr, M., and Frankel, L. (1958). *J. Am. Med. Assoc.* **168**, 1996.

Schlüssel, H. (1965). *Med. Welt* **3**, 145.

Schoop, W. (1964). *Med. Welt* **10**, 502.

Siperstein, M., and Chaikoff, I. (1955). *Federation Proc.* **14**, 767.

Skinner, J. S., and Strandness, D. E., Jr. (1967a). *Circulation* **36**, 15.

Skinner, J. S., and Strandness, D. E., Jr. (1967b). *Circulation* **36**, 23.

Skinner, J. S., Holloszy, J., and Cureton, T. K. (1964). *Am. J. Cardiol.* **14**, 747.

Skinner, J. S., Benson, H., McDonough, J., and Hames, C. (1966). *J. Chronic Diseases* **19**, 773.

Smith, D., and Levine, R. (1964). *Med. Clin. N. Am.* **48**, 1387.

Spain, D., and Bradess, V. (1957). *Arch. Internal Med.* **100**, 228.

Spain, D., and Bradess, V. (1960). *Circulation* **22**, 239.

Stamler, J., Lindberg, H., Berkson, D., Shaffer, A., Miller, W., and Poindexter, A. (1960). *J. Chronic Diseases* **11**, 405.

Starr, I., and Wood, F. (1961). *Circulation* **23**, 714.

Sterky, G. (1963). *Acta Paediat.* **52**, 1.

Stevenson, J., Feleki, V., Rechnitzer, P., and Beaton, J. (1964). *Circulation Res.* **15**, 265.

Taylor, H. L., Anderson, J. T., and Keys, A. (1961). *Circulation* **24**, 1055.

Taylor, H. L., Klepetar, E., Keys, A., Blackburn, H., and Puchner, T. (1962). *Am. J. Public Health* **52**, 1697.

Tepperman, J., and Pearlman, D. (1961). *Circulation Res.* **9**, 576.

Toor, M., Katchalsky, A., Agmon, J., and Allalouf, D. (1960). *Circulation* **22**, 265.

Walker, W., Lawry, E., Mann, G., Levine, S., and Stare, F. (1953). *Am. J. Med.* **14**, 654.

Whyte, H. M. (1965). *Am. J. Cardiol.* **15**, 66.

Wisham, L., Abramson, A., and Ebel, A. (1953). *J. Am. Med. Assoc.* **153**, 10.

Yalow, R., Glick, S., Roth, J., and Berson, S. (1965). *Ann. N. Y. Acad. Sci.* **131**, 357.

Zsotér, T., Fam, W., and McGregor, M. (1964). *Can. Med. Assoc. J.* **90**, 1203.

Zukel, W., Lewis, R., Enterline, P., Painter, R., Ralston, L., Fawcett, R., Meredith, A., and Peterson, B. (1959). *Am. J. Public Health* **49**, 1630.

9

VARIATION IN ALTITUDE AND ITS EFFECTS ON EXERCISE PERFORMANCE

Bruno Balke

The fundament of organic life on earth is the existence of oxygen in the atmosphere. The air around us, as light as it feels, nevertheless has considerable weight. At sea level (S.L.), it exerts the pressure of 1 atm, which is equivalent to the pressure of a mercury column of 760 mm/cm², or 14 lb to the square inch. Approximately one-fifth of the atmospheric gas mixture consists of oxygen. Accordingly, the partial pressure of oxygen at S.L. is approximately 150 mm Hg. Man's lungs, blood, heart, brain, muscles, and other organs have, over millions of years, adjusted to receive and to utilize the amount of oxygen which is available at this pressure. Any change to lower or higher oxygen tensions requires particular physiological adjustments to re-store or to maintain the internal equilibrium of oxygen exchange. In this chapter, only the physiological effects of decreasing atmospheric pressure or increasing altitude will be discussed.

I. Man at Altitude

Great areas on our globe are covered with high and rugged mountains, presenting conditions adverse to human, animal, and plant life. In addition to the loneliness and cold climate of the high altitude regions, the thinned at-mosphere contributes greatly to the discomfort of man. Sven Hedin, the Swedish explorer of the high plateau of Central Asia, was often impressed "by the silence of death which was enhanced by the cold" (Hedin, 1899). Under-standably man avoided the encounter with such an unfriendly climate. How-ever, in prehistoric times hermits and special groups of people were apparently attracted by the challenges the harder life on the mountains had to offer, and settled at elevations up to around 4500 m on the central highlands of Asia, as in Tibet, Nepal, and Southern Mongolia. Amazingly, just about on the other side of the globe, people of nearly identical appearance settled in the high mountainous areas of the South American continent. Some of the loftiest permanent dwellings in the Himalayas as well as in the Andes were built and inhabited by members of religious sects, monks, and priests. On both con-tinents these settlements of probably the most educated people of their time became the centers of mystic-religious and highly civilized states, as Tibet under the rule of the Dalai Lama, and the empire of the Incas in Peru and adjacent high countries, from Ecuador in the north to Central Chile in the south.

At the present time these areas are populated up to altitudes of nearly 5000 m. The life of some six million Indians in the high mountain regions of Ecuador, Bolivia, and Peru has changed little for thousands of years (Johnson, 1965).

The soil is poor, the climate is hostile, and the air is thin. Nobody knows why people did settle there. Today, the richness of this mountain territory in precious minerals and ores constitutes a practical reason for attracting a great number of altitude dwellers. Had this been of any importance in more ancient times?

In spite of the adverse environmental conditions, especially in regard to the relative lack of oxygen, these altitude dwellers meet the great physical demands of their daily life with adequate functional capacities. One can only be amazed by the fact that Peruvian miners, after a grinding 8-hr shift of hard physical work in a mine, at an elevation of 5700 m, can still enjoy a 1-hr soccer game after returning home. At the little mining village of Ticklio, where the central highway from Lima crosses the first Andean mountain chain at an elevation of 4800 m, four soccer fields along both sides of the highway are occupied by playing teams during the afternoon hours of almost any day. The newcomer to this altitude, after a 4-hr drive from Lima, most probably even feels too sick to enjoy the view of the gigantic scenery of snow and ice-covered-mountains.

While ascending gradually to higher elevations, one encounters distinctly different stages of functional responses to the increasing lack of oxygen. At moderate levels of elevation life apparently goes on without complications. With increasing altitude, symptoms of discomfort gradually develop in severity. At any given altitude they are usually more severe during physical activity than at rest. Table I provides a quick orientation to the progression of symptoms from stage to stage, whereby the stages are defined by a decline of the atmospheric pressure in steps of one-tenth of 1 atm. At elevations up to 2000 m, a great number of people live in complete comfort. At this altitude the unaccustomed traveler from a low country will notice effects of the thinner air only during strenuous exercise. On the other hand, at an elevation of 5600 m where the barometric pressure has fallen off to one-half its S.L. value, the same traveler would suffer greatly during rest and would be unable to perform any appreciable amount of work. At an altitude of 7000 m, with only

TABLE I

PHYSIOLOGICAL CONSEQUENCES OF DIMINISHING ATMOSPHERIC PRESSURE

Atm	Barometric pressure (mm Hg)	Altitude (m)	$P_{I_{O_2}}$ (mm Hg)	Symptoms[a] Rest	Work	$P_{A_{O_2}}$ (rest)	O_2 Saturation (%)
1.0	760	0	149	−	−	105	97
0.9	680	1000	142	−	−	94	96
0.8	600	2000	125	−	+	78	94
0.7	530	3100	111	+	+	62	90
0.6	450	4300	94	+ +	+ + +	51	86
0.5	380	5600	75	+ + +	+ + + +	42	80
0.4	305	7000	64	+ + + +	×	31	63
0.3	230	9000	48	†		19	30

[a] Key to symbols: −, no symptoms; +, moderate dyspnea; + +, lightheadedness, nausea, restlessness, dyspnea; + + +, headache, painful tiredness, food repulsion, great breathing difficulties; + + + +, lethargy, disturbed judgment, general weakness—approaching unconsciousness.

× inability to sustain minimum effort.

† death.

two-fifths of the normal atmospheric pressure remaining, no man can survive beyond a very short period of time—unless he had been exposed to sufficiently high altitudes for weeks or months. The fact that mountain climbers have reached peak altitudes of 8600 m (28,600 ft) without the support of additional oxygen breathing (Norton, 1925) is evidence for the great capacity of the human organism to become adapted to adverse environmental conditions. In the sport of mountaineering, man has met the challenge of subjecting himself to the limits of tolerance for physical exertion, for hypoxia, and for cold. The astronaut of the future might need and use the knowledge gained from the mountaineer's experiences when beginning to explore the universe.

II. Physical Considerations of Gas Tensions in the Atmosphere and in the Lungs

The exponential decrease of air pressure with increasing distance from the earth's surface parallels a decrease in air density. For the performance of man at altitude, the diminished air density offers some mechanical advantage. The reduction of air resistance should favor faster velocities in running and should allow the achievement of better performances in throwing events (Fenn, 1954). Also, the moving of thinner air through the narrow passages of the respiratory tract causes less turbulence and slightly reduces the work of breathing (Fenn, 1954; Rahn and Otis, 1949). However, the physiological disadvantages of diminished air density usually outweigh the mechanical advantages.

The composition of ambient air is the same at all levels of elevation, namely, approximately 79% gaseous nitrogen, 20.95% oxygen, 0.04% carbon dioxide and traces of the rare gases.

When fresh air is drawn into the lungs it becomes saturated with water vapor at the body temperature of 37°C. Within the lungs the inhaled air is further mixed with the alveolar air, a gas mixture resulting from the gas exchange across the alveolar-capillary membrane. The composition of the alveolar air is kept relatively constant despite the continuous diffusion of oxygen from the alveoli to the blood and of carbon dioxide in reversed direction. The relative constancy of alveolar air is usually maintained by an adequate amount of fresh air brought in by pulmonary ventilation, a process geared to keep the carbon dioxide level at approximately 5.5 to 6%. At an assumed barometric pressure of 747 mm Hg and at the alveolar water vapor tension of 47 mm Hg, which remains constant at all levels of elevation as long as body temperature stays at 37°C, the alveolar O_2 tension ($P_{A_{O_2}}$) would be $747 - 47 \times (0.2095 - 0.0595) = 105$ mm Hg, approximately.

The intrathoracic space of an individual has nearly constant physical dimensions at given phases of ventilatory involvement. Hence, the atmospheric pressure determines the number of gas molecules present within this intrathoracic air space. For example, at an elevation of 5600 m, where the barometric pressure is reduced to one-half its S.L. value, only half the number of oxygen molecules are inhaled with one breath, which involves the same diaphragmatic movement and rib cage expansion as at sea level. Since the oxygen requirements for given energy expenditures remain the same at all altitudes, these requirements can be fulfilled only by an augmentation of the bellows action of the chest to increase pulmonary ventilation. Either the depth of breathing or the respiratory frequency, or both factors simultaneously, are augmented.

III. Physiological Effects of Altitude

A. GENERAL

It follows, then, that an increase of pulmonary ventilation must be the basic functional mechanism for adaptation to altitude. The increased ventilation serves the purpose of bringing sufficient atmospheric oxygen into the lungs as well as eliminating the carbon dioxide produced in amounts concomitant with the given metabolic rate. The failure to ventilate sufficiently, as frequently observed in people on their first acute exposure to higher elevations, results in diminishing alveolar oxygen but increasing alveolar carbon dioxide tensions. Sooner or later, however, either the accumulation of carbon dioxide or the ensuing hypoxia triggers the respiratory centers, and hyperventilation is instigated.

The supply of adequate amounts of oxygen to the active tissue over a wide range of metabolic demands is a complex process, encompassing:

1. The availability of sufficient O_2 in the inspired air
2. The mixing of fresh air within the lungs to maintain an optimum oxygen pressure in the alveoli
3. The diffusion of oxygen through the alveolar-capillary membrane into the blood
4. The chemical binding of oxygen with hemoglobin, the oxygen carrying pigment of the red blood cell
5. A blood flow through the lungs properly geared to pick up and to carry the oxygen required for given metabolic processes
6. The unloading of the oxygen from the tissue capillaries to the cells in exchange for the metabolic waste products, especially carbon dioxide
7. The same complex mechanism, in reverse, for the elimination of CO_2

One can visualize that a temporary or permanent breakdown of any of these factors would have to be compensated for by a more efficient utilization of one or more of the other mechanisms. As long as submaximal metabolic demands do not require the engagement of all these mechanisms to full capacity, a definite limitation of the total functional adaptability may not be realized. Only if one of the oxygen supplying functions is severely impaired, and the other mechanisms have already become engaged at a maximum rate in a compensatory effort, would performance capacity be expected to be affected. A discussion of the effects of altitude on physical performance capacity requires, therefore, a critical evaluation of the functional limitations of all the major components contributing to maximum oxygen transport.

B. Acute Hypoxia

According to observations by Rahn and Otis (1949), no measurable increase in pulmonary ventilation occurs in the nonacclimatized resting man during acute exposure to altitudes up to 3000 to 3600 m, with a mean atmospheric pressure close to 500 mm Hg. Under such conditions, the alveolar CO_2 tension would be maintained close to its "normal" value of 38–40 mm Hg while the $P_{A_{O_2}}$ would drop to slightly less than 60 mm Hg. Correspondingly, the CO_2 fraction in the alveolar air would be approximately 0.085 and that of O_2 about 0.125.

The transport of oxygen to the active tissue is a function of the hemoglobin (Hb). The amount of Hb in the blood determines the potential capacity of the blood for carrying oxygen. With a 100% oxygen saturation in the blood the maximum oxygen carrying capacity for 1 gm of Hb is 1.34 ml of oxygen. Assuming an average value of 15 gm Hb in 100 ml of blood the oxygen carrying capacity of "normal" blood is approximately 20 vol %.

By equilibrating blood experimentally with gas mixtures of various oxygen tensions at body temperature, and then determining the oxygen content in the blood, an S-shaped curve is established as shown in Fig. 1. The relationship between the oxygen carrying capacity and the actual content in the blood at the various equilibration pressures is expressed as the oxygen saturation. The long, nearly flat upper part of the oxyhemoglobin dissociation curve indicates that a relatively high oxygen saturation of the arterial blood is assured even at the relatively low oxygen tension of 55 mm Hg which might be found at an altitude between 3000–3600 m. The following steeper slope of the curve indicates that while the unloading of oxygen to the tissue becomes enhanced, the capacity for oxygen transport is reduced at very high altitudes.

The arrows on the oxygen dissociation curve shown in Fig. 1 are directed toward oxygen saturations which would be found in individuals acutely exposed to elevations of 3100, 4300, 5600, 7000, and 9000 m, and would be associated with the symptoms described in Table I. They point out that a drop of the arterial oxygen saturation to 80% of its normal value will cause severe symptoms of hypoxia known as "mountain sickness." At the "critical" alveolar oxygen pressure of 30 mm Hg (Christensen and Krogh, 1936), corresponding to an arterial P_{O_2} of approximately 27–28 mm Hg, nonacclimatized individuals fall unconscious. At this point the arterial oxygen saturation has reached a value of 60%. For the brain tissue the critical oxygen tension compatible with sufficient brain function has been established at 19 mm Hg (Noell and Schneider, 1944). The heart appears to have a critical tissue oxygen tension very close to that of the brain (Balke, 1964).

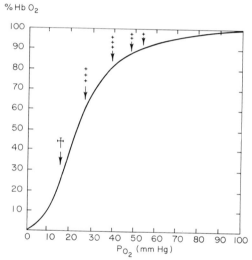

Fig. 1. A typical oxyhemoglobin dissociation curve of a sea-level resident. Arrows point to the oxygen saturations found at elevations of 3100, 4300, 5600, 7000, and 9000 m.

A logical consequence of any reduction in arterial oxygen content below the level of normalcy ought to be a compensatory increase of the blood flow. In fact, determinations of cardiac output at rest and in exercise during acute hypoxia confirmed this hypothesis (Beard *et al.*, 1951; Christensen and Forbes, 1937; Grollman, 1930; Marbarger *et al.*, 1954; Opitz, 1941). The only dispute to arise centered around the role of the two factors involved, namely, which of these factors—increase in heart rate or increase in stroke volume—may be of greater relative magnitude when cardiac output becomes larger in acute hypoxia. The divergent reports on this matter which had also been reviewed by Van Liere and Stickney (1963) may only be the result of different experimental conditions, methods and test subjects.

C. HEART RATE

The heart rate increases in proportion with the severity of acute hypoxia, but even during severe lack of oxygen at rest the normal heart rate is rarely doubled. When lack of oxygen approaches the level of critical hypoxia, the imminent state of unconsciousness is occasionally preceded by an abrupt fall of the heart rate, a phenomenon quickly reversed after application of oxygen-enriched air. This "critical" fall of the heart rate has been explained as a consequence of central vagal stimulation (Greene and Gilbert, 1921).

During physical exercise at fixed work loads, the heart rate is always higher in acute exposure to high elevations than it is at lower altitudes. The maximal heart rate, therefore, is attained at work intensity levels below those attainable at S.L.

D. STROKE VOLUME

The usual procedure for estimating stroke volume requires the determination of cardiac output and of heart rate. The difficulties involved in routinely obtaining a great number of reliable results on cardiac output under resting and working conditions, even in well-equipped laboratories near S.L., explain the scarcity of such data reported from high altitude experiments. Many of the results procured with methods requiring an absolute "steady state" cannot be considered sufficiently reliable because a true steady state is not readily attained during the first few hours of altitude exposure.

Because of the difficulties involved in obtaining direct measurements of stroke volume, blood pressure measurements have been used frequently as an indirect method for an estimation of relative changes in stroke volume. According to Hamilton (1960), the predictions of stroke volume made from the pulse pressure can be used with accuracy in man.

E. BLOOD PRESSURE DURING REST AND EXERCISE

Apparently there is no typical response of blood pressure to hypoxia. In addition to individual differences, the degree of hypoxia appears as a distinct factor in affecting the type of reaction (Van Liere and Stickney, 1963). A frequently observed slight fall in diastolic pressure is considered a significant factor in the regulation of circulation during hypoxia and is brought about by a decrease in peripheral resistance (Comroe and Dripps, 1945). In sudden exposure to very severe degrees of hypoxia, equivalent to an elevation of 8000 m, considerable increases in systolic pressure accompanied by slight rises in diastolic pressure have been observed (Opitz, 1941). When, at such altitude, critical alveolar-arterial oxygen tensions were attained, the sudden slowing of heart rate was accompanied by an abrupt decline in both systolic and diastolic pressure, indicating the development of a cardiac crisis which is presumably a coronary crisis (Wiggers, 1941).

During physical exercise, blood pressure adjustments to given work loads are rather consistent in a given individual. Changes of environmental conditions, such as alterations in degree and duration of hypoxia, have a specific impact on blood pressures during exercise. When 6 men were tested on a bicycle ergometer with gradually increasing work, first under normal atmospheric conditions and then in a low pressure chamber at a simulated altitude of 4200 m, the identical work intensities in acute hypoxia not only required 15 to 18 heart beats per minute more, but the systolic pressures were 5–10 mm Hg higher and the diastolic pressures about the same amounts lower (Wells *et al.*, 1956).

F. Metabolic Oxygen Requirements

In vitro, the oxygen consumption of the living cell has been found constant even at oxygen tensions as low as 10 mm Hg in the nutritive medium (Warburg, 1914). *In vivo* observations on basal energy metabolism have been conflicting. For obvious reasons a decrease of the metabolic rate should be of advantage for survival under severe hypoxic conditions. For albino rats such "advantageous" adjustments have actually been observed (F. G. Hall, 1960). However, in this case the body temperature fell markedly as a side effect of hypoxia. Thus, the apparent decrement in oxygen requirements must have been a consequence of the developing hypothermia. When body temperatures were prevented from falling, the rats could not survive such extreme hypoxic conditions as before. In man, body temperature is not significantly affected in an oxygen-poor atmosphere unless the latter is coupled to a cold environment. Therefore, a reduction in metabolic rate usually does not occur. On the contrary, the thermoregulatory mechanisms in the colder environment at high elevations tend to raise the metabolic rate by the mechanisms of shivering or by unnoticed muscle tensions. A slight elevation of the basal energy expenditure, even under most carefully controlled experimental conditions, should theoretically exist because of the ensuing hyperventilation at high altitude and the concomitantly increased work of breathing. The greater work demands on the heart in acute hypoxia should also favor a slightly higher total metabolic rate.

G. Chronic Hypoxia and Altitude Acclimatization

A continuation of the discussion on the effects of altitude on the metabolic rate becomes more sensible if altitude exposures of longer duration are considered. In spite of ample evidence that the energy expenditure during rest and work is practically the same at all elevations (Barcroft, 1925; Herxheimer *et al.*, 1933; Hurtado, 1965), substantially increased values have been reported in the literature (Delius *et al.*, 1942; Ewig and Hinsberg, 1931; Zuntz *et al.*, 1906). Not only the cold temperatures in high altitude laboratories but also such factors as greater evaporative water loss, temporarily restricted fluid intake, loss of appetite, unbalanced diets, physical sluggishness, and quick fatigability may upset the normal energy metabolism. Hasselbalch and Lindhard (1915), in low pressure chamber experiments of several days' duration, found basal metabolic rates increased by about 8% on the morning following a day of moderately strenuous work. In another study of the basal metabolic rate under strictly controlled conditions (Balke, 1945), the respiratory gas exchange was noticeably increased at the elevation of 3000 m on the days following strenuous mountain climbs. No such delayed recovery was observed in trained individuals performing similarly strenuous work at lower elevations. It appears to be a common experience of people who have stabilized their weight during regular physical training at low elevations to lose considerable weight when they continue nearly equal physical training efforts at high altitude, even with the caloric intake remaining unchanged. The long periods of increased metabolic rate during the recovery phases at high—in contrast to moderate—altitudes might contribute, in part, to this weight loss.

The physical sufferings and subjective discomforts which make life miserable for the first few days and nights at high altitude usually disappear after a week's time. At that time, physiological processes of acclimatization gradually begin to substitute for the previously initiated acute adaptive mechanisms. A perfect achievement of natural acclimatization is displayed by the natives of high mountain areas who were born and have lived and worked there for centuries. Hurtado (1964) classifies the main mechanisms of natural acclimatization into two categories: those which result in a marked economy of the oxygen transport from the oxygen deficient atmosphere to the body tissue, and those which are present at the tissue level.

An individual only temporarily exposed to the high altitude environment will also, within weeks or months, achieve a state of acclimatization which enables him to live apparently unaffected by hypoxia. However, he never reaches the same level of economy in the transport and utilization of oxygen as the native resident. This was brought out in experiments conducted by Velásquez (1959) who determined the duration of the time of consciousness in natives during simulated ascents to very high altitudes in a low pressure chamber. A great number of the natives remained conscious when exposed to a simulated altitude of slightly more than 9000 m (30,000 ft) and maintained their writing ability for a practically indefinite period of time. Although a similar level of altitude tolerance was achieved by a "newcomer" after 5 weeks of mountaineering and acclimatization at elevations between 4500 and

5300 m, there was a considerable difference in the functional response by which consciousness was maintained. The pulmonary ventilation of the natives increased only slightly and unconsciousness did not set in before the alveolar oxygen tension had fallen to about 21 mm Hg. The temporarily acclimatized newcomer, on the other hand, reacted with a much greater increase of pulmonary ventilation at the more extreme altitude levels, as Fig. 2 demonstrates (Velásquez and Balke, 1956). By doing so he prevented the alveolar oxygen tension from falling below the critical level which had been lowered

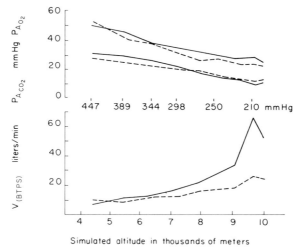

Simulated altitude in thousands of meters

Fig. 2. Differences in pulmonary ventilation and alveolar gas tensions between native residents of Morococha, Peru (dashed line), and a Caucasian newcomer (solid line) after 5 weeks of physical training at altitude. The ventilatory responses were elicited by gradual "ascents" in a low pressure chamber stationed at an elevation of 4500 m.

from 30 to 25 mm Hg during the 4-week period of altitude training. Although there were qualitative differences in the perfection of acclimatization, the basic mechanisms of adaptation were the same. These mechanisms are: increased pulmonary ventilation with accompanying changes of the acid-base balance of the blood, improved diffusing capacity for oxygen in the lungs as manifested by a decrease in the alveolar-arterial (A-a) gradient for oxygen, and the increase of the red blood cell count as well as of the hemoglobin content of the blood.

H. Increased Pulmonary Ventilation

It has been mentioned before that an individual without previous altitude experience does not increase his resting ventilatory volume on acute exposure to hypoxia unless he ascends to an altitude in excess of 3500 m. Since the resting metabolic rate is essentially the same at both low and high elevations, a lesser amount of oxygen is brought into the lungs than is consumed by the body tissues. The alveolar oxygen content, therefore, decreases slowly while the content of carbon dioxide, which is produced and released into the lung alveoli at a normal rate, rises. There can be no doubt that this disproportion of oxygen and carbon dioxide tensions in the alveoli and in the arterial blood must affect the regulatory centers for pulmonary ventilation. Luft (1965) is probably correct in stating that the hyperpnea induced by hypoxia is mediated exclusively through a reflex pathway originating in the chemoreceptors of the carotid sinus and aortic bodies, which are specifically susceptible to changes in the oxygen tension of arterial blood. On the other hand, the simultaneously occurring CO_2 accumulation should not be discarded as a very potent stimulus for respiration in hypoxia. Whatever the more appropriate stimulus, hyperventilation finally ensues in the form of a few gasping deep breaths. With such few breaths sufficient CO_2 is washed out from the lungs, or sufficient oxygen is restored, to reduce the respiratory drive to a trickle, frequently to such an extent that a period of apnea follows. During that time and during the next few shallow breaths the same process of alveolar oxygen deprivation and carbon dioxide enrichment repeats itself and invariably leads to the same cycle of gasping and then dying ventilation as before. This type of periodic breathing (Douglas and Haldane, 1909), experienced by nearly everyone temporarily exposed to high altitude, may last for several days before gradually converting into a continuous hyperventilation.

I. Altitude Hyperventilation

There has been considerable speculation about the possible interference of hyperventilation with the tolerance for hypoxia. In voluntary or involuntary hyperventilation, more carbon dioxide is exhaled than metabolically produced. Usually the resulting hypocapnia leads to muscle spasms and to vasoconstrictions. Such narrowing of capillaries in the brain may result in symptoms very similar to those of hypoxia. It was assumed, therefore, that hypocapnia would rather potentiate the effects of natural hypoxia. Altitude tolerance tests of well-acclimatized individuals have clearly demonstrated, however, that even extreme hypocapnia must not have an additionally detrimental effect (Opitz, 1941). The vasodilatation which accompanies hypoxia apparently outweighs the vasoconstriction of hypocapnia. Since frequent practice of hyperventilation renders an individual nearly immune to incapacitating symptoms of hypocapnia (Balke et al., 1958), the method of voluntary overbreathing during exposure to very low atmospheric pressures can increase altitude tolerance considerably.

A definite limitation for the tolerance of very low barometric pressures is the presence of water vapor in the lungs. At an altitude of 15,000 m (50,000 ft) where the barometric pressure is 87 mm Hg, an aviator breathing 100% oxygen for several hours would only have a pressure of 40 mm Hg available in the alveoli for oxygen and CO_2 combined because a pressure of 47 mm Hg is exerted by water vapor. A well-acclimatized aviator may survive this situation if he can lower the CO_2 tension sufficiently to make way for an oxygen tension slightly above the critical level. The experimental evidence for the achievement of such hypoxia tolerance through temporary altitude acclimatization has been established by simulating such a condition in the low pressure chamber (Velásquez and Balke, 1956).

The development of a permanent hyperventilation at high elevations causes a change in the biochemistry of the blood. The reduction of CO_2 in the alveolar air leads to an increased diffusion of this gas from the venous blood to the alveoli and, retrograde, from the tissues to the blood. The elimination of carbon dioxide, a weak acid, from the body stores leads to a disturbance of the acid-base balance of the blood and body fluids with the pH shifting to the alkaline side. This disturbance of the acid-base balance during the first few days of altitude exposure is probably the main reason for the transient period of "mountain sickness" experienced by nearly all newcomers. The low O_2 and high pH appear to have deleterious effects upon cellular function, and acclimatization to altitude seems to be a matter of adaptation to a low P_{CO_2} as well as to low P_{O_2} (Riley et al., 1954).

Over a period of days the acid-base balance of the body fluids is restored as a consequence of increased base excretion through the kidneys. This base excretion terminates when the blood pH is restored to its normal value of 7.4. As hyperventilation then becomes possible without much further lowering of the alveolar P_{CO_2} and increased alkalinity of the blood, the periodic breathing ceases. An important consequence of the increase in ventilation and lowering of the P_{CO_2} is the accompanying elevation of alveolar P_{O_2} (Riley et al., 1954).

J. DIFFUSING CAPACITY FOR OXYGEN IN THE LUNGS

In man at sea level the oxygen pressure in the arterial blood is usually about 9 mm Hg lower than in the alveolar air. In the native resident of the high mountain country in Peru, Hurtado (1964) observed an oxygen pressure gradient of only 2 mm Hg across the alveolar-capillary membrane. At such a low pressure gradient, adequate gas diffusion can only be maintained if the other factors involved in the diffusion capacity of the lungs have altered their properties toward an enhancement of the oxygen transfer. Thus the entire surface area available for diffusion might have become slightly enlarged as a consequence of the increased pulmonary ventilation and of an increase in the amount of air contained in the dilated alveoli of the residual volume (Hurtado, 1964). Man residing at altitude also shows a permanent dilation of the lung capillaries (Compos and Iglesias, 1964). This in combination with the enlargement of the alveoli should result in a thinning of the alveoli-capillary membrane, favoring the oxygen exchange between alveolar air and circulating blood. Also, a major factor permitting the reduction of the alveolar-arterial oxygen pressure gradient would be a slower blood flow through widened lung capillaries. This improvement of conditions for gas diffusion actually appears to take place.

It has been shown that hypoxia produces pulmonary hypertension in animals (von Euler and Liljestrand, 1946) and in men (Motley et al., 1947). In cattle this condition was found as brisket disease at altitudes from 2400 to 3600 m (Hecht et al., 1962); in man it was not observed in residents of altitudes up to 3100 m but was commonly found at elevations of 3700 m and above (Rotta, 1961). The cause of pulmonary hypertension during acute hypoxia is still not well understood. Several authors (P. W. Hall, 1953; Riviera-Estrada et al., 1958; Wiggers et al., 1953) feel that a resistance must develop peripheral to the pulmonary alveolar capillaries. Fitting into this concept are the findings of increased blood volume in the lungs. Rotta (1961) reported the following observations on permanent residents of the Peruvian Andes at altitudes of 3700 m and above. (1) Teleroentgenograms showed a 20% increase of the transverse heart diameter in 70% of 400 natives living at high altitude compared to an almost equally large number of residents at sea level. More detailed studies indicated that the right ventricle was responsible for this enlargement. (2) Catheterization of the right heart furnished pulmonary arterial pressures of 38/15 mm Hg, which are consistently higher in the altitude group than in people at sea level. (3) A greater quantity of blood was contained in the lungs. (4) There was soon evidence that during physical activity pulmonary hypertension would greatly increase.

K. BLOOD PROPERTIES

1. Red Blood Cells

Since the early work of Viault (1890) the augmentation of the red blood cell count at high altitude has been confirmed over and over. The average number of erythrocytes to be expected in the blood of residents at various altitudes has been tabulated by Keys (1938) from various sources as shown in the following tabulation:

Altitude (m):	S.L.	1000	1500	2500	3500	4500	5500	6500
RBC (millions/ml):	5.3	5.4	5.5	5.8	6.2	6.6	7.3	8.2[a]

[a]Luft (1941).

Controversies might still exist about the speed at which erythrocytes are formed. The immediate rise in acute hypoxia must be caused by hemo-concentration (Van Liere and Stickney, 1963), i.e., by plasma loss. Usually a true increase of red blood cells becomes apparent after three to four days at altitudes above 3000 m. In men living for several months at an altitude near the limit for acclimatization (approximately 6000 m), erythropoiesis was not found inhibited as has been suggested (Pugh, 1964). Values as high as 8.3 to 8.7 million erythrocytes per milliliter have been observed in mountain climbers after several days above 7000 m (Hartmann et al., 1941).

2. Hemoglobin

The formation of new hemoglobin appears to be retarded compared with the course of erythropoiesis (Luft, 1941). There appears to be a quick rise of red blood cell mass and hemoglobin during the first few days at altitude because of a decrease in plasma volume (Luft, 1941; Buskirk et al., 1967). Such changes in plasma volume seem to play a major part in the quick adaptation of the blood to hypoxia; a greater amount of oxygen can then be carried within the same volume of blood. Interestingly enough, in older men Dill et al. (1963) found a decreased hemoglobin concentration during the first days at altitude. They speculated that plasma volume increased faster than red cell volume. During the process of acclimatization, a really new formation of hemoglobin reestablishes the normal oxygen content of the arterial blood despite the lowered oxygen saturation (Hurtado et al., 1945; Hurtado, 1964; Luft, 1941). This essential factor in altitude acclimatization is of the same magnitude in residents at high altitudes as it is in mountaineers after an 8- to 10-week period of living at nearly equivalent levels of elevation. Table II, composed of reported data (Dill et al., 1937; Hurtado, 1956; Luft, 1941; Rotta, 1961), demonstrates the ability of the organism to restore blood oxygen content to normalcy.

TABLE II
BLOOD PROPERTIES AT VARIOUS ALTITUDES

Altitude (m)	Blood volume (ml/kg)	Hb (gm/ 100 ml)	O_2 Capacity (vol %)	O_2 Saturation (%)	Art. O_2 content (vol %)	References
S.L.	79.6	15.3	20.6	97	20.0	Hurtado (1965)
3100	83	16.8	22.5	91	20.5	Rotta (1961)
3600	96	18.8	25.2	87	21.9	Rotta (1961)
4600	100.5	20.13	27.0	80.5	21.7	Hurtado (1965)
4600	104	20.7	27.8	80.5	22.4	Rotta (1961)
5340	—	22.9	30.8	—	—	Dill et al. (1937)
6500	—	24.8	33.3	~65	21.7	Luft (1941)

3. Blood Volume

Changes of blood volume in acute exposure to high altitude had been observed during the Anglo-American Pikes Peak Expedition by Douglas *et al.* (1913). After an initial decrease during the first few days at an altitude of about 4200 m, the blood volume returned to normal. Similar results were reported by Asmussen and Consolazio (1941). During a Himalayan expedition in 1960–1961 the plasma volume of the mountaineers was 29% below the S.L. control value during the first few weeks, but later rose as the red cell mass increased. Concomitantly, blood volume was reduced in the early part of the expedition, but rose eventually to values ranging from 0 to 21% above the S.L. control values (Pugh, 1964). In well-trained runners who were studied over a period of several weeks during acclimatization to an elevation of 3900 m, plasma volume was reduced about 16% at the eighth day at altitude, and remained at this level for the next 3 to 4 weeks (Buskirk *et al.*, 1967). At that time the total blood volume, although still below the control value, had slightly increased with respect to the value obtained initially at altitude. The initial decrease in plasma volume could be a consequence of dehydration resulting from water loss in hyperventilation or in insensible sweating, particularly in the absence of adequate water supply. A definite decrease in blood volume was also observed after 8 days of living at a simulated altitude of approximately 4000 m in a low pressure chamber. In that case the very moderately active experimental subjects lost 4 kg of body weight—presumably most of it from water loss (Balke, 1959). On Mt. Norikura (3000 m) in Japan the circulating blood volume increased from the second through the eighth day after ascent. The plasma volume was increased on the second day but decreased somewhat toward the eighth day (Oda, 1965). The initial increase of total circulating blood volume was considered the result of a plasma increase while at the later stage an increase of the red cell mass was held responsible. Apparently there is no consistent course in the adaptation of the blood volume to altitude. However, in the final stage of altitude acclimatization total blood volume is undoubtedly increased (see Table II).·

4. Blood Viscosity

The hemoconcentration initially observed during altitude acclimatization and the later following true increase of red blood cells cause the blood to become more viscous. A greatly increased blood viscosity is generally assumed to interfere with most efficient hemodynamics by virtue of the increased peripheral resistance. However, if the high blood viscosity encountered under chronic hypoxic conditions would seriously increase the capillary resistance, an increase of blood pressure should be observed at altitude. The observation on miners in the High Andes (Hurtado, 1956; Talbott and Dill, 1936) that those with the highest hematocrits had the lowest resting blood pressures almost rules out the seriousness of the high-viscosity problem. The theory has been advanced (Fahrens and Lindquist, 1931) that in the smallest capillaries the red blood cells move relatively freely in an axial flow within a slower moving plasma sleeve. The main reason for the low blood pressure of natives living permanently at high altitudes with relatively high hematocrit values must be the very effective vasodilation in all major areas. Even in acclimatizing newcomers a decrease of peripheral resistance was observed at altitude (Reichel, 1944). The trend toward a development of lower blood pressures could have reflected changes in the elastic characteristics of the arterial walls.

Hypoxia is presumably the most potent physiological stimulus for evoking relaxation of the coronary arteries (Berne, 1964), brain capillaries (Noell and Schneider, 1944), and probably of all major capillary beds. Without such compensatory mechanisms at high altitude the increased blood volume and blood viscosity, the low oxygen saturation and the increased pulmonary artery pressure, would throw a tremendous burden upon the work of the heart. The high altitude dweller's relatively great capacity for physical work and the mountain climber's experiences at elevations between 7000 to 8000 m do not favor the theory that a high blood viscosity is a serious physiological handicap at altitude.

IV. Physical Performance Capacity at Altitude

Until a few years ago, interest in man's capacity to do physical work at altitude was mainly stimulated by the experiences encountered in mountaineering. Since mountain climbing is a noncompetitive sports activity in which the time–distance factor does not play a major role in judging performances, the cardiorespiratory adaptive capacity is not usually utilized to maximum extent. Only when the mountaineer in keeping up his normal pace exceeds certain levels of elevation, does he realize difficulties in breathing, a pounding heart beat and unusual local muscular fatigue. The fact that major discomfort does not become obvious until an altitude of 3000 m is approached may be looked upon as the reason that for many years scientists did not bother to study the physiological effects of altitude on work capacity at levels much lower than 3000 m. In more recent years, however, a number of athletic competitions were held in cities located at more moderate elevations between 1600 to 2300 m, and the performances in some events turned out substandard when compared with the achievements under conditions of normal atmospheric pressure.

Before discussing the effects of any altitude on the capacity for performing maximum physical work, the components of work capacity must be defined:

(1) Nearly everyone has experienced the fact that a maximum physical all-out effort can only be maintained for a very short period of time, certainly not longer than about 40 sec. After that time the power output, or the speed of movements, drops off considerably. This phase or component of the total work capacity is the so-called "anaerobic work capacity" because the actual oxygen requirements for the energy expenditure exceed by far the amount of oxygen supplied during that period of time. The human organism has the ability to incur an oxygen debt, the size of which mostly depends on such factors as quality and quantity of muscle mass, myoglobin content, buffering capacity, age and training state. (2) At the beginning of any physical effort the oxygen supply lags behind the demands and an oxygen debt is contracted and carried along even when the adequate supply has caught up with the demands. The latter can only come to pass as long as the demands do not exceed the maximum aerobic work capacity, that is, the maximum amount of oxygen which can be delivered to the working tissues through combined cardio-respiratory accommodations. Theoretically, physical efforts at this crest-load of aerobic metabolism could be maintained for a considerable length of time, at least for 1 or 2 hr. Any effort continued beyond the maximum aerobic capacity must lead to an exhaustion of the oxygen debt capacity, setting a limit to the performance in a much shorter period of time. (3) Finally, the maximum metabolic capacity for performing strenuous work at a sub-maximal level near the aerobic limit is largely dependent upon the fuel reserves in the form of glycogen and fatty acids, and upon the synergetic relationship in the utilization of these 2 types of fuel.

Selecting examples from track competition for the illustration of these three components of maximum work capacity, we can consider distances up to the 400 m run as the representatives of the maximum anaerobic type; the distances from 800 to about 3000 m or 2 mi require the quickest possible attainment of the maximally possible oxygen supply but still depend to a large extent on the oxygen debt capacity, more so in the shorter than in the longer runs. In the 5000 and 10,000 m races the maintenance of a speed engaging the maximum aerobic capacity is the most important tactical consideration of the runner; the rest of the oxygen debt capacity not yet exhausted during the relatively fast start or in following spurts for better positioning usually does not permit more than a relatively short final "kick." In races of the distance and duration of a marathon run success or failure rests with the pace which can be held near the aerobic capacity at the most efficient mobilization and utilization of metabolic substrates. A complete exhaustion of carbohydrates with the finish line in sight might turn out a disastrous disappointment to the runner who looked like the undisputed winner of the race.

A. Effects of Altitude on the Maximum Anaerobic Work Capacity

Muscular strength and power for short maximal efforts remain practically unaffected upon ascent to altitude (Christensen and Nielsen, 1936) or when breathing low oxygen gas mixtures (Hollmann and Venrath, 1966). Therefore, a deterioration of performance does not occur in events of short duration. Bicycle-ergometer work at an overload of 2500 kpm/min, which is sufficiently high to lead to complete exhaustion within 76 to 120 sec, was maintained by trained experimental subjects for the same duration of time at both low and high elevation (Balke et al., 1965). The maximum power output in sprint races over 100 and 200 m is practically the same at S.L. and at moderate altitude. In some of the competitions held in cities at higher elevations, as in Mexico City, Albuquerque, Johannesburg, etc., sprinting performances have even been slightly better because of the reduced air density.

B. Maximum Aerobic Capacity

There is complete agreement among all investigators who have studied the effects of various altitudes on physical performances that the capacity for maximum oxygen intake decreases with the reduction of the atmospheric pressure. Discrepancies with regard to the extent at which deterioration takes place can merely be considered indications of great inter- and intra-individual variability enhanced by experimental situations. The use of the maximum oxygen intake as a measure for the adaptability to the hypoxic environment does not reveal a common pattern of response. Neither does youth insure a high degree of success, nor does age bar successful adaptation to work at high altitude (Dill et al., 1964). Although a high degree of physical conditioning, involving especially the cardiorespiratory systems, appears of benefit for maximum hypoxia tolerance in the resting state (Balke and Wells, 1958), it does not ensure superiority in achieving a performance closest to the maximum aerobic level.

A great unsolved problem is the apparent unpredictability of success or failure of altitude training for achieving at higher elevations performances which are either close to or as consistent as the individual's performances at S.L.

C. Effect of Various Activity Levels at Altitude on Work Capacity

An essential prerequisite for evaluating the effects of the lowered atmospheric pressure upon maximum work capacity during a period of altitude training is the frequent monitoring of physiological responses to submaximal and maximal work while undergoing a preceding training under normal atmospheric conditions. Only when an asymptote in functional adaptive capacity has been established, can the factors of training and of high elevation be separated during a continuation of the training at altitude. Even then the results might be misleading on occasion because sudden jumps to new levels of performance capacity—lower or higher—have been observed during extremely long periods of training with stagnating performance capacity. Athletes who have won the reputation of being persistent performers near the recognized absolute records for events which require the maximum engagement of aerobic and anaerobic working capacity should be considered the most reliable subjects for appropriate studies. However, the enlistment of such athletes for altitude studies has rather complicated the issue. There is now considerable divergence of experimental facts on the extent to which maximum work capacity at altitude might "recover" from its initially reduced level, with time. A review of observations made during several altitude training studies might be helpful in analyzing the different results obtained.

The author conducted training studies at low and high altitude in 1942–1943 in the Alps (Balke, 1945). The training consisted essentially of covering long uphill grades of varying steepness at the greatest possible speed. Daily training efforts of a continuous type of work lasted from a minimum of 20 to 30 min to a maximum of 2 hr per session. When the aerobic capacity had reached an apparent maximum level after about 8 weeks of such training at low altitude, the base of experimental operations was transferred to a laboratory station at an elevation of 3000 m. There maximum aerobic working capacity was reduced initially by about 10 to 15%. After 24 days of continued hard training the maximum oxygen intake was nearly the same as in the control experiments at low altitude. However, between this value and the one attained in the following days after return to the low elevation, there was again a difference of 10 to 15%. In other words, the altitude training had improved the maximum aerobic capacity considerably. Since this improvement slowly receded during the following 8 weeks toward the pre-altitude performance level, in spite of continued training, the temporary gain in maximum work capacity was not considered purely another training effect but an altitude effect.

In another study (Wells et al., 1956), the leveling-off of maximum aerobic capacity was attained toward the end of an 8-week training which consisted of interval and continuous work in cross-country running, grade walking on the treadmill, and bicycling on an electrically braked ergometer. Then work capacity was measured (1) at normal atmospheric pressure, (2) during acute exposure to a simulated altitude of 4200 m in a low pressure chamber and (3) repeatedly, during a 6-week period of acclimatization to the same altitude on Mt. Evans, Colorado. In the low pressure chamber the average reduction of the maximum aerobic capacity in six individuals was 27%. The 6-week period of acclimatization to 4200 m was not sufficient to raise this performance level perceptibly. Immediately after return from the mountain, physical performance was improved above the controls and the capacity for maximum oxygen uptake was increased. During the stay at altitude no special training efforts had been made beyond daily hikes at a comfortable pace. Most likely, the intensity of physical activity during acclimatization might be an important factor in influencing work capacity at altitude.

This assumption seemed to be confirmed in a study on White Mountain, California (Dill *et al.*, 1964), in which two individuals attained 76% and 79%, respectively, of their "normal" maximum aerobic capacity at an elevation of 3800 m after about 10 days at altitude. While one of the subjects continued his normal daily activities, the other spent many hours in climbing steep slopes as rapidly as possible. After 4 weeks of acclimatization to mainly the level of 3800 m, work capacity was tested at the elevation of 4200 m and was found reduced by 27% in the former subject but only by 18% in the latter. The reduction of 27% in both the Mt. Evans and the White Mountain study for the same altitude of 4200 m is remarkable. Only very strenuous training efforts appear to affect physiological acclimatization processes toward a restitution of more "normal" work capacity. This was partly borne out by the effect the sojourn to the higher elevation had on the maximum aerobic capacity of subject Dill when he returned to the lower elevation of 3800 m; it was now 86% of "normal" compared to 76% attained previously. Thus a substantial improvement of work capacity appears to be within reach even at considerable elevations.

These experiences were confirmed at the more moderate altitude of 2400 m (Balke *et al.*, 1965). With maximal workouts in laboratory tests and with time trials in sprints as well as in middle distance runs beginning immediately after arrival at altitude, maximum aerobic capacity as well as performance in running improved during a 10-day altitude training. On the second day at altitude, the timed mile run was 8% slower than under normal barometric conditions; on the tenth day it was only 4% slower. The performances after return to the low elevation were 5% better than originally. None of the runners had ever made similar quick improvements during a rather long athletic career.

Experiments carried out in 1965 at an elevation of 2300 m furnished new observations. There was an initial performance loss of 23 sec in the mile run. At the end of two weeks of training at altitude the difference from the control values was only 13 sec. One more week of training at altitude did not result in any further improvement. Upon return to S.L. all performances were better than in the controls. When the athletes were re-exposed to altitude within a period of 1 to 3 weeks, the performances were now practically identical with those established at the original controls. Upon final return to normal atmospheric conditions, performance reached a new peak. Compared with this new peak, the most recent performances at altitude were 3 to 5% off (Balke *et al.*, 1966).

Recently other investigators from the U.S. (Klausen *et al.*, 1966), Japan (Asahina *et al.*, 1960) and Russia (Zimkin, 1966) reported similar results from altitude training. In several other investigations, however, the altitude training was not found effective in restoring some of the work capacity initially lost. Nor was there an improvement beyond the original performance level after return to low elevation. These "negative" findings are of equal interest with the "positive" results.

In one of these studies (Buskirk *et al.*, 1967), well-trained college distance runners were taken to an elevation of 3900 m in Peru. There, maximum aerobic capacity was reduced 30% during the first week, and still 26% after 6 to 7 weeks. After return to S.L., not even the original control level of max $\dot{V}_{O_2}$ was attained. Similarly, performances in the mile and 2-mi run were 20 to 24% slower on the forty-seventh day at 3900 m, 5 to 8% slower at the elevation of 2300 m on the return trip home, and still 3 to 4% slower on the home track, 3 to 15 days after return. Buskirk *et al.* (1967) made the very careful statement that "training at altitude had apparently no deleterious effects on subsequent performance at lower altitude although it is conceivable that some detraining occurred at 13,000 ft because the intensity and duration of training activities were somewhat reduced." He conceded that "certain runners may perform in a superior fashion following return from altitude for reasons that are not clear." Two of the athletes showed outstanding performances in cross-country training and races which began soon after return from altitude.

In a similar study (Grover and Reeves, 1966), high school athletes at the peak of training were taken from Lexington, Kentucky, to Leadville, Colorado (3100 m). Maximum oxygen intake was reduced an average of 25% shortly after arrival and no measurable improvement occurred with continued residence. There was no evidence that the altitude episode had an effect on performance after return to S.L. Athletes residing at Leadville had a maximum aerobic capacity of 27% less at 3100 m than at S.L. Of great interest—and very useful for further consideration—was the observation that in every running event the Lexington athlete was faster than the Leadville man, at both low and high elevation. From the laboratory testing of work capacity such a result was not anticipated.

All these and other study reports (Owen and Pugh, 1966; Saltin, 1966) point to the possibility that modifications of altitude training might be the essential factor in the great variability of observation made.

V. Altitude Training

For optimum success of training at altitude the factors of duration and intensity of training appear as important as the level of altitude at which the training takes place. Success or failure of training becomes most evident in competitive events which are measured by tape or by the stop watch. In such events the records and performance standards are known and competition is usually equally important as a race against time or distance as against the opponents. This is especially true for the modern Olympic games in which everyone looks forward to seeing existing record marks shattered. This attitude is the actual handicap of any athletic championship held under abnormal environmental conditions. There has never been great concern about the effects of altitude on skiers who may compete above the 3000 m level. Here man still competes against man, and the time as an absolute measure is not of so much importance because identical conditions of terrain, snow weather, etc., can never be guaranteed. For a stadium running track, however, such variability of conditions does not exist and everyone therefore expects world class performances from a field of world class runners. Thus, for many people some of the results in the next Olympic Games in Mexico City (2300 m) may appear disappointing. It does not take much courage to predict that the achievement of new Olympic records in the middle and long distances is out of reach for our best specialists in these events.

For any contestant in an athletic event lasting longer than 2 min, a period of training at altitude is a necessity. Without such training the really fastest man might suffer most because he might find it hardest to adjust his pace to the limitations set by the environment.

With regard to the duration of time required for sufficient accommodation to a level of 2300 m, most investigators agree that physiologically important countermeasures are usually developed within 2 or 3 weeks. Owen and Pugh (1966) and Saltin (1966), however, reported that the performances of their European athletes in Mexico City in 1965 were still improving at the end of the fourth week. In this case, the physiological adjustments for maximum performance might have been affected or delayed by the 6- to 7-hr time shift from Europe to Mexico. And again, the mode of training may have been of some influence.

With regard to the intensity of training at altitude, Owen and Pugh's advice (1966) appears sound, namely, that during the first week at altitude the work intensities should be rather light and then build up slowly. However, other experiences indicate that time trials early in the first week had no ill effect on the athlete, introduced him quickly to the need for changes in pace and breathing pattern and served as psychological reinforcement. Furthermore, logical reasoning suggests that in altitude training the maintenance of the greatest possible speed or power output must be emphasized. Since the oxygen lack at altitude interferes with such exertion, the intervals of hard work must be shortened somewhat and the recovery periods slightly extended. If highly trained athletes adjust to the greater physiological demands at altitude by reducing their pace consistently below their former power output, a sort of power loss can be expected. The muscles have achieved maximum power by adapting, in quality and quantity, to the repeated maximum demands in training under optimum atmospheric conditions—in step with the development of maximal respiratory and circulatory functions. At altitude, however, the same maximum of functional efforts cannot be sustained. The insufficient oxygen supply is prohibitive in attaining the former level of muscular work. Therefore, in spite of greater general strain the muscles work at reduced power. Thus, for a runner in record form, a longer period of altitude exposure might become rather detrimental to his performance capacity because of a slight muscular detraining.

What is the most efficient elevation for an altitude training toward competition at a level of 2300 m? A simple answer could be the elevation which results in a physiological enhancement of the capacity for oxygen transport and utilization. Conceivably, at an elevation of about 3000 m this should happen quicker and more efficiently. However, the following arguments must be raised: (1) At the elevation of 3000 m a permanent hyperventilation will develop within a few days and the consequent changes in the acid-base balance lead to a temporarily diminished buffering capacity of the blood. (2) This elevation is sufficiently high to interfere with such training efforts as necessary to achieve or to maintain the extraordinary performances to which we have become accustomed.

For these reasons training at the more moderate altitude of 2000 to 2400 m appears preferable. At this elevation the increased physiological demands during extreme physical efforts are sufficient to stimulate the development of additional adaptive mechanisms. Work can still be performed at a maximum rate for periods long enough to maintain full muscle power. And finally, the need for increased breathing exists practically only during work and not during rest. Changes in the acid-base balance are therefore minimized and performance is less impeded by changes in buffer capacity.

A combination of the normal training at moderate altitude with frequent hikes to higher elevations at a fast pace appears to have merit. Another combination, consisting of training periods repeatedly changing between two or even three different levels of elevation—low, moderate, high—might be most promising in achieving ultimate performances at any given elevation, low or high.

VI. Ultimate Performance Achievement through Altitude Training?

The question has been raised whether or not top athletes who are at the peak of physiological capacity after extensive training under normal atmospheric conditions might be able to improve further by a sophisticated altitude training program. The contention is that extensive athletic training, especially for distance running or similar types of sport activities, leads to similar compensatory adaptive mechanisms as evoked by hypoxia. Not only the mechanisms involved in the oxygen transport, e.g., pulmonary aeration, diffusion of oxygen in the lungs, cardiac work, and blood flow, but also cellular mechanisms become most efficient during hard physical training. Muscles acquire a redder coloration which is related not only to the increase in vascularization but also to the increase in cellular myoglobin (Delachaux and Tissieres, 1946). Myoglobin is not only the acceptor of stored oxygen in the tissues but also the catalyst of the oxidizing processes (Biörck, 1949). Under the influence of muscular training, just as under the action of hypoxia, an activation of the oxidizing–reducing processes appears to occur in the cells (Barbashova, 1965). The opinion has been expressed that further physiological improvement could not be expected through any type of training. But what is the ultimate achievement in human efforts? It appears most likely that with a careful utilization of altitude hypoxia in the training program an increase of the hemoglobin and myoglobin content, of total blood volume, of ventilatory capacity, and of maximum cardiac output could be attained. As a consequence, the performance capacity achievable by training exclusively at S.L. should be slightly surpassed.

REFERENCES

Asahina, K., Ikai, M., Oqaua, S., and Kuroda, U. (1966). *Schweiz. Wochschr. Sportmed.* **14**, 240.

Asmussen, E., and Consolazio, C. F. (1941). *Am. J. Physiol.* **132**, 555.

Balke, B. (1945). Habilitation Thesis, Universität Leipzig.

Balke, B. (1959). *In* "Bioastronautics, Advances in Research," p. 161. U.S.A.F. School of Aviation Med., Randolph Field, Texas.

Balke, B. (1964). *Am. J. Cardiol.* **14**, 796.

Balke, B., and Wells, J. G. (1958). *J. Aviation Med.* **29**, 40.

Balke, B., Ellis, J. P., and Wells, J. G. (1958). *J. Appl. Physiol.* **12**, 269.

Balke, B., Nagle, F. J., and Daniels, J. T. (1965). *J. Am. Med. Assoc.* **194**, 646.

Balke, B., Faulkner, J. A., and Daniels, J. T. (1966). *Schweiz. Wochschr. Sportmed.* **14**, 106.

Barbashova, Z. I. (1965). *In* "Handbook of Physiology" (D. B. Dill, E. F. Adolph, and C. G. Wilber, eds.), Sect. 4, pp. 37–54. Williams & Wilkins, Baltimore, Maryland.

Barcroft, J. (1925). "The Respiratory Function of the Blood. Part I. Lessons from High Altitudes." Univ. of Cambridge Press, London and New York.

Beard, E. F., Alexander, D. J., Howell, T. W., and Reissmann, K. R. (1951). "Dynamics of Blood Flow Under Abnormal Pressure," Proj. No. 21-23-019, Rept. I. U.S.A.F. School of Aviation Med., Randolph Field, Texas.

Berne, R. M. (1964). *Physiol. Rev.* **44**, 1.

Biörck, G. (1949). *Acta Med. Scand.* Suppl. 226, 133.

Buskirk, E. R., Kollias, J., Picon-Reatique, E., Akers, R., Prokop, E., and Baker, P. (1967). *In* "International Symposium on the Effects of Altitude on Physical Performance" (R. F. Goddard, ed.), pp. 65–71. Athletic Inst., Chicago, Illinois.

Christensen, E. H., and Forbes, W. H. (1937). *Skand. Arch. Physiol.* **76**, 75.

Christensen, E. H., and Krogh, A. (1936). *Skand. Arch. Physiol.* **73**, 315.

Christensen, E. H., and Nielsen, H. E. (1936). *Skand. Arch. Physiol.* **74**, 272.

Compos, J., and Iglesias, B. (1956). "Mechanisms of Natural Acclimatization. Preliminary Report on Anatomic Studies at High Altitudes," Rept. No. 55-97. U.S.A.F. School of Aviation Med., Randolph Field, Texas.

Comroe, J. H., and Dripps, R. D. (1945). *Ann. Rev. Physiol.* **7**, 653.

Delachaux, A., and Tissieres, A. (1946). *Helv. Med. Acta* **13**, 333.

Delius, L., Opitz, E., and Schoedel, W. (1942). *Luftfahrtmed.* **6**, 213.

Dill, D. B., Talbott, J. H., and Consolazio, C. F. (1937). *J. Biol. Chem.* **118**, 649.

Dill, D. B., Terman, J. W., and Hall, F. G. (1963). *Clin. Chem.* **9**, 710.

Dill, D. B., Robinson, S., Balke, B., and Newton, J. L. (1964). *J. Appl. Physiol.* **19**, 483.

Douglas, C. G., and Haldane, J. S. (1909). *J. Physiol. (London)* **38**, 401.

Douglas, C. G., Haldane, J. S., Henderson, Y., and Schneider, E. C. (1913). *Phil. Trans. Roy. Soc. London* **B203**, 185.

Ewig, W., and Hinsberg, K. (1931). *Z. Klin. Med.* **115**, 732.

Fahrens, R., and Lindquist, T. (1931). *Am. J. Physiol.* **96**, 562.

Fenn, W. O. (1954). *In* "Handbook of Respiratory Physiology" (W. M. Boothby, ed.), pp. 19–27. Air University, U.S.A.F. School of Aviation Med., San Antonio, Texas.

Greene, C. W., and Gilbert, N. C. (1921). *A.M.A. Arch. Internal Med.* **27**, 517.

Grollman, A. (1930). *Am. J. Physiol.* **93**, 19.

Grover, R. F., and Reeves, J. T. (1966). *Schweiz. Wochschr. Sportmed.* **14**, 130.

Hall, F. G. (1960). *J. Aviation Med.* **31**, 649.

Hall, P. W., III. (1953). *Circulation Res.* **1**, 238.

Hamilton, W. F. (1960). *In* "Medical Physics" (O. Glaser, ed.), p. 119. Year Book Publ., Chicago, Illinois.

Hartmann, H., Hepp, G., and Luft, U. C. (1941). *Luftfahrtmed.* **6**, 1.

Hasselbalch, K. A., and Lindhard, J. (1915). *Biochem. Z.* **68**, 295.

Hecht, H. H., Kuida, H., Lange, R. L., Thorne, J. L., and Brown, A. M. (1962). *Am. J. Med.* **31**, 171.

Hedin, S. (1899). Durch Asiens Wüsten, Leipzig.

Herxheimer, H., Kost, R., and Ryjaczek, K. (1933). *Arbeitsphysiol.* **7**, 308.

Hollmann, W., and Venrath, H. (1966). *Schweiz. Wochschr. Sportmed.* **14**, 27.

Hurtado, A. (1956). "Mechanism of Natural Acclimatization," Rept. No. 56-1. U.S.A.F. School of Aviation Med., Randolph Field, Texas.

Hurtado, A. (1964). *In* "Handbook of Physiology" (D. B. Dill, E. F. Adolph, and C. G. Wilber, eds.), Sect. 4, pp. 843–860. Williams & Wilkins, Baltimore, Maryland.

Hurtado, A., Merino, C., and Delgado, E. (1945). *A.M.A. Arch. Internal Med.* **75**, 284.

Johnson, W. W. (1965). "The Andean Republics." *Life World Library*, Time Inc., New York.

Keys, A. (1938). *Ergeb. Inn. Med. Kinderheilk.* **54**, 585.

Klausen, K., Robinson, S., Michael, E. D., and Myhre, L. G. (1966). *J. Appl. Physiol.* **21** 1191.

Luft, U. C. (1941). *Ergeb. Physiol., Biol. Chem. Exptl. Pharmakol.* **44**, 256.

Luft, U. C. (1965). *In* "Handbook of Physiology" (Wallace O. Fenn and H. Rahn, eds.), Vol. 3, pp. 1099–1146. Williams & Wilkins, Baltimore, Maryland.

Marbarger, J. P., Weichselberg, P. H., Pestel, C. V., Vawter, G. F., and Franzblau, S. A. (1954). "Altitude Stress in Subjects with Impaired Cardio-Respiratory Function," Proj. No. 21-23-019, Rept. 4. U.S.A.F. School of Aviation Med., Randolph Field, Texas.

Motley, H. L., Gournand, A., Werkö, L., Himmelstein, A., and Dresdale, D. (1947). *Am. J. Physiol.* **150**, 315.

Noell, W., and Schneider, M. (1944). *Pfl. Arch. Ges. Physiol.* **247**, 514.

Norton, E. F. (1925). "The Fight for Everest, 1924." Longmans, Green, New York.

Oda, T. (1965). *Osaka City Med. J.* **11**, 59.

Opitz, E. (1941). *Ergeb. Physiol., Biol. Chem. Exptl. Pharmakol.* **44**, 315.

Owen, J. R., and Pugh, L. G. C. (1966). "Report of Medical Research Project into Effects of Altitude in Mexico City." Brit. Olympic Assoc., London.

Pugh, L. G. C. (1964). *In* "Handbook of Physiology" (D. B. Dill, E. F. Adolph, and C. G. Wilber, eds.), Sect. 4, pp. 861–868. Williams & Wilkins, Baltimore, Maryland.

Rahn, H., and Otis, A. B. (1949). *Am. J. Physiol.* **157**, 445.

Reichel, H. (1944). *Klin. Wochschr.* **23**, 235.

Riley, R. L., Otis, A. B., and Houston, C. S. (1954). *In* "Handbook of Respiratory Physiology" (W. M. Boothby, ed.), pp. 143–157. Air University, U.S.A.F. School of Aviation Med., San Antonio, Texas.

Riviera-Estrada, C., Saltzman, P. W., Singer, D., and Katz, L. N. (1958). *Circulation Res.* **6**, 10.

Rotta, A. (1961). *In* "Cardiology. An Encyclopedia of the Cardiovascular System" (A. A. Luisada, ed.), Vol. 5, Part 25, p. 3. McGraw-Hill, New York.

Saltin, B. (1966). *Schweiz. Wochschr. Sportmed.* **14**, 81.

Talbott, J. H., and Dill, D. B. (1936). *Am. J. Med. Sci.* **192**, 626.

Van Liere, E. J., and Stickney, J. C. (1963). "Hypoxia." Univ. of Chicago Press, Chicago, Illinois.

Velásquez, T. (1959). *J. Appl. Physiol.* **14**, 357.

Velásquez, T., and Balke, B. (1956). Unpublished data.

Viault, F. (1890). *Compt. Rend.* **111**, 917.

von Euler, U.S., and Liljestrand, G. (1946). *Acta Physiol. Scand.* **12**, 301.

Warburg, O. (1914). *Ergeb. Physiol., Exptl. Pharmakol.* **14**, 253.

Wells, J. G., Ellis, J. P., and Balke, B. (1956). *Federation Proc.* **15**, 1.

Wiggers, C. J. (1941). *Ann. Internal Med.* **14**, 1237.

Wiggers, C. J., Hurlimann, A., and Hall, P. W., III. (1953). *Science* **117**, 473.

Zimkin, N. V. (1966). Personal communication.

Zuntz, N., Loewy, A., Müller, F., and Caspari, W. (1906). "Höhenklima und Bergwanderungen in ihren Wirkungen auf den Menschen." Deutsches Verlagshaus Bong & Co., Berlin.

10

THE RELATIVE ENERGY REQUIREMENTS OF PHYSICAL ACTIVITY

E. W. Banister and S. R. Brown

I. Introduction

The prime source of energy for man and animals is the sun. Through the intermediary of green plants, energy from the sun, water, carbon dioxide, and the elements is synthesized to food. Man may then use this food to provide the energy for his metabolic processes and the performance of external work. This energetic cycle perpetuates itself and is manifest in molecular disintegrations, rearrangements and resyntheses and leads finally to the operation of those processes controlling the central nervous, endocrine, respiratory, cardiovascular, excretory, locomotive, and reproductive systems of the body.

Although man is subject to many other energetic interactions in his environment, his major source of energy is food and its major transforms heat and mechanical work.

Mechanisms on which energy transformations are based have been conceived from the earliest times as residing, ultimately, in atomic movements. Thus, as early as the fifth century BC, the Greek philosopher Democritus speculated on a universe composed of countless infinitesimal balls called atoms.

Through the work of such men as Bernouilli, Boyle, Charles, Gay-Lussac, Avogadro, Maxwell, Lavoisier and many others, the laws basic to the calculation of energy transformations were laid down and the nature of combustion understood. A practical approach to the study of heat exchanges was made by Carnot with his investigation of the ideal steam engine, emphasizing a basic physical law, the Second Law of Thermodynamics, that heat will not flow of its own accord from a cold to a hot body.

A sober fact of all energy transformations is that some energy of such processes is always dissipated as heat, never again able to do useful work. This unidirectional flow of energy leads to the conclusion that once the energy of the universe ceases to exist there will remain no potential source for energy transformations and the performance of useful work. A state of what is termed maximum entropy will result. Entropy, the Greek word "change," is thus a measure of how level the energy of the universe is. When the sink of energy dissipated reaches the level of the potential energy source, no more work may be done. Although the final temperature of the universe may be very hot, intermediate, or very cold, it will be perfectly homogeneous and unavailable for energy transformations.

Besides investigations of the purely physical manifestations of energy in the form of chemical, heat, light, electrical, mechanical, and acoustical energy, the bioenergetic changes which occur in man have been increasingly studied. Beginning with those processes which are grossly evident in the respiration (oxygen uptake and carbon dioxide elimination), and body temperature (heat), there has been constant refinement in the techniques of experimentation and the collaboration of many disciplines so that now the processes taking place at molecular levels are better understood, although this is not the substance of this chapter. A variety of methods have been developed to study man's energetic interactions with his environment and these will now be discussed.

II. Calorimetric Methods

A. Direct Methods—Heat Exchange Calorimeter

1. Bomb Calorimetry

The nutritional value of food has been determined using the bomb calorimeter, Fig. 1(II). In this method a weighed amount of substance is placed in the bomb and weighed again with it. After placing the calorimeter in a weighed amount of water, oxygen is admitted under high pressure and the whole ignited. The mass of water and the temperature rise are measures of the heat evolved in the combustion after certain corrections are made. This classic method, although highly reproducible, is hardly applicable to the study of the heat exchanges in living organisms under normal conditions of temperature and pressure.

2. Animal Calorimetry

First adaptations of the bomb calorimeter principle to the study of living organisms were those of de Laplace and Lavoisier in the eighteenth century where the heat production of animals melted ice surrounding the calorimeter. Heat production was the product of the weight of ice melted and its latent heat.

3. Adiabatic Calorimetry

Modifications in this simple method insured no heat was gained or lost by the walls of the calorimeter chamber during the experiment. This was done by collecting the heat produced in water circulating through pipes on one side of a double walled calorimeter. The temperature gradient between the two walls of the calorimeter was maintained at zero by heating or cooling the outside

DIRECT CALORIMETRY

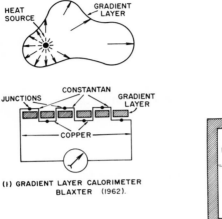

(I) GRADIENT LAYER CALORIMETER
BLAXTER (1962).

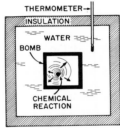

(II) BOMB CALORIMETER

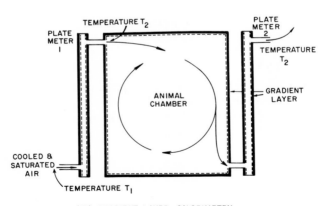

(III) GRADIENT LAYER CALORIMETRY

Fig. 1. Evolution of metabolic energy evaluation methods. (Segments reprinted with permission of cited authors and their publishers.)

EVALUATION

OPEN CIRCUIT RESPIROMETRY

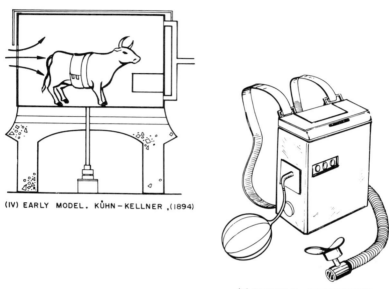

(IV) EARLY MODEL, KÜHN–KELLNER ,(1894)

(V) PORTABLE RESPIROMETER
KOFRANYI-MICHAELIS-MÜLLER
(1941)

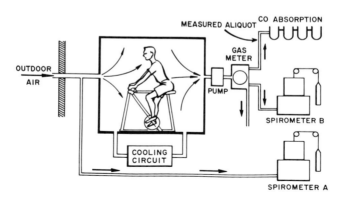

(VI) FIXED OPEN CIRCUIT RESPIROMETER, BLAXTER (1962)

Fig. 1. (*Continued*)

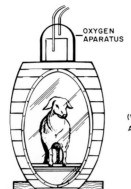

OXYGEN
APARATUS

(VII) EARLY MODEL REGNAULT
AND REISET (1849)

(VIII) CLOSED CIRCUIT RESPIROMETER, BLAXTER (1962)

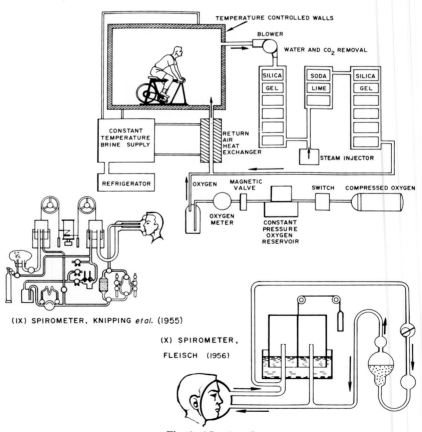

TEMPERATURE CONTROLLED WALLS

BLOWER

WATER AND CO_2 REMOVAL

SILICA GEL

SODA LIME

SILICA GEL

CONSTANT
TEMPERATURE
BRINE SUPPLY

RETURN
AIR
HEAT
EXCHANGER

STEAM INJECTOR

REFRIGERATOR

OXYGEN

MAGNETIC
VALVE

SWITCH

COMPRESSED OXYGEN

OXYGEN
METER

CONSTANT
PRESSURE
OXYGEN
RESERVOIR

(IX) SPIROMETER, KNIPPING *et al.* (1955)

(X) SPIROMETER,

FLEISCH (1956)

Fig. 1. (*Continued*)

EVALUATION·

RESPIROMETRY

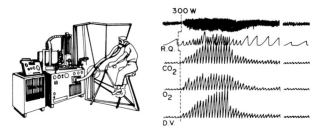

(XI) METABULATOR — ERGOMETER, FLEISCH ,(1956)

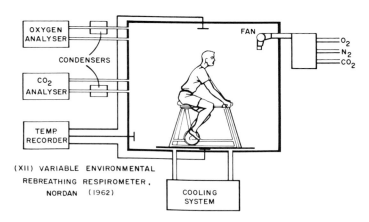

(XII) VARIABLE ENVIRONMENTAL
REBREATHING RESPIROMETER,
NORDAN (1962)

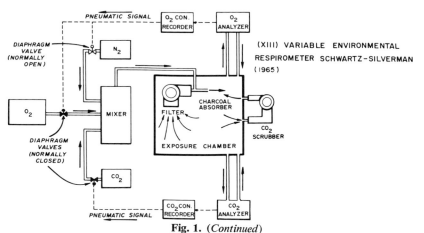

(XIII) VARIABLE ENVIRONMENTAL
RESPIROMETER SCHWARTZ—SILVERMAN
(1965)

Fig. 1. (*Continued*)

wall appropriately and thus all the heat produced was collected by the circulating water. After correction for the heat lost by the animal in vaporizing water and adding to the humidity and temperature of the air flow ventilating the chamber, the heat exchange due to convection and radiation could be calculated.

4. Gradient Layer Calorimetry

The rate of heat flow through the containing wall of a calorimeter chamber, Fig. 1(I), is given by Eq. (1):

$$dH/dt = \lambda S(T_i - T_o)t \tag{1}$$

where:
λ = thermal conductivity of the wall
S = surface area of wall
t = thickness
dH/dt = rate of heat flow
$T_i - T_o$ = temperature gradient between the inside and outside

By measuring the temperature gradient at the surface of the calorimeter with thermoelectrically active junctions (copper-constantan) and a galvonometer circuit, the rate of heat flow at the surface, due to the contents of the chamber, may be estimated. Care must be taken to keep the outermost wall of the calorimeter at a precise temperature. The heat content of the ventilating air which is necessarily increased by the animal respirations must also be determined in order to obtain the complete heat balance, Fig. 1(III). A complication of this method is the variable heat content of objects contained in the chamber. This type of apparatus has been constructed to such a degree of precision and sensitivity as to record the heat emission from a hen's egg during incubation. The types of apparatus outlined above have been mainly used in studying the heat exchanges in animals and have been profitably used in collecting a large amount of data in animal science (Brody, 1945; Kleiber, 1961; Blaxter, 1962). The elegance of the methods, however, could well be examined and exploited by the human work physiologist.

B. INDIRECT METHODS

Since direct methods of estimating heat exchanges in animals and man in response to food consumption require expensive and extensive instrumentation, indirect methods have been applied. These methods, and the subsequent computation of heat produced, are based on the measurement of oxygen consumed, carbon dioxide eliminated, and nitrogen excreted in the urine. The three main foodstuffs considered as energy sources are carbohydrate, fat, and protein, and the heat produced is calculated according to Eq. (2):

$$\text{Heat produced} = a\text{O}_2 \text{ consumed} + b\text{CO}_2 \text{ produced} - c\text{N excreted} \quad (2)$$
$$\quad\quad \text{(kcal)} \quad\quad\quad\quad \text{(liters)} \quad\quad\quad\quad \text{(liters)} \quad\quad\quad \text{(gm)}$$

where the value of the coefficients a, b, c, are 3.9141, 1.106, and 2.17, respectively, calculated by Weir (1949), and 3.941, 1.106, and 2.13, calculated by Boyd (1954), as they are applied to man.

Heat retained in terms of carbon and nitrogen balance has been expressed by Blaxter and Rook (1953) for animals as Eq. 3:

$$\text{kcal energy retained} = 12.55 \times \text{gm C retained} - 6.90 \times \text{gm N retained} \quad (3)$$

Thus, if the heat energy of the food eaten is calculated and the heat of combustion of substances which are stored in and lost to the body are estimated, the overall energy production is the difference between the two.

Although it must be emphasized that these indirect methods are imprecise in the absolute sense, they have been found to be in good agreement with animal heat production estimates from direct methods (Forbes *et al.*, 1928).

The design of apparatus to measure the rate of exchange of the respiratory gases between the test subject and his environment—essential to the indirect determination of heat balance—has taken two main forms.

1. Open Circuit Respirometry

Outdoor air passes through the respirometry chamber, Fig. 1(IV), and changes are measured in the concentration of the outflow gases. If the total volume of the air circulated is known, and the change in concentration of its constituents (oxygen and carbon dioxide) due to the respiration of the test subject is also known, the oxygen consumption and carbon dioxide elimination may be calculated. The measurement of the air volume in this type of respirometer must be very precise; true samples of the inflowing and outflowing gases must be obtained and their analysis very accurately performed.

The form of the respirometer chamber may take several shapes. It may be a permanent structure large enough to house animal farmstock, Fig 1(VI), or it may simply consist of a valve mouthpiece connected through rubber hose to a Douglas bag. Portable modifications of the instrument are the Kofranyi-Michaelis (K-M) meter, Fig. 1(V), and the integrating motor pneumotachograph (Wolff, 1958). The K-M meter is capable of monitoring up to 80 liters of ventilation per minute without serious error and removing aliquot samples of the respired air for later analysis.

The technical problems of air hoseways and breathing valves are associated with the increased difficulty of breathing at high ventilation rates and the accumulation of carbon dioxide in the breathing space at low rates although improved high velocity valves are now obtainable (Bannister and Cormak, 1954). Correction to the volume of the respired gas has to be applied since rates are usually referred to standard temperature and pressure after correcting for the water vapor added to the air by the subject and atmospheric humidity (STPD). These corrections are made from tables (Carpenter, 1948) based on the following equation:

$$V_{STPD} = 273V (P_B - P_{H_2O})/(273 + t) 760 \text{ liters}$$

V = volume of air in liters under experimental conditions
760 = standard atmospheric pressure in mm Hg
273 = degrees standard temperature in Absolute scale
t = ambient temperature °C
P_B = atmospheric pressure mm Hg
P_{H_2O} = pressure of saturated water vapor at the ambient temperature

2. Closed Circuit Respirometry

In this method [Fig. 1(VII)] air is circulated continuously both through the experimental chamber and through oxygen and carbon dioxide analyzers. In most cases the carbon dioxide is absorbed and determined gravimetrically while the partial pressure of oxygen is maintained by admitting oxygen to the chamber in the amount that it is being used by the subject. Careful control of the chamber temperature and pressure is essential and the gross dimensions of the chamber become a limiting factor in the absolute accuracy of the calculations (Kleiber, 1961). Unless carbon dioxide is removed, its accumulation could affect the normal ventilatory pattern although accumulations up to 1% of carbon dioxide have not, in the authors' experience, caused errors of this nature. The advantages to free movement of the subject within the chamber unhampered by attachments to air hoses or collection apparatus is apparent, Fig. 1(VIII). European developments have been adapted to cranking machines or bicycle ergometers, Figs. 1(X and XI). The difficulties inherent in long air hoses and face masks have been overcome to a large extent by the double capacity of the respirometer tanks, Fig. 1(IX), and the high air flow rate maintained through the face mask. Continuous registration of the respired gases is made on a recording kymograph.

3. Closed Circuit Rebreathing Respirometer

This type of apparatus, Fig. 1(XII), has been used for short-duration experiments and consists of a conventional closed circuit apparatus without the additional modifications needed to maintain atmospheric proportions of oxygen and carbon dioxide. Thus carbon dioxide accumulates in the chamber and oxygen diminishes from the fixed initial level. However, these changes have not seemed to be a complicating factor when the oxygen level does not fall below 18% and the carbon dioxide level does not exceed 1%. Table I

(Banister, 1966) indicates the reproducibility of data in one such type of respirometer in nine successive bicycle ergometer rides at the same work task for
one subject.

Closed circuit respirometers offer the additional facility of manipulating
the environmental air so that any desired partial pressure of oxygen or carbon
dioxide may be achieved inside the chamber. The respirometers of Schwartz
and Silverman (1965), Fig. 1(XIII), and Nordan (1962) are suited to this
purpose.

TABLE I

STANDARD DEVIATION OF OXYGEN CONSUMPTION IN CLOSED CIRCUIT
REBREATHING RESPIROMETRY

Time course of work and recovery (min)	Gross V_{O_2} (liters)	$\dot{V}_{O_2}$ (liters/min)	$\ddot{V}_{O_2}$ (liters/min^2)
2	3.71 ± 12.7%	2.14 ± 18.7%	0.384 ± 34.2%
8	19.90 ± 5.5%	2.61 ± 6.7%	0.146 ± 100.0%
15	41.76 ± 3.3%	2.51 ± 9.2%	−0.681 ± 25.1%
20	48.44 ± 3.5%	0.57 ± 18.6%	−0.256 ± 38.0%

Regardless of the method of arranging the course, or the collection of the
gas flow, the analysis of the gases resulting from the respiratory exchanges has
to be accurately measured. Extensive research utilizing the methods of the
physical sciences has seen developed a large variety of apparatus for analyzing
respiratory gases.

4. Methods of Analyzing Respiratory Gases

a. Gravimetric Methods. Early use was made of the fact that carbon dioxide
may be absorbed in soda lime. The gas absorbed from the outflow of a
respiratory chamber may thus be absorbed and determined by weighing,
Fig. 2 (I,a,1).

Similarly, by carefully removing water vapor and carbon dioxide from the
air stream into the respiration chamber and absorbing carbon dioxide and
water vapor produced by respiration in it, a gravimetric determination of the
oxygen absorbed and carbon dioxide produced may be made, Fig. 2 (I,a,2).

b. Volumetric–Chemical Analysis. Great precision in the analysis of
respiratory gases may be made by selective absorption of oxygen and carbon
dioxide in a known volume of air by chemical absorbents. The absorption
produces volume decrements in the initial volume which may be expressed in
terms of the percentage of oxygen and carbon dioxide in the original sample.

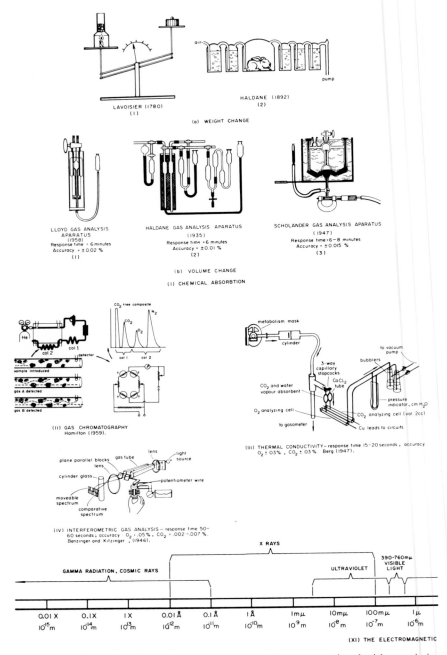

LAVOISIER (1780)
(1)

HALDANE (1892)
(2)

(a) WEIGHT CHANGE

LLOYD GAS ANALYSIS
APARATUS
(1958)
Response time = 6 minutes
Accuracy = ±0.02 %
(1)

HALDANE GAS ANALYSIS APARATUS
(1935)
Response time = 6 minutes
Accuracy = ±0.01 %
(2)

SCHOLANDER GAS ANALYSIS APARATUS
(1947)
Response time = 6−8 minutes
Accuracy = ±0.015 %
(3)

(b) VOLUME CHANGE

(I) CHEMICAL ABSORBTION

(II) GAS CHROMATOGRAPHY
Hamilton (1959).

(III) THERMAL CONDUCTIVITY − response time 15−20 seconds , accuracy
$O_2 \pm 03\%$, $CO_2 \pm 03\%$ Berg (1947).

(IV) INTERFEROMETRIC GAS ANALYSIS − response time 50−
60 seconds ; accuracy $O_2 \pm .05\%$, $CO_2 \pm .002 -.007\%$.
Benzinger and Kitzinger , (1946).

X RAYS

GAMMA RADIATION, COSMIC RAYS

ULTRAVIOLET

390−760mµ
VISIBLE
LIGHT

| 0.01 X | 0.1 X | 1 X | 0.01 Å | 0.1 Å | 1 Å | 1mµ | 10mµ | 100mµ | 1µ |
| 10^{15}m | 10^{14}m | 10^{13}m | 10^{12}m | 10^{11}m | 10^{10}m | 10^{9}m | 10^{8}m | 10^{7}m | 10^{6}m |

(XI) THE ELECTROMAGNETIC

Fig. 2. Methods of analysis of respiratory gases. (Segments reprinted with permission of cited authors and their publishers.)

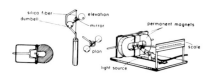

(V) MAGNETIC SUSCEPTIBILITY – PAULING GAS ANALYSER – response time 30 – 50 seconds, accuracy O₂ ± 0.01 %, suitable for continuous sampling. Pauling *et al* (1946).

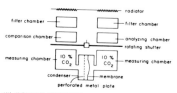

(VI) INFRARED ABSORBTION – response time 0.1 second, accuracy 0.01 – 0.02 %. Schmeiser, as presented by White *et al* (1958)

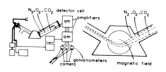

(VII) MASS SPECTROMETRY – response time (later models) 0.12 second, accuracy error less than 1% of full scale deflection, suitable for breath by breath analysis. Lilly (1950), modified from White *et al* (1958).

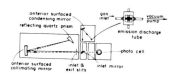

(VIII) EMISSION SPECTROSCOPY – response time 0.1 second, accuracy 0.01 – 0.02 %. White *et al* (1956).

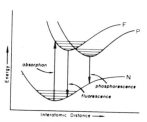

(IX) LUMINESCENCE – Response time less than 0.1 second, accuracy ± .01 %, suitable for breath by breath analysis.

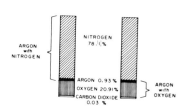

(X) CONCENTRATION OF GASES IN ATMOSPHERIC AIR

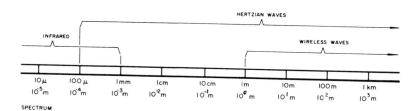

SPECTRUM

Fig. 2. (*Continued*)

i. Haldane gas analyzer. Carbon dioxide is absorbed in potassium hydroxide and oxygen is absorbed in sodium anthraquinone sulfonate solution, Fig. 2(I,b,2). The remaining gas in the sample is assumed to be nitrogen. Accuracy to a level of ± 0.02 vol % may be obtained with the instrument which has, however, the limitation that gas mixtures with high absorbable gas concentrations may not be analyzed with it. An analysis requires from 6–8 min.

ii. Scholander micrometer gas analyzer. The Scholander analyzer, Fig. 2 (I,b,3), uses the same chemical absorbents as the Haldane method. It achieves an accuracy of ± 0.015 vol % and is able to analyze samples containing from zero to over 99% of absorbable gases. The analysis time is again 6–8 min.

iii. Gallenkamp-Lloyd gas analyzer. This apparatus, Fig. 2 (I,b,1), a later modification of the original Haldane model, is accurate to ± 0.02 vol %, and is able to make an analysis in less than 6 min. It is self-compensating for temperature variations and has the merit of being compact, portable, and ideally suited to field use.

*c. Physical Methods of Analysis.** Increasing use has been made of the different physical properties of gases in determining their concentration in respired air. Although the initial calibration of this type of apparatus is usually made with known gaseous mixtures previously analyzed with the established chemical-volumetric apparatus, they offer advantages in their ease of operation, improved response time to changing gas concentrations, and their ability to give continuous records rather than single evaluations of separate samples.

i. Thermal conductivity methods. When a resistance wire is heated in the path of a gas flow, the heat generated is conducted away in a manner proportional to the thermal conductivity of the particular gas, Fig. 2 (III). Depending on the rate with which heat is conducted away, the temperature of the resistance wire will change. If the resistance is made one arm of a Wheatstone bridge arrangement, increasing temperature of the detector arm causes its resistance to increase and disbalance the bridge circuit. The electrical disbalance may finally be represented in a curve traced on an X-Y recorder where the amplitude of the vertical displacement will be proportional to the gas concentration. In practice, the test gas, from which carbon dioxide and water have been removed, is compared with air from which carbon dioxide and water have been removed. Similarly for carbon dioxide, the response of the test gas from which water vapor and carbon dioxide are removed is compared with the test gas from which water vapor has been

---

* The authors are indebted to a comprehensive review of methodology by White (1958) for much of the material in this section and to which the interested reader is referred further.

removed. These types of analyzers have a reported accuracy of ± 0.03 vol %
and a response time of 15–30 sec. They are suitable as continuous analyzers
but not for breath by breath analysis (White, 1958).

ii. Gas chromatography. The gas chromatograph, Fig. 2 (II), is an instrument incorporating the physical principles of thermal conductivity and
chromatographic separation of different gases according to their molecular
shape and size by molecular sieves. Certain aluminosilicates having the
property of acting as molecular sieves after being activated by heat, selectively
separate the several components of a gas mixture which may then be analyzed
by thermal conductivity methods. Helium gas is usually used as a carrier to
transport the test gas through the chromatographic columns. Since helium
has a high thermal conductivity, an ability to keep the thermistors at a steady
temperature and the bridge system in balance, the introduction of a
contaminant gas in the carrier stream will cause a disbalance of the system proportional to the concentration of the contaminant. An analysis may be performed in 4–7 min with an accuracy of 0.01 vol %. A particular complication
of gas chromatography which has to be allowed for is the preferential
analysis of argon in combination with oxygen. No practical chromatographic column effectively separates argon (present in the respired gases)
from oxygen.

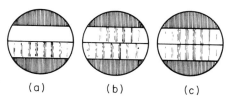

(a)   (b)   (c)

Fig. 3. Interference patterns in interferometric gas analysis. (Reprinted with permission from Mellerowicz, 1962.)

iii. Interferometry. If light is passed through a narrow slit it produces interference patterns which may be directed through a column of reference gas,
Fig. 2 (IV). A similar diffraction pattern viewed through a column of the test
gas will be latterly displaced on a screen proportionately with the concentration of the test gas, Fig. 3. The extent of replacement necessary for super-
position of the test interference pattern on the reference pattern may be made
proportional to a resistance change and recorded as a variable voltage. The
method is free from temperature and pressure effects and possesses extreme
stability. The accuracy of the method ranges from ± 0.05 vol % of oxygen to
± 0.007 vol % for carbon dioxide with a time response of 50–60 sec (White,
1958).

iv. Acoustic analyzers. Some use has been made of the variation of the velocity of sound in different gases to construct an analyzing apparatus, although it is doubtful if the method will find extensive application in the analysis of the respiratory gases (White, 1958).

v. Paramagnetic analyzers. The partial pressure of oxygen in the respired air will be preferentially estimated in this type of analyzer, Fig. 2 (V), since the volume magnetic susceptibility of oxygen, on which it depends, is much larger for oxygen than for other gases. Any element containing unpaired electrons will align itself in the direction of a magnetic field surrounding it. The resultant force on glass spheres, surrounded by the oxygen test gas when placed in a homogeneous magnetic field, produces a measure of the gas concentration. Rotation of the spheres may be made to displace a light beam for direct recording. The method is fast and accurate with a response time as low as 10 to 15 sec and an accuracy equal to that of the Haldane method. The instrument may also be used to meter water vapor and carbon dioxide.

vi. Spectroscopic methods. Visible light is only a small part of the energy spectrum, Fig. 2 (XI), called electromagnetic radiation, which is propagated as a wave phenomenon characterized by a frequency η, a wavelength λ, and a constant velocity c in a vacuum.

When light penetrates matter it may pass directly through or be absorbed. If the light is absorbed totally or in part, energy is imparted to the substance of the absorbing medium. Depending on the characteristics of the energizing light and those of the absorbing medium, typical spectra of light absorption or emission may be observed either as energy is absorbed by or released from the medium during its excitation and subsequent return to the normal state. These physical properties are used in several methods for determining gas concentrations. Absorption in the infrared usually causes molecular vibrations whereas that in the visible and ultraviolet causes molecular excitation to new energy levels, Fig. 2 (IX) (Udenfriend, 1962).

(1). *Infrared absorption*, Fig. 2 (VI). Carbon dioxide, carbon monoxide, and water vapor absorb light strongly in the infrared region of the spectrum as shown in Table II (Spoor, 1948).

TABLE II

ABSORPTION WAVELENGTHS IN THE INFRARED

Gas	Wavelength for maximal absorption (microns)
Carbon dioxide (CO_2)	4.3
Carbon monoxide (CO)	4.7
Water vapor (H_2O)	6.0

By introducing pulses of infrared light from a source on to a sample cell and analyzer cell, carbon dioxide in the gas of the analyzer cell will result in the absorption of a larger amount of light energy proportional to the concentration of the gas in the analyzer cell. The resulting infrared beams are directed to two sides of a movable diaphragm which is part of a capacitance manometer surrounded on all sides by an infrared absorbing gas. The different infrared energy reaching each side of the diaphragm will cause pulsation in it and result in a varying condenser capacity in the capacitance manometer circuit proportional to the varying gas concentration in the analyzer cell. Modifications of the general principle have resulted in instruments for which a speed of response of 0.04 sec and an accuracy of 0.1 vol % are claimed (Young and Robinson, 1954). The specificity of this type of instrument results from the characteristic wavelengths exhibited by different gases for the maximal absorption of infrared radiation. By introducing filters through which light from the infrared source passes, any gas may thus be preferentially analyzed even in the presence of the others.

(2). *Mass spectroscopic methods*, Fig. 2 (VII). The principle of the mass spectrograph first proposed by Aston (1942) has been very successfully applied to gas analyzers. In this method, the gas mixture is ionized at low pressure and the ionized particles accelerated by electrical means and passed through a magnetic field. The ions are thus distributed throughout a spectrum according to their mass number. Collecting electrodes are situated at points in the accelerating tubes coincident with the points of deflection of the different ionized gases. The amount of ion-current collected by the electrode will be proportional to the particular gas concentration. Recent modifications of the method have reported a response time of 0.12 sec and an accuracy greater than 1% of the full-scale deflection. The chief advantages of the method are the small response time, the ability to measure the respiratory gases, each specifically and separately in one instrument within the same time period. The recent development of a mass spectrographic method having a response time of less than 0.1 sec, capable of analyzing carbon dioxide, oxygen, nitrogen, and argon simultaneously in concentrations of each gas ranging from less than 3% to an accuracy of 1 to 3% of full-scale deflection, is an outstanding contribution (Fowler and Hugh-Jones, 1957).

(3). *Emission spectroscopy*. Considerable work has recently been done by Lovelace II and White (1958) in applying the technique of emission spectroscopy to gas analysis. The light sources used for exciting the test gases were electrically energized discharge tubes around which the test gas was made to flow. When the gas absorbs energy from the light source, its molecules become excited, emitting radiation at a longer wavelength than that of absorption while some energy is dissipated as heat. Using a special instrument, the spectrophotometer, the emitted radiation can be collected by a photo-multiplier. The intensity of the emitted radiation is determined at different wavelengths. Preliminary work shows linearity of carbon dioxide emission intensity at 2896 Å (10^{-8}cm), the emission of oxygen in the near infrared 10,000 Å, and nitrogen at 7000–8000 Å. Potentially, emission spectroscopy offers the most versatile, accurate, and quick method. Limitations are presented by technical complexity and maintenance of the equipment.

III. Time and Motion Studies

A. MOTION PICTURE ANALYSIS OF ACTIVITY*

Movements involved during the expenditure of energy are particularly suited to permanent recording by motion picture film and later analysis by film projection. The technique of photography has been developed so that ultrahigh-speed cameras up to 16,000 frames/sec may be used in the recording of events (Waddell and Waddell, 1955). Particular attention to detail before and during filming is an essential of recording events for scientific analysis. Optimum subject size should be obtained in each frame by excluding unnecessary items from the picture field. Subject contrast with the background field should be emphasized and, if necessary, a calibrated background provided (McIntosh, 1958). Sufficient illumination of the subject must be retained. Several sources are available (Lester, 1954). The type of film used does not differ materially regardless of the filming speed. Black and white is most useful and its exposure time standard in photography procedures. Suggestions for camera speeds depend on the duration of the event studied, as shown by Eq. (4) (Eastman Kodak, 1953):

$$\text{Camera speed} = 40 \text{ (subject speed, inches/sec)/field width, inches} \qquad (4)$$

or by Eq. (5) (Hyzer, 1955):

$$R = (500S/W) \cos \theta \qquad (5)$$

where:

R = frames/sec
S = subject velocity ft/sec
W = field width inches
θ = angle between line of motion and film plane

Too low a repetition rate results in blurred images, too high a rate will still produce excellent pictures for frame by frame analysis.

* The authors are indebted to a review by Palmer (1958) for material in this section to which the interested reader is referred for further information.

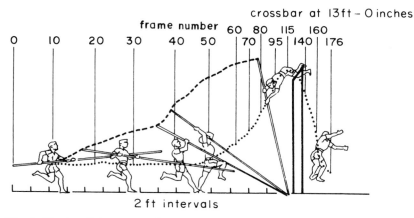

Fig. 4. Tracks of the center of gravity and of the top of the pole during a practice vault. The frame numbers refer to the position of the center of gravity which is marked with a circle every 1/16 sec (i.e., every fourth frame of film taken at 64 frames/sec). (Reprinted with permission from Fletcher *et al.*, 1960.)

Analysis of the film may be made in a variety of film readers. Probably the most versatile analytical projector is the Bell and Howell* 16-mm analyzer, allowing frame by frame analysis. Adaptation of the 3M† Filmac 400 microfilm reader-printer to film analysis would probably be advantageous. Data from frame by frame analysis of the film record is usually presented in time-displacement curves of the body center of gravity or some other body part, Fig. 4 (Fletcher *et al.*, 1960). Differentiation of this primary curve will yield

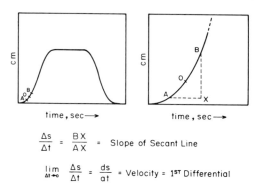

$$\frac{\Delta s}{\Delta t} = \frac{BX}{AX} = \text{Slope of Secant Line}$$

$$\lim_{\Delta t \to 0} \frac{\Delta s}{\Delta t} = \frac{ds}{dt} = \text{Velocity} = 1^{ST} \text{ Differential}$$

Fig. 5. Graphical method for obtaining the first time derivative curve. (Banister *et al.*, 1964a.)

* Bell and Howell Company, 7100 McCormick Road, Chicago 45, Illinois.
† 3M Company Microfilm Products, St. Paul, Minnesota.

the velocity as the first differential and acceleration as the second differential. Differentiation may be done graphically as in Fig. 5 (Banister, 1964a), or better by programming the original time-displacement data for computer differentiation. Integration of the area under the time-acceleration curve is in fact some measure of the energy expenditure in the movement and has been defined by Starr (1951) in units of dyne-sec. Momentary consideration will show, however, that a plot of displacement against acceleration, where corresponding acceleration-displacement points are obtained from the original time displacement curve, yields a curve whose integrated area is in the units appropriate to energy; namely, the dyne-cm or erg when multiplied by the mass of the moving object.

B. Visual Observations/Timing/Energy Estimates

Comparative studies of the calculated energy cost of any particular job together with an assessment of the quality and speed of the work performed are important to the economic aspects of industrial occupations. Estimates of energy expenditure in this type of evaluation are usually made with a K-M meter (Ganslen and Van Huss, 1953) or IMP (Zajaczkowska, 1962) or from the telemetered heart rate (Bonjer, 1962). Improved efficiency in working methods often leads to a better utilization of the energy available from the worker, Figs. 6 and 7.

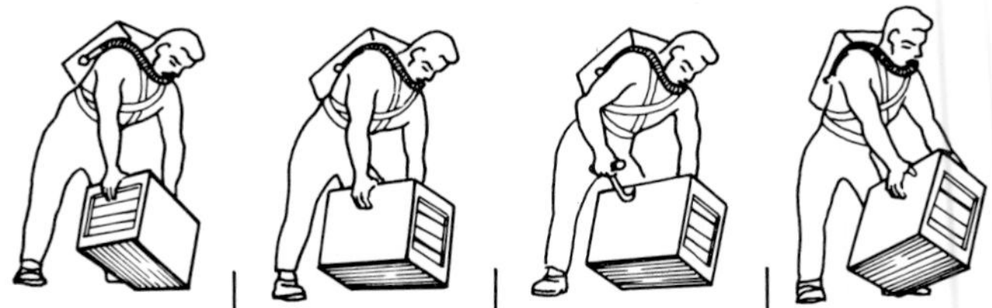

	METHOD I Tilting on short edges	METHOD II Tilting on long edges	METHOD III Tilting on long edges with hook	METHOD IV Turning on angular points
Total kcal/case	2.21	2.49	2.17	1.17
Total heartbeats /case	135	136	152	123
Mechanical work in kgm/case	111.3	107.6	107.6	71.4
Gross efficiency in %	11.8	10.1	11.6	14.3

Fig. 6. Four different methods of handling a packing case in a ship's hold. Note the K-M respirometer on the subject's back. (Reprinted with permission from Bonjer, 1962.)

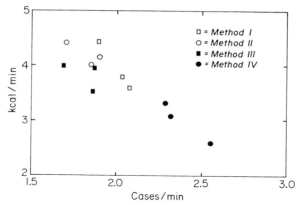

Fig. 7. Dock-workers' experiment: diagram showing energy expenditure per minute plotted against production rate. The table at the bottom of Fig. 6 shows the energy expenditure, the number of heart beats, and the mechanical work required for the transportation of one case. The gross mechanical efficiency has been computed for each of the four methods. (Reprinted with permission from Bonjer, 1962.)

C. ANALYTICAL DIARY METHODS

Only rarely has a determined attempt been made to carry out the task of estimating energy output over an extended period of time, including both the occupational and leisure activity of the individual together with the assessment of his dietary habits and nutritional state. Reiff *et al.* (1964) have made an important contribution in this respect with their development of a physical activity recall record. Previous studies (Pearl, 1924) had made attempts ranging from qualitative estimates to comprehensive quantitative estimates of the energy expenditure of occupational jobs (Passmore and Durnin, 1955). In this last regard, it is germane to the economics of industry that the idea of the "cost price of food calories," essentially a European idea, be fully evaluated, standardized, and paid for before consideration is given to remuneration for other aspects of the job (Kerkhoven, 1962).

IV. The Force Platform

The first force platform was designed by Lauru (1954) to establish the relations between physiological cost and bodily movement by means of the reaction forces imposed on the platform by the movement. Several modifications of the instrument have been developed (Barany and Whetsel, 1962; Carlsöö, 1962). Essentially, the device, Fig. 8, performs a similar analysis to that which can be obtained from motion pictures. The final presentation of force-time curves due to the reactions on the platform by movement in three

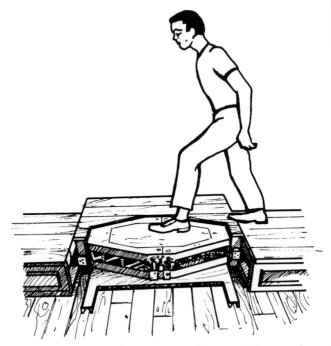

Fig. 8. Force platform method for studying walking on different surfaces. (Reprinted with permission from Carlsöö, 1962.)

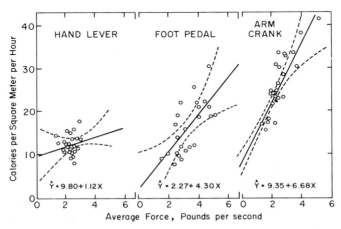

Fig. 9. Regression of average force exerted per second on caloric cost for one subject and three tasks. (Reprinted with permission from Yoder *et al.*, 1964.)

directions, frontal, lateral and vertical, while not in the conventional formulation of work (force-distance), is representative of the work involved. Thus, rather complex movements may be studied if they can be performed within the rather restricted area of the force platform, which is usually of the order of 25 × 25 × 5 inches. Using the technique of Yoder *et al.* (1964), Fig. 9, the regression of caloric output on applied force may be obtained. Figure 10 (Brouha, 1959) serves to illustrate that the external production of

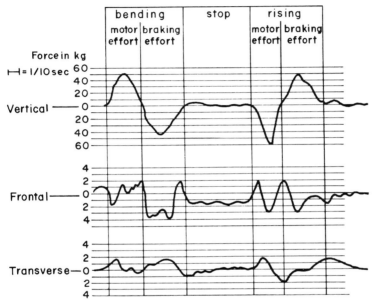

Fig. 10. Forces involved in bending the knees and straightening up as recorded by the Lauru platform in the vertical, frontal, and transversal components. Note scale change for vertical force. (Reprinted with permission from Brouha, 1959.)

work is only one factor in the total physiological cost of activity and that the constant accelerative and decelerative movements of the limbs and body contribute significantly to the energy cost of activity and the onset of fatigue.

V. Regression of Energy Expenditure on Heart Rate, Oxygen Intake, and Ventilation

It is logical to assume and has been verified in practice that energy expenditure, except at maximal work rates, is linearly related to heart rate, oxygen uptake, and ventilation. Thus, these parameters may be used in estimating the amount of work being done in any given task. Perhaps the

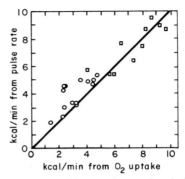

Fig. 11. Work calories as determined from pulse rate in relation to calories determined from oxygen uptake. (Reprinted with permission from Poulsen and Asmussen, 1962.)

most useful of these parameters is the heart rate since it poses relatively little problem to record continuously by radio telemetry (Rose, 1965) during the work task. This method has been used by Poulsen and Asmussen (1962) for job classification. In this method, heart rate is recorded in a typical job situation and also while working at a known rate on a bicycle ergometer, as shown in Eq. (6):

$$\frac{\text{Pulse increase on job}}{\text{Pulse increase ergometer test}} = \frac{\text{work equivalence job}}{\text{cycle work}} \tag{6}$$

Since all values in the formula are known except the job work, it may be estimated. The relationship is shown in Fig. 11.

Similar relationships exist between energy expenditure and oxygen uptake (except near maximal values where linearity curves to asymptotic values), and

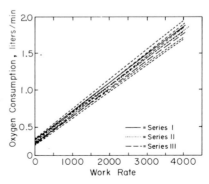

Fig. 12. Regression of work rate on oxygen consumption. Series I is performance of native labor on recruitment; Series II after 1 month of work; Series III after a further 3 months of work. (Reprinted with permission from Maritz *et al.*, 1961.)

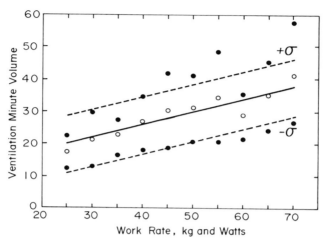

Fig. 13. Regression of ventilation (min vol) on work rate (kg and watt) for 185, 7 to 17-year-old boys performing 1 watt of work per kilogram of body weight. (Reprinted with permission from Mellerowicz, 1962.)

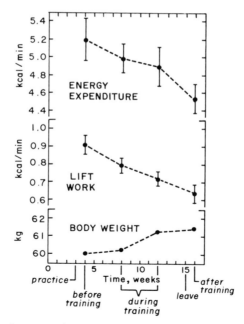

Fig. 14. Mean values, with standard errors, for energy expenditure, lift work, and body weight of 10 subjects walking at 3½ mph on four occasions over a period of training. (Reprinted with permission from Coates and Meade, 1960.)

energy expenditure-ventilation (Maritz *et al.*, 1961). These relationships are shown in Figs. 12 and 13. Care must be taken, however, in using them since it appears that a family of such curves exist. The point of entry into the curves is determined by the age of the subject, his degree of fitness, and the environmental conditions, Figs. 14, 15 (Coates and Meade, 1960; Sjöstrand, 1950).

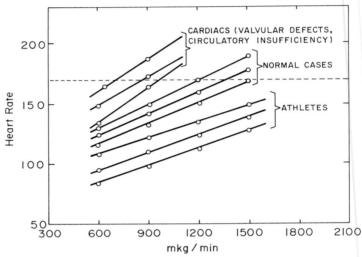

Fig. 15. Dependence of heart rate response on the degree of physical fitness. (Reprinted with permission from Sjöstrand, 1950.)

VI. Theoretical Considerations

A. Positive and Negative Work

It has been described in Section IV how the forces involved in complex movements against gravity are a combination of both accelerative and decelerative processes. The energy of both types of movement must be met out of the overall metabolism and without direct inquiry into the two processes, separately, the demands of each on the physiological reserves cannot be estimated, nor can their individual contribution to the efficiency of the total movement be stated. Now, this is of no moment if our desire is an uncritical evaluation of the gross energy expenditure of different work tasks, but if it is our purpose to modify or even alleviate the metabolic demands of a certain activity then the separate contribution of accelerative and decelerative movements, and the characteristics of muscle working in a positive (concentric) or a negative (eccentric) manner, deserve consideration.

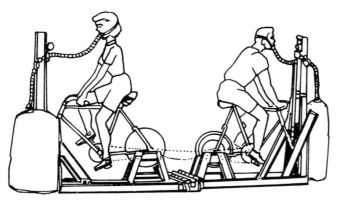

Fig. 16. Two bicycle ergometers coupled together in opposition. The girl back-pedaled (negative work) in opposition to the forward pedaling male. The male subject was soon exhausted. (Reprinted with permission from Abbott *et al.*, 1952.)

Antagonists (Klieber, 1961) to the theory that eccentric contractions make a significant contribution to the energy requirements of a movement at a low physiological cost, discount the fact that if none of these actions occurred, in work against gravity, the body would many times be deposited in an unceremonious manner on the ground.

A. V. Hill (1960) has postulated the reversal of chemical processes in the muscle in eccentric contractions where a contracting muscle is forcibly stretched. Abbott *et al.* (1952) elegantly and amusingly demonstrated the low

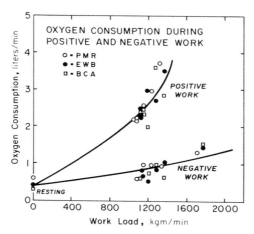

Fig. 17. Oxygen consumption during positive and negative work performed by stepping in two different directions and maintaining body position on a moving escalator (Banister *et al.*, 1964a).

physiological cost of negative work before the Physiological Society, Fig. 16. Several authors have demonstrated the high efficiency of movements of a stepping nature performed against gravity and the wide difference in physio- logical cost of positive and negative work (Asmussen, 1953). Figure 17 (Banister et al., 1964a) shows graphically this difference when the positive and negative movements of stepping are separated by performing the work task on a moving escalator. The arrangement of work tasks to take advantage of this apparent "physiological conservation" merits the serious consideration of those engaged in human engineering research. Cavagna et al. (1965) have recently demonstrated, Fig. 18, in isolated muscle preparations, the bene- ficial effect on positive work of negative work immediately preceding it.

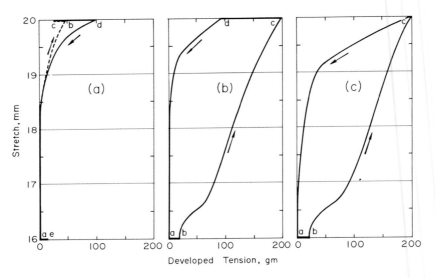

Fig. 18. Graph (a) represents an isolated frog gastrocnemius of length indicated in the ordinate (18 mm), stretched from 16 to 20 mm in the relaxed state (dashed line, a-b-c). It is then stimulated isometrically (full line, c-d) and allowed to shorten (d-a). At the end of shortening, the tension rises (a-e). The spread of stretching and shortening is 11.25 mm/sec. On the abscissa, the tension developed is given in grams. Positive work per- formed: 3.94 gm-cm. Graph (b) represents the same muscle as in (a). The muscle is stimulated isometrically at length 16 mm (a-b); then, when maximal tension is reached, it is stretched to a length of 20 mm (b-c). The tension then subsides in about 5 sec (c-d). The muscle is then allowed to shorten to the original length (d-a). The other indications are the same as for (a). Positive work performed: 4.65 gm-cm. Graph (c) represents the same indications as in (b), the only difference being that no delay is allowed between stretching and shortening, this last being described by (c-a). Positive work performed: 13.04 gm-cm. (Reprinted with permission from Cavagna et al., 1965.)

B. Empirical Relationships

Almost all the relationships derived between the physiological cost of different activities and their dependence on such variables as heart rate, ventilation, oxygen uptake, and rest allowances have been derived in an empirical manner being most commonly described in Eqs. (7)–(12):

$$H = \alpha_1 + \beta_1 W_R \text{ (Maritz et al., 1961)} \tag{7}$$

$$O = \alpha_2 + \beta_2 W_R \text{ (Maritz et al., 1961)} \tag{8}$$

$$V = \alpha_3 + \beta_3 W_R \text{ (Maritz et al., 1961)} \tag{9}$$

$$\dot{A} = [(\log 5700 - \log t)/3.1]a \text{ (Bink, 1962)} \tag{10}$$

$$RA = [(\text{kcal per min}/4) - 1]100 \text{ (Christensen, 1962)} \tag{11}$$

$$B = 70 \ W^{\frac{3}{4}} \text{ (Kleiber, 1961)} \tag{12}$$

where:

H = heart rate, beats/min
W_R = work rate, kcal/min
O = oxygen uptake, liter/min
V = ventilation, liter/min
$\dot{A}$ = physical work capacity, kcal/min
a = aerobic capacity, kcal/min
RA = rest allowance, % of work time
B = basal metabolic rate, kcal/min
W = weight, kg

Equations as described above cannot be sustained in terms of strict dimensional analysis (Baird, 1962) and provide only the beginning to further and complete understanding of the physiological significance underlying them. As Kleiber (1950) has said: "The theoretical significance of empirical regression equations expressing physiological relations is as a rule limited. Such equations should therefore be the start rather than an end to a physiologist's further reasoning and calculating . . . .. In general, ratios of equidimensional terms furnish the simplest and most general expressions for physiological relations. Other ratios are, however, also justified and may be best suited for particular problems."

One of the significant examples of "further reasoning and calculating" to appear in the recent literature (Margaria et al., 1965) is the relationship drawn between the acceleration of oxygen uptake and the increasing severity of the work task expressed by Eq. (13):

$$d\dot{V}_{O_2}/dt = b(10^a - \dot{V}_{O_2}) \tag{13}$$

where:

10^a = oxygen equivalent of the task, liter/min

V_{O_2} = oxygen uptake, liter/min, at any time t from the onset of the work task

b = velocity constant

VII. Computer Technology in the Analysis of Physical Activity

The application of computer techniques to the analysis of data, prediction of relations, and the construction of models of biological systems for discrete manipulation and study represent but a few ways this research tool may be expected to influence the study of bioenergetics (Barry, 1962; Bell, 1962).

The expression of limiting characteristic human factors and their inter-action with the man-machine systems of this era is most effectively made by multivariate analysis of experimental data. It may be expected, however, that unifying concepts of man's energetic interaction with his environment (to be derived from the comprehensive analyses made possible by the computer) will be in direct proportion to the store of well-planned, searching experiments submitted to it.

COMPARISONS OF VARIOUS SPORTS AND OTHER EXERCISE ACTIVITIES AS TO ENERGY REQUIREMENTS

VIII. Comparative Units

The performance of work requires energy in an amount directly proportional to the duration and rate of work and to the mechanical efficiency.

The heat equivalent of mechanical work is expressed in kcal, i.e., 1 kcal is the amount of heat necessary to raise the temperature of 1 kg of water 1°C. The mechanical equivalent of 1 kcal of heat is 4184 joules.

The relationship between units of force, work, and power are shown as follows (Mellerowicz, 1962):

Force

Force = mass × acceleration

1 dyne = the force which imparts an acceleration of 1 (1 cm/sec^2) to a grammass of 1 (1 gramweight = 981 dynes)

Work

Work = force × distance

1 erg = the work which a dyne performs when it moves a body in the direction of the force by 1 cm

10^7 ergs = 1 joule

1 kgm = 9.81 joules (427 kgm are equivalent to 1 kcal)

Power

$$\text{Power} = \text{work/time}$$
$$1 \text{ joule/sec} = 1 \text{ watt}$$
$$1 \text{ kgm/sec} = 9.81 \text{ watts}$$
$$1 \text{ kgm/min} = 0.1635 \text{ watts}$$
$$1 \text{ hp} = 736 \text{ watts}$$
$$= 75 \text{ kgm/sec}$$
$$= 4500 \text{ kgm/min}$$

In some bicycle work tests, the rate of work is expressed in kpm/min (kilo-pond meters per minute). 1 kp is the force acting on the mass of 1 kg at normal acceleration of gravity.

$$100 \text{ kpm/min} = 723 \text{ ft-lb/min}$$
$$= 16.35 \text{ watts}$$

IX. Man as a Source of Mechanical Power

A. GENERAL CONSIDERATIONS

If external work can be measured, it can be converted into kilocalorie equivalents. When man is a source of mechanical energy, the net caloric cost (gross cost minus basal or resting requirement) of performing the work can be obtained indirectly by determining the oxygen consumption and converting this to kilocalories. In metabolic work it is conventional practice to ignore protein metabolism and to use the value of 4.9 or 5.0 kcal as the caloric equivalent per liter of oxygen uptake.

Mechanical efficiency may be expressed as the percentage relationship between the caloric cost of work and the caloric equivalent of the mechanical work output. The mechanical work output can be measured by machines under laboratory conditions or under work conditions by time-motion, force platform, or cinematographic analysis methods. Usually, however, the measurement of mechanical work is either impossible or much too difficult to make the undertaking worthwhile.

The conventional formula (H. L. Taylor, 1960) for the calculation of mechanical efficiency is shown in Eq. (14):

$$\text{M.E. (\%)} = \frac{100 \text{ (kcal external work produced)}}{\text{(kcal net energy used)}} \tag{14}$$

There are problems associated with the denominator as well as with the numerator of this equation. Usually the net energy is measured by subtracting the basal metabolic oxygen consumption from the total oxygen consumed during work and recovery. Three types of work efficiency equations are in use (Procter *et al.*, 1934).

$$\text{Gross efficiency} = A/H$$
$$\text{Net efficiency} = A/(H - H_2)$$
$$\text{Absolute efficiency} = A/(H - H_w)$$

where:

H_2 = metabolic rate × duration of resting (lying or standing)
H_w = metabolic rate × duration of walking at same speed as when working but without load

Example:

A man pedaling on a bicycle ergometer at a rate of 600 kgm/min has an O_2 consumption of 1.48 liter/min = 7.4 kcal/min. The heat equivalent of 600 kgm/min = 1.4 kcal/min. Gross mechanical efficiency = (1.4 kcal/7.4 kcal)100 = 18.9%.

Durnin (1955) described two methods for calculating the metabolic cost of hill climbing. In one method the metabolic cost of walking on the level is deducted from the total metabolic cost of the activity and in the other (Orsini and Passmore, 1951) the energy expended when walking downhill is deducted from the total. In Durnin's opinion, "any method of calculating the mechanical efficiency is open to criticism" and "no particular usefulness is served by quoting efficiencies other than the gross efficiency." The mechanical efficiency of work depends on the following.

1. The Nature of the Task

Values have been reported in the literature, ranging from 40.3% for grade-walking on the treadmill corrected for horizontal energy (Erickson *et al.*, 1946) to 2.0% (Goff *et al.*, 1957) for swimming. Accurate calculation of the external work done is often impossible due to the difficulty in estimating the work of accelerating and decelerating limbs (Wilkie, 1960) in maintaining static loads, in lowering loads against gravity (negative work), overcoming wind resistance and estimating energy absorbed in frictional heat loss. In activities involving horizontal progression, the amount of measurable external work performed against gravity is small.

2. Economy of Movement

Improvement in skill reduces the energy expenditure. (See Fig. 14.)

3. Speed of Muscular Contraction in Relation to Load

With a high velocity of shortening the available force is small, although the maintenance heat of contraction is also small. When a muscle moves slowly, the force is large but maintenance heat of contraction is also large. Intermediate velocities of contraction will give maximum efficiency, i.e., when the

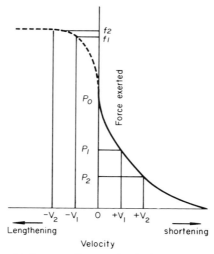

Fig. 19. The relationship between force and velocity of shortening for human muscle: P_1 and P_2 are the forces exerted by a single fiber shortening at velocities V_1 and V_2; f_1 and f_2 are the forces when the fiber is being stretched at the same velocities V_1 and V_2; P_0 represents the isometric tension of the fiber. (Reprinted with permission from Abbot *et al.*, 1952.)

force is about one-half of maximum value and speed about one-quarter of maximum value. This matches the load to the muscles so as to exploit fully the intrinsic force-velocity relationship, Fig. 19 (Abbott *et al.*, 1952).

4. Diet

Men fed on a high carbohydrate diet will consume less oxygen per unit of work than men fed on a high fat diet.

5. The Physical Condition of the Subject

This is important at oxygen intakes above 2 liters/min. Balke (1963b) has advanced the concept of "manpower" as a useful method of classifying various levels of work intensity. One horsepower equals 4500 kgm/min. At a mechanical efficiency of 26.8%, this would represent an oxygen consumption of 8 liters/min (40 kcal/min). The maximum oxygen intake of a horse is estimated to be 28.6 liters/min. Over a period of 8–9 hr maximum effort, a horse trotting 80 to 100 mi at a velocity of 300 m/min would have an oxygen intake of 24 liters/min. Thus, the horse works at a rate of 3 hp per minute. The maximum oxygen intake determined in man is approximately 5 liters/min. A first-class marathon runner, in completing the course in $2\frac{1}{2}$ hr, runs at a velocity of 300 m/min and has a $\dot{V}_{O_2}$ of approximately 4.5 liters/min. If this rate of energy expenditure is also considered to be equivalent to 3 manpower, then 1 manpower is equal to a $\dot{V}_{O_2}$ of 1.5 liters/min (7.5 kcal/min) which permits work to be carried out at a rate of 840 kgm/min. Thus, for people at the top level of fitness, "the potential physical performance capacity is about 3 manpower; at the average level—2 manpower; and at the lowest end of the scale of 'normals,' slightly better than 1 manpower . . . People in a state of 'very poor' physical fitness cannot exceed the daily working rate of 0.3 manpower output. . . ."

Wilkie (1960) has described the mechanical output of man in conventional terms of horsepower. "Since 1 liter of oxygen yields about 0.1 hp/min of mechanical work under optimal conditions, the steady state power output must be limited to 0.40–0.54 hp, depending on whether we are considering fit ordinary men or champion athletes." These values are based on oxygen consumptions of 4.0 liters/min for a fit young man and Don Lash's record of 5.35 liters/min (Robinson *et al.*, 1937), plus the assumption that 1 liter of oxygen yields 0.1 hp/min (applicable at a mechanical efficiency of 21.4%). In long term work lasting all day, the power output would probably be limited to 0.2 hp.

B. Work Output—Intensity in Relation to Duration (in Work, Industry, and Sport)

1. Integrated Whole Body Response

The intensity of work which can be tolerated depends upon environmental conditions and upon the age, sex, and physical fitness of the worker. All other things being equal, there will be a distinct contrast between the responses of relatively fit and unfit people at all levels of work intensity. The fit person will have a higher maximal working capacity, greater endurance at submaximal rates of work, and will perform work at any combination of intensity and duration at a lower physiological cost than a person who is less fit. Work performed at the highest possible metabolic rate will be chiefly anaerobic and thus of brief duration. Many sports activities involve short bouts of anaerobic work separated by recovery periods. If these are repeated sufficiently often, the result will be a steady accumulation of fatigue. The same effect will result from performance of aerobic work of relatively high intensity if continued for lengthy periods.

Temporary exhaustion arising from all-out effort is a normal and accepted by-product of participation in some sports but in nearly all other forms of human activity considerable attention is paid to reducing the level of fatigue.

Figure 20 (Wilkie, 1960) shows the relationship between power output at maximum intensity of work and time for which a given constant output would be maintained.

An expenditure of 4800 kcal/day has been considered the maximal energy output for a man working at the same task on a year round basis (Lehman, 1953). If a value of 2300 kcal is subtracted for basal metabolism plus eating, dressing, leisure activities and travel to and from work, this leaves 2500 kcal for 8 hr of work. This is a maximal value and 2000 kcal could be considered normal, i.e., a suitable load for heavy workers. This gives an average rate of energy expenditure of 4.2 kcal/min, although some jobs will require a higher expenditure and this should be compensated for by suitable rest pauses. Others have considered 4000 kcal energy expenditure to be maximal for industrial and outdoor workers.

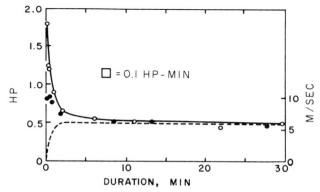

Fig. 20. Left-hand ordinate: circles, maximal external mechanical power produced by champion athletes. Right-hand ordinate: dots, running speed, world records (Guinness, 1956). Abscissa: total duration of exercise (not time elapsed since the beginning of exercise). The broken line shows the energy available from oxidative processes. To this is added 0.58 hp/min of work from anaerobic (hydrolytic) sources, to give the theoretical curve, full line. Note: 1 hp = 0.746 kg-wt meter sec^{-1}. (Reprinted with permission from Wilkie, 1960.)

Balke (1963b) has described the relationship between maximal aerobic capacity (crest load) and ability to work at certain levels of energy expenditure. It has been demonstrated under laboratory conditions that it is possible for very fit individuals to work for as long as 8 hr at a rate which would give a total 24-hr energy expenditure of 5700 kcal. For a 75-kg man this rate of energy expenditure would require 38.5% of a crest load $\dot{V}_{O_2}$ of 4.5 liters/ min and would be possible only for a person in superb physical condition. People in very poor physical condition cannot work at an energy expenditure higher than 2500 kcal/day which is equivalent to 20% of 2.25 liters/min (75-kg man). People in "average" condition can work for 8 hr at a rate which will use 3200 kcal for 24 hr and this, for a 75-kg man, is 25% of a crest load $\dot{V}_{O_2}$ of 3.0 liters/min. It is thus obvious that as fitness becomes progressively worse not only does the aerobic capacity diminish but also there is a distinct reduction in the proportion of aerobic capacity which the worker is able to use in continuous work without incurring fatigue.

The work of I. Åstrand et al. (1959) showed that 50% of the maximal aerobic capacity is the upper limit of the optimal work load for a 1-hr period, i.e., without disturbance in physiological equilibrium. Work continued at this rate for 7 hr, with 10 min rest pauses per hour, resulted in a high caloric expenditure of 4250 kcal in one subject (corresponding to approximately 6400 kcal for the 24 hr day (I. Astrand, 1960).

TABLE III

CLASSIFICATION OF INDUSTRIAL TASKS BY ENERGY REQUIRED PER MINUTE

	Energy expenditure over	
Task classification	kcal/min	$\dot{V}_{O_2}$ (liters/min)
Unduly heavy	12.5	2.5
Very heavy	10	2
Heavy	7.5	1.5
Moderate	5	1.0
Light	2.5	0.5

In order to permit daily tasks to be carried out without harm and difficulty, there should be reasonable margin between working and maximal oxygen intakes. The maximal oxygen intake should not be less than 1.4–1.6 liters/min (Hollman and Knipping, 1961). Müller (1962) has suggested that the occupational working capacity, i.e., the highest work level permissible in one's daily occupation, should be about one-fifth of the maximal working capacity at age 30 or less. After 30 years of age maximal work capacity falls off but occupational work capacity remains the same.

Pulse rate and/or body temperature have been used to estimate the energy cost of industrial work (Lundgren, 1946; Berggren and Christensen, 1950). However, the assessment of energy expenditure from post-work pulse rates or body temperature or their increments during work in the heat can be misleading since the degree of acclimatization may affect the values recorded. A more accurate method is to correct the post-work pulse rates for level of body temperature, since body temperature will reflect the degree of acclimatization to a given heat load (Edholm et al., 1962).

The measurement of physiological response to work has been used to determine the suitability of the job for the worker and the worker for the job. Measurement of heart rate during work (Adolph et al., 1947) and immediately following a work task (Brouha, 1959) provides a simple and effective means of assessing the physiological cost and fatigue effect of work. This method, together with the time-motion study (Lehman, 1958), permits a detailed job analysis to be made for the express purpose of promoting the maximal comfort and efficiency of the worker.

Table III represents Christensen's (1953) classification of work loads in terms of caloric equivalents and oxygen consumption.

2. Local or Peripheral Response of Isolated Muscles or Muscle Groups

Monod and Scherrer (1965) have demonstrated that the maximum work of muscles is apparently related to the use of an energetic reserve and an energy of reconstruction. This same interpretation has been given for general exercise; A. V. Hill (1927) and others (Margaria *et al.*, 1965) have shown that in exercise of the whole body, energy is available as a function of a fixed amount plus a rate of supply dependent on circulatory mechanisms. Monod and Scherrer (1965) devised dynamic, static, and intermittent static effort tests in order to investigate the relationship between work time and work rate to the point where work was terminated abruptly. This point was reached when a drop-off in amplitude or frequency of performance (dynamic work) occurred, or when a load could be sustained no longer (static work). From the linear (dynamic) and curvilinear (static) relationships between total work accomplished and time spent in work at different rates, it is possible to determine the critical power for dynamic work and critical force for static work. These are the points at or below which muscular work can be continued indefinitely without fatigue. There is general agreement that the critical force in continuous static effort is about 15% of the maximum force (Rohmert, 1960; Caldwell, 1963). In intermittent static effort, the level of the critical force depends on the time apportionment between the duration of the contraction phases and the duration of the effort. When the former is 50% of the latter, the critical force is 40% of the maximal force. This fact has a number of important applications in industry, rehabilitation medicine, physical education, and other areas of applied work or effort.

Bouisset *et al.* (1965) analyzed the problem of selecting physiological variables which would distinguish between differences in physiological cost of light muscular work and found that measurement of heart rate and oxygen consumption could be used to do this if values above basal or resting level were used rather than values which included the basal or resting rates. It was their opinion that in light muscular work, the necessity for visual control of the work field may transcend considerations of physiological cost; in most instances, however, biomechanical criteria should be paramount. They defined light muscular work according to three criteria: the muscular mass set to work must be less than a third of the whole muscle mass; the metabolic rate increase must not exceed resting $\dot{V}_{O_2}$ values by more than 250 ml/min; the percentage of maximum available force employed should not be more than 40% if the static component is significant; and rest pauses should not be less than 50% of the contraction time. Under these conditions, work can be continued indefinitely without fatigue.

C. Energy Requirements in Relationship to Age and Sex

Differences between the sexes and age groups in working capacity are much less apparent during submaximal work than during maximal work. Certain tasks are impossible or contraindicated for very young or older people because of limitations imposed by inadequacies of strength, aerobic capacity, and health. Some factors which influence mechanical efficiency may be related to sex and age differences. Older workers may be more highly skilled than younger workers and thus able to work at a lower caloric expenditure. Stronger people may be able to work at optimal velocities of muscular contraction and therefore at a lower caloric cost than people who are less strong.

Women who are physically fit may attain similar or higher maximal aerobic capacities than unfit men (Metheny *et al.*, 1942). As men and women increase in age they are more suited for jobs or sport requiring skill, endurance, and coordination, whereas work or sports activities with the emphasis on speed and strength are more suited to younger men and women (Dill and Consolazio, 1962).

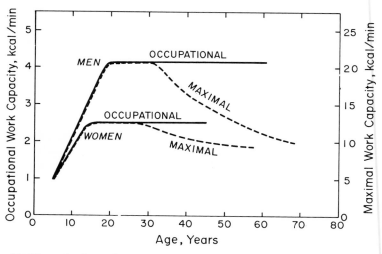

Fig. 21. Normal values of maximal and occupational physical work capacity of men (♂) and women (♀) at different ages. (Reprinted with permission from Müller, 1962).

The average maximal and occupational working capacities of young adult males are higher than those of young women or of children and adolescents of both sexes (Fig. 21). The two measurements go together in these groups since, by definition, occupational work capacity is approximately one-fifth of the maximal work capacity up to the age of 30. The rate of rise of maximal work capacity in adolescence is less for girls than for boys, but female adult performance is attained at an earlier age (Müller, 1962). The average maximal oxygen intake—corrected for body weight—of fit young adult female subjects was 17% below the average value for fit young adult males (P. O. Åstrand, 1952). This difference in maximal aerobic capacity between physically fit young men and women may be related to sexual differences in active tissue—body weight ratios linked with corresponding proportional cardiac outputs.

The gradual decline in maximal $\dot{V}_{O_2}$ which occurs in both sexes after the age of 30 is relatively more rapid in the male (Müller, 1962). Since women have lower strength and maximal aerobic capacities than men, the limits of the energy costs for female occupational work tasks are set correspondingly lower. However, many industrial tasks for which males are employed (Hellerstein and Ford, 1959) require energy expenditures which are not any higher than the female occupational work capacity (Müller, 1962); women doing housework may, in fact, expend more energy than men engaged in industry, Fig. 22.

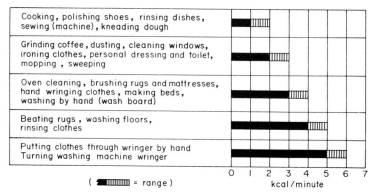

Fig. 22. The average kilocalorie expenditure per minute by housewives in domestic work.

X. Typical Energy Costs of Graded Intensities of Work

Information about the energy requirements of specific tasks has a variety of important applications in the promotion of human welfare and efficiency.

The most common method of determining energy requirements for different work loads is by oxygen consumption methods, although many tasks do not lend themselves at all to analysis by this method. Analysis of energy costs of complex or simple movements of brief duration may be more suitably done by the force-platform, time-motion study, or the cinematographic method.

Values for total energy expended over the working day or for the duration of exercise do not adequately describe the functional requirements of many complex tasks, jobs, or activities. It is often necessary also to know the pattern of rise and fall in energy output throughout the working period and especially to know the metabolic cost of "peak" loads.

A. CLASSIFICATION OF ENERGY REQUIREMENTS

Several different but related units of measurement can be used in reporting energy requirements. The most commonly used are: kcal/unit of time; $\dot{V}_{O_2}$ liter/unit of time; $\dot{V}_{O_2}$ ml/kg body weight/unit of time; multiples of basal metabolic rate (Met). Energy requirements expressed in kilocalories are meaningful to nutritionists; for many purposes, however, oxygen intake is preferable to the caloric equivalent.

Many tables appearing in the literature lack certain desirable refinements. They may show average values without reference to the numbers of subjects tested or to the variabilities of the measurements. In many instances the averages are not adjusted for subject differences in body weight or surface area. Ideally any table of energy requirements for increasing intensity of work should be based on tests on the same subjects done under the same environmental conditions. Many tables have been published without any adequate description of the subjects. Unfortunately, some of the tables in this chapter are, of necessity, reproduced without these refinements.

Of the several different methods of classifying energy requirements of different intensities of work, the method of Dill (1936) has several advantages. Differentiating energy requirements of activities in terms of multiples of BMR takes into account individual differences due to body size, age, and sex, and the classification of activities into broad categories is conceptually appealing and inherently meaningful. In Dill's classification, hard work is encompassed within multiples of three to eight times BMR and moderate work up to three times BMR. The cardiovascular and respiratory systems are engaged fully in maximal work and limits are set by the physical condition of the individual. The limits for an unfit subject may be ten times BMR, and for a highly trained man twenty times BMR. Christensen's (1953) classification of industrial tasks is based upon oxygen consumption and corresponding caloric equivalents.

B. Graded Intensities of Work

In order to compare energy requirements, it is first necessary to describe as precisely as possible the nature of the relevant tasks. Precise description is possible for activities such as walking or runnning on the level or up a grade at a prescribed rate, riding a bicycle ergometer at fixed work loads, or lifting weights under standardized conditions. Even these activities provide certain difficulties. The reliability of measurements of oxygen uptake is higher for walking than for running (Erickson *et al.*, 1930). Different values for maximal oxygen intake will be obtained in different laboratories with different bicycle ergometers and with different tests (Damoiseau *et al.*, 1963). Differences in levels of skill will influence the oxygen consumption of individuals performing the same task (Dill *et al.*, 1930).

Tasks with such vague descriptions as "shoveling snow" or "rowing for pleasure" are examples of self-regulating activities in which the rate of work and the frequency and duration of rest periods for each person will depend in large measure upon physical fitness. Thus the amounts of energy expended by different individuals in these activities will be quite variable (Fig. 23).

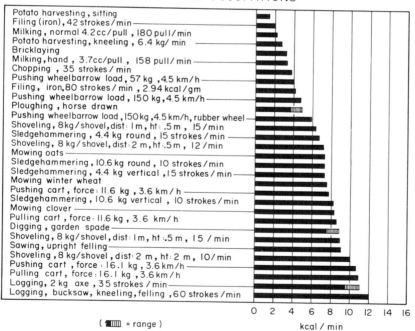

INDUSTRIAL OCCUPATIONS

(▰▭ = range)

kcal / min

Fig. 23. The average kilocalorie energy expenditure per minute in some industrial occupations.

C. COMPARATIVE ENERGY COSTS OF PHYSICAL ACTIVITY

1. Pathological and Sedentary

The rehabilitation of cardiac patients may involve an initial period of complete rest followed by gradual progression in activity to the stage where return to normal life is possible. It is important, therefore, to so order the hospital routine that these conditions are not violated by the introduction of sudden exertion or transient disturbances in metabolic or cardiac equilibrium. It is thus essential to know what the metabolic and cardiac demands of routine hospital and rehabilitation procedures are. Few studies for the purpose of obtaining this data have been carried out.

Kubicek *et al.* (1959) and others studied the effects upon circulation, respiration, and metabolism of various hospital activities using nurses as subjects. The obtained values for metabolic and cardiac index increase over supine resting values are shown in Table IV.

TABLE IV

A COMPARISON OF METABOLIC RATE AND CARDIAC INDEX

Activity	Metabolism percentage increase over supine[a]	Cardiac index percentage increase over supine[a]
Reclining at 45° angle	3.21	7.60
Sitting on a chair	6.62	−6.80
Sitting on edge of bed, feet supported	10.98	−7.60
Leather tooling in bed 45° angle	16.54	22.80
Chip carving, sitting on chair	54.08	15.60
Getting into and out of bed	64.44	39.60
Printing press (working at)	141.54	70.00

[a] Supine resting value = 33.97 kcal/m²/hr.

Thirty-six Cleveland industrial workers with recognized heart disease and employed at a wide variety of jobs had average sustained energy expenditures during work of only 2 kcal/min and average peak expenditures of 3.45 kcal/min (Hellerstein and Ford, 1959). These values were no different from those of control subjects doing similar jobs considered typical of those held by at least one-third of the working population of the city. These values were considered to lie in the lower range of possible sustained energy output, and possibly lower than energy expenditure during nonworking hours. The Master's Two-Step Test, by contrast, requires an expenditure of 8.5 kcal/min.

2. Military

There are various studies presenting energy costs of marching and maneuvering at various speeds with or without packs and rifles but there are few values for energy expenditure obtained under conditions simulating combat where control was exerted solely by seasoned infantry commanders rather than by the scientists involved in collecting data. Values reported by Goldman (1965) for heat-acclimatized troops in good physical condition carrying out a series of tactical maneuvers over dry hilly terrain and in a jungle are presented in Table V. Oxygen intake was measured by means of the Müller-Franz respirometry air meter. The maneuvers were carried out in protective clothing in the 83WBGT index environment and thus the resultant heat load and possible dehydration may have increased the energy cost slightly. The energy cost

TABLE V

THE ENERGY COST OF VARIOUS TACTICAL TASKS

Task situation	Mean energy cost (kcal/min)	Number of measures (*n*)	Range (kcal/min)
Rifleman resting on top of final objective 2 min after assault	2.2	2	±0.3
Mine clearance of road			
Probing	2.3	1	
Squad leader c radio	2.6	1	
Mine sweeper operator	2.9	1	
Infantry litter bearers—in jungle patrol	3.4	2	±0.03
Rifleman—in jungle patrol	3.8	4	±0.5
Rifleman—in jungle patrol as pointman	4.8	2	±0.1
Infantry radio telephone operator			
—on approach road march	4.0	2	±0.2
Rifleman—digging foxhole in rear area	4.1	2	±0.1
M-60 machine gunner—on approach road march	4.7	1	
M-60 machine gunner—on jungle patrol	5.0	2	±0.3
Litter bearers—littering 80 kg casualty on road	6.7	3	±0.3
Rifleman—in assault	6.9	2	±0.1
Rifleman—digging foxhole in forward area	7.0	3	±0.6
81mm mortarman—machine to emplace in jungle	7.0	4	±0.4
Company Commander—trooping ride line positions	7.3	1	
Rifleman—in fire fight in jungle	7.3	1	
90mm recoilless rifleman—in assault	7.6	1	
81mm mortarman—road march to emplace	8.0/10.1[a]	2	
M-60 machine gunner—in fire fight in jungle	8.0	1	

[a] At point of exhaustion, rectal temperature 30.5°C (103°F); could not continue.

SPORTING ACTIVITIES

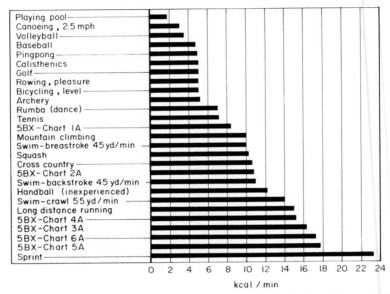

Fig. 24. The kilocalorie energy expenditure per minute for typical sporting activities.

MAXIMAL OXYGEN UPTAKE IN VARIOUS PHYSICAL ACTIVITIES

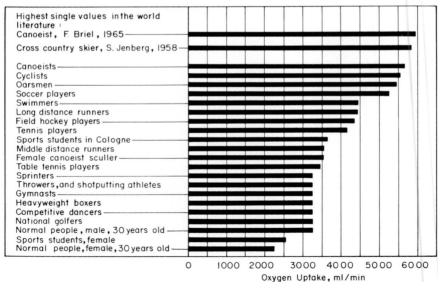

Fig. 25. Comparative maximal oxygen uptake values for some recreational and highly competitive sporting activities. (Reprinted with permission, Hollmann, 1965.)

values for different soldiers carrying out similar tasks in different terrain were quite similar, indicating that the soldiers appeared to adjust their pace to compensate for the tactical difficulties encountered. Maneuvers which produced energy expenditure rates in excess of 7.0 kcal/min seldom lasted more than 10 min.

3. Sports

The range of human activities encompassed within the realms of "sports" is very wide and includes events which require the highest attainable levels of oxygen consumption and those which would scarcely tax the reserves of an ambulatory hospital patient (Fig. 24). In comparing energy costs of different sports activities, data for highly competent or champion performers would appear to be most suitable for the purpose. Some activities are possible only for an elite of highly trained people and it seems pointless to compare the energy costs of such people in one activity with the energy costs of indifferent

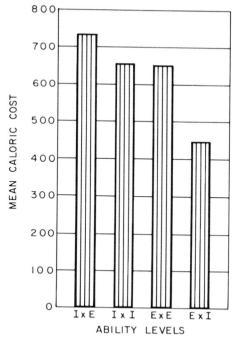

Fig. 26. Total mean caloric cost per hour of experienced players (E) and inexperienced players (I) playing against a player of their own ability and also one of either superior or inferior ability (Banister *et al.*, 1964b).

or mediocre performers in other activities (Fig. 25). It may, however, be a matter of some interest and importance to compare the energy costs of people of different levels of ability performing the same activity.

In competitive games, people who are not closely matched in ability may expend quite different amounts of energy from those amounts which they will expend when matched more closely. This is shown in Fig. 26 from a study carried out by Banister *et al.* (1964b) on handball players. A champion swimmer uses much less energy than an inexpert swimmer traveling at the same speed (Karpovich and Millman, 1947).

Some activities lend themselves more readily than others to measurement of energy requirements since the encumbrance of even light metabolic equipment such as the Müller-Franz respirometer may render performance impossible or may so grossly distort its nature that estimates of energy cost will be misleading. As a consequence, the available information on the energy cost of competitive team games is either completely lacking or very meager. On the other hand, there is a good supply of information available on the energy requirements of running at various speeds and distances.

XI. Effect of Environmental Variations on the Energy Cost of Physical Activity

Conditions producing heat or cold stress may elevate the energy expenditure values for activities above those usually obtained at thermally neutral ambient temperatures and humidities.

This additional caloric cost will reflect the amount of activity of the biological mechanisms which regulate the internal temperature. Changes in atmospheric pressure (at altitude or underwater) may alter the work of breathing, although this will normally represent only a fraction of the energy cost of external work. Differences in environment may affect endurance, maximal aerobic capacity, and heart rate. The variation in these parameters caused by changes in environmental conditions will depend upon individual differences in age, sex, and physical fitness.

Some specific problems of work and energy expenditure under different environmental conditions are discussed below.

A. Arctic

A number of widely different daily caloric requirement values have been reported for men living in the Arctic. Rodahl's (1955) study of servicemen in Alaska showed that an average gross consumption of 3000 kcal to 3500 kcal per man per day was sufficient to maintain weight balance and good health. These figures were similar to caloric consumption values for Eskimos and trappers in Greenland. Eskimos in Alaska were found to consume an average of approximately 3100 kcal per day, with 2700 kcal estimated for energy expenditure. It seems, therefore, that the energy requirements for men living in the Arctic are very similar to the requirements for men living in temperate or tropical zones (Le Blanc, 1961). Caloric requirements in the Arctic (or Antarctic) will depend upon regional variations in weather conditions, the amount of wind chill, the amount of outside work possible under different environmental conditions, the type of clothing worn, the nature of the terrain, and the degree of skill shown in using equipment.

Gray *et al.* (1951) found the caloric requirement for a given amount of external work performed in a given outfit of clothes decreased about 2% as the temperature rose from −15° to +60°F. Johnson and Kark (1947) found that an increase in caloric intake with falling environmental temperature could not be accounted for by differences in basal metabolism and that the restrictions in movement caused by the heavier clothing worn in the colder environment was partly responsible for the increase in caloric intake. The work of Gray *et al.* (1951) supports this conclusion. Men who performed the same work at the same environmental temperature in light clothing, increased their caloric requirement 5% when they put on Arctic clothing. Walking on Arctic tundra or in loose deep snow will require more energy than walking on firm ground. The energy requirements for cross-country travel on skis or snow shoes will vary according to the amount of training and skill of the men using the equipment.

Under most circumstances, Eskimos and servicemen in the Arctic are not actually exposed to cold and, therefore, do not have to elevate their metabolism. There is conflicting evidence about the effect of Arctic living upon the basal metabolic rate; some investigators have found no effect and some have found an increase of BMR. Modern Arctic clothing will provide enough insulation under windless conditions to prevent a resting man from suffering heat loss at environmental temperatures down to −40°F. With such clothing the limiting factor of work capacity in the Arctic might well be that of heat stress. If, however, men are subjected to repeated cold exposure, a decline or extinction of shivering occurs with no change in heart rate or oxygen consumption and this "offers a valuable means of observing and defining the presence of cold acclimatization" (Joy *et al.*, 1962). It is possible that cold acclimatization initiates another source of heat production to replace that due to the muscular work of shivering and that this is due to heightened tissue response to normal levels of circulating calorigenic humoral agents.

B. DESERT

Human efficiency and integrity of function depends upon the body's ability to maintain its core temperature within narrow limits. The process by which this is accomplished depends upon the thermal gradient between the body and the surrounding environment. If there is a large thermal gradient from the body to the surroundings, heat must be conserved and the amount of heat conveyed to the surface will be reduced by means of a diminished peripheral circulation. If this is insufficient to prevent heat loss, the level of heat production can be increased by involuntary shivering or by voluntary exercise. Normally, the need for increasing heat by either of these methods can be avoided by wearing protective clothing and living under adequate shelter.

The resting metabolism produces sufficient heat to maintain the core temperature at 99°F. The skin temperature is usually somewhat cooler, i.e., approximately 92°F. If the heat produced to maintain core temperature is not transferred into the surrounding environment, body core temperature increases more than 2°F in 1 hr (Adolph et al., 1947). The body must, therefore, lose heat or fever will result. In a warm environment, where the surrounding air temperature is several degrees or more above body surface temperature, it becomes essential to lose heat by the mechanism of sweat evaporation. The problem for man working in a hot environment is to dissipate the heat of resting metabolism, the heat produced by working, and the heat gained from the surroundings against a heat gradient. Sweating will permit him to do this but he can also improve matters by creating conditions in which the heat gain is minimized. In all hot environments, heat is gained from the air by convection. In the desert, heat is also gained by radiation from the sun, sky, ground, and other reflecting surfaces. The provision of shade or wearing of white clothing will reduce the amount of heat gain by radiation.

At 100°F the average clothed man in the desert sun will acquire slightly more than 200 kcal/hr from the surroundings. If he removes his clothing he will gain an additional 100 to 140 kcal/hr. At 110°F his environmental heat gain while clothed is over 300 kcal/hr. This contrasts greatly with the heat gain of 90 kcal/hr in a laboratory hot room with wall and air temperatures of 100°F.

A number of investigators have used a work rate of 250 kcal/hr in hot chamber experiments in order to determine the upper limits of heat stress beyond which men cannot maintain thermal balance. For nude subjects, the upper limits were bounded by 120°F dry bulb (D.B.) and 94°F wet bulb (W.B.) temperatures (Eichna et al., 1945); for men in herringbone twill uniforms the upper limits were D.B. 120°F, W.B. 90°F (Shelley et al., 1945).

The power output of man in the desert is limited both by the temperature of his surroundings and his state of dehydration. These impose an additive and cumulative circulatory strain which is reflected in a rising pulse rate and core temperature. At an air temperature of 110°F, a man in the desert sunshine will require, for the dissipation of heat gain alone, the evaporation of

530 gm of water per hour. It is obvious that even at rest the possibility of acute water loss by dehydration is an important problem and can only be managed by letting men drink as often and as much as they are able. When men at work sweat so freely that their skins become covered with water, they must soon rest or reduce their rates of work, for at this point evaporative cooling cannot proceed fast enough and a rise in core temperature will ensue.

Men who have become adapted to a hot environment or who are physically fit, or both, can perform the same amount of work as unacclimatized or less fit men at lower pulse rates and lower core temperatures (Edholm *et al.*, 1962). They can also tolerate higher environmental temperatures and can work at higher intensities at a given temperature than unacclimatized or less fit men. An important reason for this difference is that they perspire more freely (Wyndham *et al.*, 1965) than men who have not become adapted through sufficient heat exposure. Men who are trained for endurance running or a similarly intensive continuous activity are already heat adapted; adaptation otherwise takes three to four days of living in the hot environment.

Men conditioned to working for 1 hr a day in a hot chamber (D.B. 120°F, W.B. 93°F), at an energy expenditure of 250 kcal/hr were fully acclimatized to a similar work load at any lower heat stress and were partially or completely acclimatized for much longer periods of work at lower wet bulb temperatures. Men can thus be trained to work efficiently at industrial tasks in moderate heat by being first conditioned at higher levels of heat (Horvath and Shelley, 1946).

C. ALTITUDE

Several investigators (Douglas *et al.*, 1913; Dill *et al.*, 1931; Christensen, 1937; Balke, 1963a) have shown that the oxygen intake at identical work intensity is practically unaffected by variation in altitude. However, the barometric pressure and degree of acclimatization to altitude will impose limitations on the rate of work possible. Mountain climbers working at their own natural pace, can maintain an oxygen consumption at 15,000–20,000 ft (Pugh, 1958) which is close to values obtained for climbers near sea level (Durnin, 1955). The increased ventilatory work at lower barometric pressures is partially offset by the reduced resistance of the respiratory passages to air of reduced density and can virtually be discarded in measurement of oxygen consumption made in the field (Pugh, 1958).

Men climbing at their own habitual pace at various altitudes, during the 1953 Everest Expedition, demonstrated oxygen intakes ranging from 1.45 to 2.18 liters/min (depending upon body size, difficulty of terrain and fitness). These values agree closely with those obtained by Durnin (1955) for men walking uphill at their own pace on Ben Lomond. Durnin estimated that subjects ascending Ben Lomond with a 5-kg load had an approximate rate of energy expenditure of 700 kcal/hr. It is not uncommon for a day's climb, including rest pauses, to occupy 10 hr. Climbing, with periods of downhill or level walking, might then result in an expenditure of between 4400 and 5800 kcal. With normal requirements added for the remaining 14 hr, this amounts to a 24-hr expenditure of between 5900 and 7300 kcal, i.e., mountain climbing is very hard work.

Sea level dwellers doing work capacity tests at altitude cannot reproduce maximal oxygen intakes demonstrated at sea level. In tests done at 20,500 ft on Mount Everest, maximal oxygen intakes for members of the 1953 expedition were approximately one-half their sea level values (Pugh, 1958). Christensen (1937) reported his own maximal oxygen intake data at sea level and after successive 10-day stays at different altitudes. His maximal values demonstrated a progressive fall with decreasing barometric pressure down to 48% of the sea level value at 401 mm Hg (approximately 17,000 ft). Similar records have been reported by Dill and others (1964).

Balke (1963a) reported average maximal oxygen intakes of five Morococha natives (14,900 ft) during a stepwise treadmill test as 36.6 ml/kg/min, which was below average compared with standards for "normals" at sea level (Balke, 1963b). This value was no different from the average maximal oxygen intake of a group of physically conditioned men who normally lived at sea level and who had been living at a similar altitude to the Peruvian subjects for 6 weeks when they were tested. It is apparent that men living permanently at altitude are not necessarily superior in working capacity to subchronically acclimatized but fit men.

Physical training at altitude appears to effect an immediate improvement in endurance performance on return to sea level. Highly conditioned track athletes, after two weeks acclimatization and training at altitude (9180 ft), demonstrated higher values of maximal work capacity, maximal heart frequency, pulmonary ventilation, and better 440 yd and mile run times (Balke, 1965).

D. Submarine

The problems associated with submarine life stem not so much from the excessive energetic demands of the tasks involved in maintaining submarine routines, but rather from the stresses imposed by the abnormal atmosphere which has to be sustained for long periods and with the absence of certain stimuli regulating normal biological rhythms.

Ionic concentrations (Schaefer, 1959), nitrogen narcosis (Behnke *et al.*, 1935), vagotonia (Schaefer, 1949), are but a few of the many problems which may be attendant on submarine life. Experiments, such as those recently concluded in Sealab II and Precontinent III, will provide essential information about the ability of man to conduct a submarine life.

E. Space

The amount of available data on the energetic requirements of sustained space flight are as yet necessarily meager. There is no reason to suppose, however, that the physiologic demands are high, but that they are related to the complexity of the flight task, the skill level, and experience of the pilot. Table VI (Dryden *et al.*, 1958) lists the energy requirements of some specific flight tasks in conventional flying machines. The toxic hazards associated with gaseous buildup in a sealed cabin have been computed by E. R. Taylor

TABLE VI

VENTILATION RELATED TO VARIOUS FLIGHT TASKS

Task	Type of plane	$\dot{V}_{O_2}$(ml/min)	Ratio to rest rate
Rest		270	1.0
Take off and land	DC3	580	2.14
	DC4	542	2.00
ILS landing	DC3	446	1.65
	DC4	440	1.63
Taxiing	DC3	590	2.18
	DC4	465	1.72
Cross-country flight	DC3	350	1.30
	DC4	360	1.33

TABLE VII

TOXIC HAZARDS FROM PHYSIOLOGICAL FUNCTION (FLATUS) IN A SEALED CABIN[a]

Substance	Maximable allowable concentration	Effect	Time (days)
H_2S	20 ppm	Nausea, tears	420
H_2	4.1%	Explosive	124
CH_4	5.3%	Explosive	166
CO_2	0.5%	Mild hyperventilation	28
CO_2	3.0%	Respiratory disability	174

[a] Data for one person at 1 g in 100 ft³ sealed cabin.

(1958). One of the many human engineering problems presented by sustained manned space flight is the reconciliation of efficient regeneration and elimination systems with pay load or weight penalty. Experiments under conditions simulating all types of stresses likely to be encountered in space flight have indicated that subjects with high physiological reserves can withstand them. The importance of effective physical training during long continued flights has also been indicated (Clark, 1962).

XII. Future Developments

The review of methodology, and the categorization and quantification of activities and jobs in terms of their energy cost outlined above, indicates the diversity of approach to the single problem of estimating man's energetic interaction with his environment.

Since man is no longer content to habitate those regions of the universe naturally compatible with him, the techniques of energy estimation will be increasingly used to probe alien environments. Inevitably, human systems engineering must follow the results of basic research for the stable long term solution of problems, although interim solutions may be quickly found.

In some cases, the entire presently accepted methodology of evaluating the living environment may have to be changed. In the event that this environment presents unknown hazards or extends the responses of man to their known tolerance limits, the initial explorations may have to be done by simulation under carefully controlled conditions. Computers may be used to extrapolate from known responses to the unknown. Extensive use may be made of model systems to make estimates of the effect of new environments upon man.

The immediate need of the work physiologist, however, is the standardization of laboratory methods and the refinement of field techniques for making estimates of energy expenditure. If these goals can be attained, then he has an important and continuing part to play in long term epidemiological studies of the effects of cultural living patterns on health. No less important is the development of an itemized body of knowledge on the energy cost of physical activity which can be made readily available as a guide for physical recreational habits and the delimitation of industrial working conditions.

REFERENCES

Abbott, B. C., Bigland, B., and Ritchie, J. M. (1952). *J. Physiol. (London)* **117**, 380.
Adolph, E. F., Brown, A. H., Goddard, D. R., Gosselyn, R. E., Kelly, J. J., Molnar, G. W., Rahn, H., Rothstein, A., Towbin, E. J., Wills, J. H., and Wolf, A. V. (1947). "Physiology of Man in the Desert." Wiley (Interscience), New York.
Asmussen, E. (1953). *Acta Physiol. Scand.* **28**, 364.

Aston, F. W. (1942). "Mass Spectra and Isotopes." Arnold, London.
Åstrand, I. (1960). *Acta Physiol. Scand.* **48**, 448.
Åstrand, I., Åstrand, P. O., and Rodahl, K. J. (1959). *J. Appl. Physiol.* **14**, 562.
Åstrand, P. O. (1952). "Experimental Studies of Physical Working Capacity in Relation to Sex and Age." Munksgaard, Copenhagen.
Baird, D. C. (1962). "Experimentation: An Introduction to Measurement Theory and Experimental Design." Prentice-Hall, Englewood Cliffs, New Jersey.
Balke, B. (1963a). *Symp. Physiol. Effects High Altitude, Interlaken, 1962*, pp. 233–240. Pergamon Press, Oxford.
Balke, B. (1963b). *Proc. 1st Can. Fitness Seminar, Saskatoon, Saskatchewan, 1963*, pp. 5–14.
Balke, B. (1965). *J. Am. Med. Assoc.* **194**, 646.
Banister, E. W. (1966). Progress Report Committee Research University of British Columbia, Research Grant 68-0714/686694.
Banister, E. W., Ribisl, P. M., and Abbott, B. C. (1964a). Positive and Negative Work. AAHPER Convention, Research Section Presentation, Washington, D.C.
Banister, E. W., Ribisl, P. M., Porter, G. H., and Cillo, A. R. (1964b). *Res. Quart.* **35**, 236.
Bannister, R. G., and Cormack, R. S. (1954). *J. Physiol. (London)* **124**, 4.
Barany, J. W., and Whetsel, R. G. (1962). Report to National Science Foundation, Grant Number G17738, Purdue University, Lafayette, Indiana.
Barry, A. J. (1962). *Australian J. Phys. Educ.* **25**, 20.
Bell, D. A. (1962). "Intelligent Machines." Ginn (Blaisdell), Boston, Massachusetts.
Behnke, A. R., Thomson, R. M., and Motley, E. P. (1935). *Am. J. Physiol.* **112**, 554.
Benzinger, T., and Kitzinger, C. (1946). "Photographische Registrierung interfero metrischer Gasanlyser" (Translation 06-46-36), Aero-Med. Center HQ 3D Central Med. Establ., U.S. Army.
Benzinger, T. H., and Kitzinger, C. (1949). *Rev. Sci. Instr.* **20**, 849.
Berg, W. E. (1947). *Am. J. Physiol.* **149**, 597–610.
Berggren, G., and Christensen, E. H. (1950). *Intern. Z. Angew Physiol. Arbeit.* **14**, 255.
Bink, B. (1962). *Ergonomics* **5**, 25.
Blaxter, K. L. (1962). "The Energy Metabolism of Ruminants." Hutchinson, London.
Blaxter, K. L., and Rook, J. A. F. (1953). *Brit. J. Nutr.* **7**, 83.
Bonjer, F. H. (1962). *Ergonomics* **5**, 254.
Bouisset, S., Monod, H., and Pertuzon, E. (1965). *Intern. Z. Angew. Physiol.* **21**, 74.
Boyd, W. C. (1954). *J. Appl. Physiol.* **6**, 711.
Brody, S. (1945). "Bioenergetics and Growth." Reinhold, New York.
Brouha, L. (1959). *In* "Work and the Heart" (F. F. Rosenbaum and E. L. Belknap, eds.), pp. 180–195. Harper (Hoeber), New York.
Caldwell, L. S. (1963). *J. Eng. Psychol.* **2**, 155.
Carlsöö, S. (1962). *Ergonomics* **5**, 271.
Carpenter, T. M. (1948). *Carnegie Inst. Wash. Pub.* **303C**.
Cavagna, G. A., Saibene, F. P., and Margaria, R. (1965). *J. Appl. Physiol.* **20**, 157.
Christensen, E. H. (1937). *Skand. Arch. Physiol.* **76**, 88.
Christensen, E. H. (1953). *In* "Ergonomics Soc. Symposium of Fatigue" (W. F. Floyd and A. T. Welford, eds.), pp. 93–108. Lewis, London.
Christensen, E. H. (1962). *Ergonomics* **5**, 7.
Clark, R. T. (1962). *In* "Man's Dependence on the Earthly Atmosphere" (K. E. Schaefer, ed.), pp. 3–11. Macmillan, New York.
Coates, J. E., and Meade, F. (1960). *Ergonomics* **3**, 97.

Damoiseau, J., Devoanne, R., and Petit, J. M. (1963). *Arch. Intern. Physiol. Biochem.* **71**, 225.

Dill, D. B. (1936). *Physiol. Rev.* **16**, 263.

Dill, D. B., and Consolazio, C. F. (1962). *J. Appl. Physiol.* **17**, 645.

Dill, D. B., Talbott, J. H., and Edwards, H. T. (1930). *J. Physiol. (London)* **69**, 267.

Dill, D. B., Folling, A., and Obeg, S. A. (1931). *J. Physiol. (London)* **71**, 47.

Dill, D. B., Robinson, S., Balke, B., and Newton, J. L. (1964). *J. Appl. Physiol.* **19**, 483.

Douglas, G. S., Haldane, J. S., Henderson, Y., and Schneider, E. C. (1913). *Phil. Trans. Roy. Soc. London* **B203**, 185.

Dryden, C. E., Lit-Sien, H., Hitchcock, F. A., and Zimmerman, R. (1958). *In* "Physical and Physiological Data for Biostronautics" (E. R. Taylor, ed.), Fig. 1.4.1.12. U.S.A.F. School of Aviation Med., Randolph Air Force Base, Texas.

Durnin, J. V. G. A. (1955). *J. Physiol. (London)* **128**, 294.

Eastman Kodak Co. (1953). "Kodak 16mm Equipment for Sports Analysis Pamphlet." Rochester, New York.

Edholm, O. G., Adam, J. M., and Fox, R. H. (1962). *Ergonomics* **5**, 545.

Eichna, L. W., Ashe, W. F., Bean, W. B., and Shelley, W. B. (1945). *J. Ind. Hyg. Toxiol.* **27**, 59.

Erickson, L., Simonson, E., Taylor, H. L., Alexander, H., and Keys, A. (1930). *Am. J. Physiol.* **93**, 433.

Erickson, L., Simonson, E., Taylor, ·H. L., Alexander, H., and Keys, A. (1946). *Am. J. Physiol.* **145**, 391.

Fleisch, A. (1956). "Neue Methoden zum Studium des gas tauches and des Lungen-funktion." Thieme, Leipzig.

Fletcher, J. G., Lewis, H. E., and Wilkie, D. R. (1960). *Ergonomics* **3**, 30.

Forbes, E. B., Braman, W. W., and Kriss, M. (1928). *J. Agr. Res.* **40**, 37.

Fowler, K. T., and Hugh-Jones, P. (1957). *Brit. Med. J.* **I**, 1205.

Ganslen, R. V., and Van Huss, W. D. (1953). *Intern. Z. Angew. Physiol.* **15**, 207.

Goff, L. G., Brubach, H. F., Specht, H. (1957). *J. Appl. Physiol.* **10**, 376.

Goldman, R. F. (1965). *Ergonomics* **8**, 322.

Gray, E., Consolazio, F. C., and Kark, R. M. (1951). *J. Appl. Physiol.* **4**, 270.

Guinness (1956). Book of Records, Guinness Superlatives. London.

Haldane, J. S. (1892). *J. Physiol. (London)* **13**, 419.

Hamilton, L. H. (1959). *Physiologist* **2** (3), 51.

Hellerstein, H. D., and Ford, A. B. (1959). *In* "Work and the Heart" (F. F. Rosenbaum and E. L. Belknap, eds.), pp. 123–131. Harper (Hoeber), New York.

Hill, A. V. (1927). "Muscular Movement in Man." McGraw-Hill, New York.

Hill, A. V. (1960). *Science* **131**, 897.

Hill, A. V., and Long, C. N. H. (1924). *Proc. Roy. Soc.* **B97**, 96.

Hollmann, W. (1965). "Korperliches Training als Pravention von Herz-Kreislauf-krankheiten." Hippokrates, Stuttgart.

Hollmann, W., and Knipping, H. W. (1961). *In* "Health and Fitness in the Modern World" (T. K. Cureton, A. J. Barry, and L. Huelster, eds.), pp. 17–30. Athletic Inst. Chicago, Illinois.

Horvath, S. M., and Shelley, W. B. (1946). *Am. J. Physiol.* **146**, 336.

Hyzer, W. G. (1955). "Machine Design." Penton Publ. (Reprint by Eastman-Kodak Co., Rochester, New York.)

Johnson, R. E., and Kark, R. M. (1947). *Science* **105**, 378.

Joy, R. T., Poe, R. H., Burman, F. R., and Davis, T. R. A. (1962). *Arch. Environ. Health* **4**, 28.

Karpovich, P. V., and Millman, N. (1947). *Am. J. Physiol.* **142**, 140.

Kerhkoven, C. L. M. (1962). *Ergonomics* **5**, 53.

Kleiber, M. (1950). *J. Appl. Physiol.* **2**, 417.

Kleiber, M. (1961). "The Fire of Life." Wiley, New York.

Knipping, H. W., Bolt, W., Valentin, H., and Venrath, H. (1955). "Untersuchung und Beurteilung des Lungen and Herzkranken." Steinkopff, Darmstadt.

Kofranyi, E., and Michaelis, H. F. (1940). *Intern. Z. Angew. Physiol.* **11**, 148.

Kofranyi, E., Michaelis, H. F., Müller (1940). *Intern. Z. Angew. Physiol.* **11**, 141.

Kubicek, W. G., Kottke, F. J., and Danz, J. N. (1959). *In* "Work and the Heart" (F. F. Rosenbaum and E. L. Belknap, eds.), pp. 215–223. Harper (Hoeber), New York.

Kühn, G., and Kellner, O. (1894). *Landw. Versuchsstationen* **44**, 257–581.

Lauru, L. (1954). *Manager* **22**, 369.

Lavoisier (1780). *In* "Elements of Chemistry." H. Regency, Chicago (1949).

Lavosier, A. L., and de Laplace, P. S. (1780). *Mem. Acad. Roy. Belg.* p. 355.

Le Blanc, J. (1961). *In* "Performance Capacity" (H. Spector, J. Brozek, and M. S. Peterson, eds.), pp. 203–294. Research and Development Command, Department of the Army.

Lehman, G. (1953). "Praktishe Arbeitsphysiologie." Thieme, Stuttgart.

Lehman, G. (1958). *Ergonomics* **1**, 328.

Lester H. M. (1954). "Photo-Lab-Index," Sect. 10, Illumination. Morgan & Lester, New York.

Lilly, J. C. (1950). *In* "Medical Physics" (W. O. Glasser, ed.), Vol. II, pp. 845–855. Year Book Publ., Chicago, Illinois.

Lloyd, B. B. (1958). *J. Physiol. (London)* **143**, 5.

Lundgren, N. P. V. (1946). *Acta Physiol. Scand.* **13**, 1.

McIntosh, P. C. (1958). *J. Phys. Educ. Assoc. Gt. Britain and Northern Ireland* **50**, 7.

Margaria, R., Mangili, F., Cuttica, F., and Cerretelli, P. (1965). *Ergonomics* **8**, 49.

Maritz, J. S., Morrison, J. F., Peter, J., Strydom, N. B., and Wyndham, C. H. (1961). *Ergonomics* **4**, 97.

Mellerowicz, H. (1962). "Ergometrie." Urban & Schwarzenberg, Munich.

Metheny, E. L., Brouha, L., Johnson, R. E., and Forbes, W. H. (1942). *Am. J. Physiol.* **137**, 318.

Monod, H., and Scherrer, J. (1965). *Ergonomics* **8**, 329.

Müller, E. A. (1962). *Ergonomics* **5**, 445.

Nordan, H. C. (1962). Unpublished data. University of British Columbia, Vancouver.

Orsini, D., and Passmore, R. (1951). *J. Physiol. (London)* **115**, 95.

Palmer, M. A. (1958). *In* "Aviation Medicine: Selected Reviews" (C. S. White, W. R. Lovelace, II, and F. G. Hirsch, eds.), pp. 23–38. Pergamon Press, Oxford.

Passmore, R., and Durnin, J. V. G. A. (1955). *Physiol. Rev.* **35**, 801.

Pauling, L., Wood, R. E., and Sturdivant, J. H. (1946). *J. Am. Chem. Soc.* **68**, 795.

Pearl, R. (1924). "Studies in Human Biology." Williams & Wilkins, Baltimore, Maryland.

Poulsen, E., and Asmussen, E. (1962). *Ergonomics*, **5**, 33.

Procter, R. C., Brody, S., Jones, M. M., and Chittenden, D. W. (1934). *Missouri Univ., Agr. Expt. Sta., Res. Bul.* **209**, 1.

Pugh, L. G. C. E. (1958). *J. Physiol. (London)* **141**, 233.

Regnault, V., and Reiset, J. (1849). *Ann. Chim. Phys.* [3] **26**, 299.

Reiff, G. G., Montoye, H. J., Remington, R. D., Napier, J. A., Metzner, H. L., and Epstein, F. H. (1964). Am. Coll. Sports Med. Presentation, Hollywood. From G. G. Reiff, unpublished Ph.D. Dissertation, University of Michigan, Ann Arbor, Michigan.

Robinson, S., Edwards, H. T., and Dill, D. B. (1937). *Science* **85**, 409.

Rodahl, K. (1955). Proj. No. 7-7954, Rept. No. 1, Arctic Aeromed. Lab., Ladd Air Force Base, Alaska, Alaska Air Command.

Rohmert, W. (1960). *Intern. Z. Angew Physiol.* **18**, 123.

Rose, K. D. (1965). *Proc. Intern. Telemetering Conf., 1965.* Vol. I, pp. 225–241. F. G. McGavock Assoc., Pasadena, California.

Schaefer, K. E. (1949). *Arch. Ges. Physiol.* **251**, 689.

Schaefer, K. E. (1959). *J. Aviation Med.* **30**, 350.

Schmeiser, K. (Undated). Kaiser Wilhelm Institut, Heidelberg (quoted by White, 1958, p. 151).

Scholander, P. F. (1947). *J. Biol. Chem.* **167**, 235.

Schwartz, W. B., and Silverman, L. (1965). *J. Appl. Physiol.* **20**, 766.

Shelley, W. B., Eichna, L. W., and Horvath, S. M. (1945). *Federation Proc.* **4**, 64.

Sjöstrand, T. (1950). *Svenska Lakartidn.* **7**, 349.

Spoor, H. J. (1948). *J. Appl. Physiol.* **1**, 369.

Starr, I. (1951). *J. Appl. Physiol.* **4**, 21.

Taylor, E. R. (1958). "Physical and Physiological Data for Bioastronautics." U.S.A.F. School of Aviation Med., Randolph Air Force Base, Texas.

Taylor, H. L. (1960). *In* "Science and Medicine of Exercise and Sports" (W. R. Johnson, ed.), p. 133. Harper, New York.

Udenfriend, S. (1962). "Fluorescence Assay in Biology and Medicine." Academic Press, New York.

Waddell, J. W., and Waddell, J. H. (1955). "Photographic Motion Analysis," pp. 69–76. Industrial Laboratories, Chicago, Illinois.

Weir, J. B. de V. (1949). *J. Physiol. (London)* **109**, 1.

White, C. S. (1958). *In* "Aviation Medicine: Selected Reviews" (C. S. White, W. R. Lovelace, II, and F. G. Hirsch, eds.), pp. 125–127. Pergamon Press, Oxford.

White, C. S., and Lovelace, W. R., II (1958). *In* "Aviation Medicine: Selected Reviews" (C. S. White, W. R. Lovelace, II, and F. G. Hirsch, eds.), pp. 253–267. Pergamon Press, Oxford.

White, C. S., Watkins, L. C., Jr., and Fletcher, E. E. (1956). *J. Aviat. Med.* **27**, 414–423.

Wilkie, D. R. (1960). *Ergonomics* **3**, 1.

Wolff, H. S. (1958). *J. Physiol. (London)* **141**, 36P.

Wyndham, C. H., Strydom, N. B., and Morrison, J. F. (1965). *J. Appl. Physiol.* **20**, 37.

Yoder, T., Barany, J., and Ismail, A. H. (1964). *Am. Coll. Sports Med. Reg. Meeting, Purdue Univ., Lafayette, Indiana.*

Young, A. C., and Robinson, W. A. (1954). Reprint No. 1, Projects No. 7-7951 Arctic Aeromedical Laboratory, Ladd Air Force Base, Alaska.

Zajaczkowska, E. (1962). *Ergonomics* **5**, 337.

II

THE PHYSICIAN and EXERCISE PHYSIOLOGY

Allan J. Ryan

I. Physician's Interest in the Physiology of Exercise

The primary concern of the physician must always be to prevent disease as well as to treat the person suffering from it in whatever form it may occur. In this respect he must deal with those factors in the external environment of man which may be responsible for sickness and death, and the disorders of man's internal environment which may contribute to or even be solely responsible for such results. Since effective prevention and treatment depend on

323

understanding the causes of these disorders, and identifying the harmful factors, the scope of modern medical research and medical investigation has widened to include all the scientific disciplines.

The great contributions made toward the improvement of health and conquest of disease by science in the nineteenth century were the development of basic understandings of normal and abnormal human physiology as well as the identification of the bacterial origin of infectious diseases. The prime task of this century so far has been to amplify these understandings in order to focus the attack on degenerative disease.

The great physicians have always demonstrated a broad interest in human anatomy and physiology. They have been extremely conscious of the effects of man's activity on his state of health. Even before scientific bases had been established upon which sound recommendations could be made, their intuitive observations led many of them to advise empirically that health could better be maintained and restored by exercise rather than rest.

A. HISTORICAL CONTRIBUTIONS MADE BY PHYSICIANS

Herodicus (fifth century BC) was the first physician of whom we have knowledge to recommend exercise as a form of treatment of disease. He applied therapeutic gymnastics so excessively that he was rebuked by Hippocrates (Littre, 1839–1861). Asclepiades (126–68 BC) employed gymnastics in connection with massage and diet in his treatment of patients (Green, 1955). Rufus of Ephesus (AD 60?–120) described the differing characteristics of the pulse in health and disease and its direct relationship to the apical beat of the heart (Brock, 1939).

Galen (AD 130–200) made or recorded more fundamental contributions to exercise physiology than any physician before or since. He was the first to develop systematic descriptions of the human body. He was the first to recognize that muscle has but one action, contraction. He observed that each muscle had only one direction of action and noted the antagonistic action of different muscle groups. He identified the force of muscle contraction as coming from the brain through the nerves. He described the connections and functions of the arteries and veins and showed that arteries contained blood obtained from the right heart and air from the lungs. He described the formation of urine from the serous portion of the blood. He developed the concept of tonus as active posture. Finally, he described the conduct of a comprehensive physical examination and history taking, based on logical principles (Brock, 1916; Duckworth, 1962; Singer, 1956).

Avicenna (tenth century AD) conceived of medical gymnastics as including all healthful and health-furthering exercises (Kruger, 1962). During convalescence he advocated rest, baths, and gentle massage.

Vittorino da Feltre (ca. 1378–1446) developed a school for children under the patronage of the Duke of Mantua. When children entered at age four or five, they were tested for their capabilities and exercise was prescribed individually according to the body type, age, season, and time of day. Dietetics were practiced and a wide variety of sports employed. Gymnastics were conceived of as an integral and indispensable preliminary for educational success for the first time since Ancient Greece (McCormick, 1943, 1944).

Maffeus Vegius (1407–1458) believed in the obligatory introduction into education of gymnastics to strengthen the body and of sports for recreation. He wished to avoid exaggerated exercises and heavy athletics (Vegius, 1613). Christobal Mendez (ca. 1553) wrote in the "Book of Bodily Exercise" (Guerra, 1960), "The easiest way of all to preserve and restore health without diverse peculiarities and with greater profit than all other measures put together is to exercise well." He advocated exercise for older persons and for those who were crippled as well.

Gerolamo Mercuriale (1530–1608) published six books on the "Art of Gymnastics" (Mercuriale, 1569). He classified gymnastics into preventive for the healthy and therapeutic for the sick. He was interested in exercise principally for its medical value and recommended particularly the type which would cause strenuous breathing and vehement movement. His work set the standard of thought in this regard for more than a century.

Ambroise Pare (1510–1590) was the first to point out in his work in surgery that exercise of the limbs after the primary treatment of fractures was indispensable (Pare, 1582). Joseph Duchesne (1546–1609) wrote on exercise in his "Ars Medica Hermetica," "The essential purpose of gymnastics for the body is its deliverance from superfluous humors, the regulation of digestion, the strengthening of the heart and the joints, the opening of the pores of the skin and the stronger circulation of the blood in the lungs by strenuous breathing." He was the first to recommend swimming for strengthening the body as well as for purposes of lifesaving (J. Duchesne, 1648). Laurent Joubert (1529–1583), who was professor of medicine at Montpellier, was the first to introduce gymnastics into the medical course. He considered physicians the only ones capable of prescribing gymnastics properly. He also recommended daily exercises (Joubert, 1582). Marsilius Cagnatus (1543–1612), of Verona, in his "Preservation of Health" asked for specially educated physicians to supervise games and introduced rowing into gymnastics (Cagnatus, 1602).

Santorio Santorio (1561–1636), a close friend of Galileo in Padua, invented the weighing chair which enabled him to measure insensible perspiration and develop a basic theory of metabolic balance. He also invented a machine for measuring the pulse (Santorio, 1614). Gerolamo Cardano (1510–1576) conceived a theory of movement of muscles from a mathematical-mechanical standpoint (Cardano, 1562). Other works by physicians on the physiology of muscle movements were those of D'Acquapendente (1614), Aldrovandri (1616), Deusing (1656), and Perrault (1680). Pierre Jean Burette (1665–1747) was the first physician to write on the history of athletics, especially ball games and discus throwing (Burette, 1748).

Bernardino Ramazzini (1633–1714) wrote the first treatise on occupational diseases. He pointed out that sedentary workers suffer from ill health and recommended regular exercises for them (Wright, 1940). Nicholas Andry (1658–1742) introduced the word orthopedics to Medicine. He was interested in preventing and correcting the deformities of children's bodies by exercise (Andry, 1741).

Robert Whytt (1714–1766), a neurologist of Edinburgh, established that reflex action was mediated through the spinal cord (Ackernecht, 1955). He understood fully the mechanism and significance of reflex action.

Claude Bernard (1813–1878) showed that the body performs a physiological synthesis by breaking down chemicals and building up complex substances. He also discovered the vasoconstrictor nerves (Greene, 1927). Guillaume Duchesne de Boulogne (1806–1875), as a result of his careful and detailed studies of striated muscle, came to the conclusion that contraction of single muscles was not a normal occurrence (G. Duchesne, 1855).

William Einthoven (1860–1927) invented the string galvanometer and first appreciated the spatial relationships of the action potentials spreading through the myocardial mass, and described this in 1901. In 1903, he reported on the galvanometric registration of the human electrocardiogram (Einthoven, 1903).

John Hughlings Jackson (1835–1911) developed the concept of the hierarchy of levels in the central nervous system. He described it as a mechanism for the coordination of impressions and movements (Jackson, 1932).

R. Tait McKenzie (1867–1938), in his "Exercise in Education and Medicine" laid the ground work for the modern concept of rehabilitation. He put his ideas into practice with the Canadian Expeditionary Forces in England in 1916 (McKenzie, 1909, 1916).

Siegfried Weissbein (nineteenth and twentieth centuries) produced a two-volume work entitled "Hygiene des Sports" which was the first book to deal comprehensively with sports medicine (Weissbein, 1910).

Since that time the contributions of physicians around the world to exercise physiology and sports medicine have multiplied so rapidly that it would require an entire book to list them. It would be impossible to single out a few without doing an injustice to many others.

B. Special Qualifications of the Physician-Physiologist

The majority of the great innovators who made the basic contributions which we have reviewed were practitioners primarily who utilized the scientific means available to them in the clinic, dissecting room, or laboratory to develop and test their theories. It is not until we come down to Bernard that we find a physician forsaking the rewards of practice entirely for the laboratory and the charity patients in the hospital.

The tremendous explosion of scientific development in this century has resulted inevitably in specialization. Since the study of natural phenomena requires a knowledge of different branches of science, however, a certain amount of mixed- or cross-specialization has taken place. Today the physician who works in the field of exercise physiology does so perhaps because his preparation in physiology was originally greater than average, but more likely because his interest in the problems he would like to attack have led him to further special preparation in physiology.

Perhaps the only significant difference in the approaches of the pure physiologist and the physician-physiologist to the problems of exercise is the orientation toward pathology which the latter has acquired in his training. Many of the technical advances of modern surgery would not have been possible without the close collaboration of physicians and physiologists working together in the laboratory. Both, in turn, have had to call on another specialist, the engineer, and to learn something of his techniques and his approach themselves.

The great interest in all phases of rehabilitation which has developed in medicine today has caused a number of physicians to direct their investigations into the area where a knowledge of physiological principles and techniques of physical medicine and physical education are essential. Among other results of this collaboration of ideas has been a revolution in thinking with regard to the role of exercise in the treatment of the patient who has suffered a myocardial infarction due to coronary occlusion.

C. The Sports Physician

Galen was the first sports physician whom we know by name. For 4 years he took care of the gladiators in his home city of Pergamon before leaving for Rome in AD 161. The surgical experience he acquired was invaluable to him because there were strict laws prohibiting the dissection of dead bodies, and he had few other opportunities to learn human anatomy.

During the next 1700 years there must have been many physicians who took care of gladiators, knights at tournaments, and athletes of all sorts in many countries, but we just do not have specific records of their names and accomplishments.

In England, in 1873, Dr. John E. Morgan, a former university oarsman and a distinguished physician, attempted a comparison of the longevity of 299 former oarsmen with that of the general population (White, 1958). This was probably the first modern study in sports medicine. Two other Englishmen, J. B. Byles and Samuel Osborn, wrote a section on first-aid for athletics in "The Encyclopedia of Sport," published in New York and London in 1898. The first book on the diagnosis and treatment of sports injuries in English was by Heald (1931).

On the European continent, interest developed rapidly following the publication of "Hygiene des Sports" (Weissbein, 1910). The first medical congress dealing with sports was held in Paris in March 1915. The progress of World War I and its aftermath prevented subsequent meetings until 1928, when a scientific session was held in connection with the Olympic Winter Games at St. Moritz, Switzerland. This meeting was attended by 93 physicians from 11 nations and resulted in the establishment of the Federation Internationale de Medicine Sportive (FIMS). The first International Congress of Sports Medicine was held in Amsterdam later that year. The International Bulletin of the FIMS was established in 1934.

In 1954, the American College of Sports Medicine was founded and the American Medical Association appointed an ad hoc committee on Injuries in Sports, which has subsequently become a standing committee on the Medical Aspects of Sports. There are thousands of physicians for high school, college, professional, and other athletic teams and groups. Many of them belong to professional organizations active in sports medicine and attend regular conferences which are now numerous in this field.

The sports physician today may be a general practitioner who examines the candidates for high school teams and treats their injuries. He may be a full-time employee of a college health service who devotes most or all of his time to the medical supervision of athletes. In Europe, he may be a recognized specialist in sports medicine with a diploma or certificate indicating his special training in this field. In any case he should have not only a special interest in sports and physical education but particular knowledge in these subjects which enables him to interpret his medical supervision in terms of the peculiar requirements and circumstances of the area of physical activity. He must be thoroughly familiar with the basic concepts of the physiology of exercise. Finally he must understand the principles of safety and be familiar with the use of protective equipment and the fundamentals of physical therapy and rehabilitation.

D. Present Realization of the Dynamic View of the Patient

One of the great setbacks to medical progress occurred paradoxically around the turn of the century when new discoveries in medical and surgical treatment were beginning to appear in clusters. This was the idea that rest in bed was sovereign, no matter what other type of treatment would be offered.

Surgical patients were kept lying flat on their backs for 3 weeks following operations. When they finally got up, it took three people to help them and it was often another week before they were able to walk unassisted. Patients with coronary thrombosis were kept lying down and hardly allowed to move for 6 weeks. When they got up, some of them promptly died, and the others took another 3 weeks to be able to help themselves.

Fortunately, early ambulation was rediscovered in the 1940's and is now in full sway. Every reasonable effort is made to keep every sick patient up and active as much as is consistent with safety. Those who must remain in bed are given exercise to do there. As soon as the immediate danger of the rupture of heart muscle is passed, many coronary thrombosis patients are now exercised on treadmills and encouraged in vigorous game activities. Drug therapy has even made it possible for tuberculosis victims to exercise actively.

The basis for this reversal of thinking has been the realization that rest causes stasis of the circulation, loss of muscle tonus leading to muscular atrophy, and impaired respiratory and renal function. Good function in these systems is essential to rapid and complete recovery. Poor function may lead to a death which should not occur.

This wholesome therapeutic attitude is now carrying over into the preventive phase of medicine. Physicians now advocate exercise and all forms of physical activity as means of preventing degenerative disease and of preparing the body for the emergency which may be created by the onslaught of infectious disease or trauma.

II. The Dynamic Physical Examination

With the reestablishment of the dynamic view of the patient who is suffering from illness or injury has come the realization that it is time for a new approach to the examination of the supposedly or apparently healthy individual. The physical examination as practiced by the physician in his office, at the factory, in the clinic, or even in the athletic setting has been essentially static for many years. The individual was examined at rest, and, indeed, almost in a basal state. Unless compelled by the request of a third party (usually by an insurance company) to perform a very light exercise test of response of pulse, functional evaluations were not included in the examination. It is perhaps significant that one of the laboratory tests most favored by physicians in the past has been the basal (resting) metabolic rate.

The cardiologists were the first to reassert the value of exercise in the evaluation of the patient. This came about through their desire to differentiate angina of exercise and true coronary disease. Patients were given a provocative test of exercise and electrocardiograms recorded before and after. When these experiments were first reported, they were decried by many as too dangerous. Compared to present coronary treatments, they appear timid.

The development of surgery of the lung demanded better methods of evaluating pulmonary function. Methods were developed to give a reliable picture of the patient's response to exercise in terms of lung capacity and reserve. The traditional methods had failed to indicate properly how much lung tissue could be removed without making the patient a respiratory cripple.

Modern technology in measuring the functions of the human body during exercise has arisen partly from the demand to know more about this, but in turn has made it possible to find out much more than had been previously imagined. Techniques of telemetering, continuous monitoring of cardiac and pulmonary function and of the metabolites of the blood now make possible the construction of a continuous picture of the response of the body to exercise.

A. Scope of the Examination

In a practical sense, there is no such thing as a "complete" physical examination. No matter what points may be covered by a physician, another could easily add several more which were omitted. The purpose of any such examination is actually twofold: to uncover any significant defect or deficit which may not be suspected or which may have been concealed by the subject; and to assess the status of those organs which are a particular matter of concern to the examiner in the light of the purpose for which the examination is being made.

It cannot be stated categorically, therefore, that such and such parts of the body should be examined in this and that way or under these or those conditions as a matter of general practice. The examiner should have clearly in his mind the purposes for which the examination is given and design its structure accordingly. Even in those areas of the body which are covered, the emphasis may vary considerably.

Functional tests and tests of exercise capacity have multiplied as rapidly as investigators in the field of exercise physiology during the past 20 years. It would be almost impossible to make a complete listing of those which have been described, and it would be soon outdated by additions yet to come. In several recent publications, such as that of Fleishmann (1964), attempts have been made to establish cross-correlations between several of these tests in order to arrive at a simple set of standards for determining a person's state of physical fitness.

If the physician is to be expected to perform functional tests in his office as part of a patient's examination, those employed must be simple enough not to require elaborate equipment, not excessively time-consuming, and subject to simple analysis for practical purposes. Two examples of tests which meet these criteria will be mentioned. The first has probably found the widest acceptance of any functional test among physicians, in its original or in some modified form. The second seems to have great potentiality as a test of fitness in the person who has had a cardiac problem, because it measures some of the most important aspects of cardiac and pulmonary function at the same time and in relation to each other.

One group of investigators (Falls *et al.*, 1965; Ismail *et al.*, 1965) has defined the state of physical fitness as being dependent on 9 separate factors: (1) athletic fitness, (2) maximum metabolic rate, (3) respiratory capacity, (4) blood pressures, (5) heart response to exertion, (6) forced respiratory capacity, (7) pulse pressure, (8) force efficiency, and (9) heart rate. In order to gain a truly meaningful estimate of an individual's state of fitness, it is necessary to measure at least four of these factors, including the maximum oxygen intake related to the lean body mass. The means of measuring this latter and the time involved in such a study make it not feasible for the regular physical examination.

The version of the step test which comes closest to the original description and is most commonly used as a simple functional evaluation is as follows.

The patient steps up and down on a 20-inch bench at a rate of 30 times/ min for 5 min, unless he stops earlier because of fatigue. Upon completing the exercise, he sits quietly. Pulse counts are then taken as follows:

1 min after exercise for 30 sec
2 min after exercise for 30 sec
3 min after exercise for 30 sec

The patient's Physical Fitness Index (PFI) can then be calculated according to the formula:

$$\text{PFI} = \frac{\text{duration of exercise in seconds} \times 100}{\text{sum of pulse counts in recovery} \times 2}$$

The result is interpreted according to Table I.

For example, if a patient exercised the entire 5 min, or 300 sec, and his recovery pulse rates were 80 at $1\frac{1}{2}$ min, 60 at $2\frac{1}{2}$ min, and 40 at $3\frac{1}{2}$ min, his formula would read:

$$\text{PFI} = 300\,(100)/180\,(2) = 83$$

In a patient over 30 years of age, this would be an exceptionally high fitness index. However, if his index falls in the range of 60 or below, it may prove desirable to encourage his participation in an exercise program.

The height of the step can be varied for people of below average height, and for children. The minimum height should probably be 14 inches. During exercise, the patient should be watched for shortness of breath, undue flushing, and chest pain. If severe discomfort or chest pain occurs, the exercise should be terminated immediately. In any case, a more accurate assessment of physical fitness and prescription of a properly weighted exercise program for the patient can result.

TABLE I

STANDARDS FOR USE IN INTERPRETING THE PFI SCORE

	Age		
Score	Under 30	30–50	Over 50
90	Excellent	—	—
80–90	Good	Excellent	—
65–79	High average	Good	Excellent
55–64	Low average	Average	Good
Under 55	Poor	Poor	Poor

Another useful test is the Hyman Cardio Respiratory Index (Hyman, 1962). It requires a stop watch, a stethoscope, cuff, and manometer for measuring blood pressure, and a simple spirometer which can measure vital capacity and maximum expiratory pressure. The sum of the vital capacity (in units of 100 cm^3), breath holding time (in seconds), maximum expiratory pressure (in mm Hg), and age (in years) are divided by the sum of the systolic blood pressure (in mm Hg), the diastolic blood pressure, and the individual's age (in years). An index score of 1.000 is considered to be normal. Most athletes will score well above this level. Subjects in a poor state of physical fitness or with uncompensated cardiovascular disease may score as low as 0.500.

If a laboratory equipped for research in exercise physiology is available and time permits, more accurate determinations of physical fitness can be obtained by determining with the aid of a treadmill, or bicycle ergometer, the maximal oxygen intake in milliliters per kilogram of body weight (Balke, 1960). The correlation of these findings with exercise pulse rate, percent of lean body mass, resting diastolic blood pressure, and resting pulse pressure will give an estimate of a subject's overall state of fitness with a very high degree of reliability.

The need to include tests of blood and urine, x-ray examinations, and other studies must be decided in terms of the results sought. Certain procedures have a high yield of unexpected findings. Routine testings of urine for sugar will turn up in a cross section of the population a number of unsuspected diabetics. In a school population the number would be very small; in a home for the aged it would be relatively large. Routine chest x-rays give a fairly high yield of abnormal findings because they cover a number of different organs about which they can provide some sort of information. The absolute yield of specific disease states, such as tuberculosis, will vary tremendously with the type of population surveyed.

The combination of a physical examination directed primarily at the points which are of specific interest, according to the purpose for which the examination is being performed, with a functional test or tests, especially in relation to what is called physical fitness, is the modern approach to a dynamic physical examination. Whereas the ordinary static examination can only tell the physician a limited amount about the subject's physical condition at the moment, the dynamic examination can demonstrate and predict his response to stress, placing the individual in the correct context, that of an environment in which he acts and to which he reacts.

B. Timing of the Examination

Since physical examinations are performed for a variety of purposes, the timing must depend to a certain extent on the purpose. The annual physical examination has become an accepted feature of progressive industrial health programs. The selection of this arbitrary timing is partly a matter of convenience, partly a response to a concept which has become traditional in thought if not in general practice, and partly a concession to the necessity of dealing with numbers of employees. For athletes, it has been customary to perform an examination before the start of the competitive season. In some primary and secondary schools there is a requirement that an examination be performed every 3 years.

It may be that for any particular purpose, a physical examination should be performed every 6 weeks or as infrequently as every 6 years. The decision should be made by the examiner as objectively as possible within the limitations imposed by time, expense, and the possible availability of the subjects. In the case of athletes it may be desirable to conduct a comprehensive examination once a year, and to supplement this with periodic evaluations at the change of seasons, following an injury or illness, or when certain critical periods of competition are approaching. The supplementary examinations would be designed to bring out the points of specific interest to the examiner, allowing a comparison with the baselines obtained at the annual examination.

When the decision has been made as to calendar period in which the examination is to be conducted, care should be exercised to prevent untoward occurrences from influencing the result. The subject should not be examined when acutely ill, or during the early stages of convalescence, when unusually fatigued, or, if possible, when under any severe mental strain. There is some variation in the body's activity and response throughout the day, so that examinations made for direct and accurate comparisons should be repeated at the same hour if possible.

The results of functional tests performed shortly after eating may vary from those performed in a fasting state. In this case it may be desirable to carry them out at a different time from the remainder of the examination or on a subsequent day.

The setting of the examination should provide both the subject and examiner with the necessary privacy and freedom from noise and other distraction. On the occasion of a first examination by an unfamiliar physician, pulse and blood pressure may be considerably higher than would normally be found in the same subject.

Female subjects should not be examined during the immediate premenstrual period or the first 2 days of menstruation, if possible, for routine purposes, since significant changes in certain functional capacities may be noticed. The subject's response to the examination as a whole may also be less favorable due to irritability or depression.

C. Interpreting the Examination to the Subject

The patient in the physician's office who has just undergone an examination wants principally to know that he is "normal." The applicant for an industrial position is chiefly concerned that he will "pass." The athlete seeks to find out if he is "fit" or "in condition." Each one of these persons must be informed of the results in terms of what he wishes to learn.

Each examination provides an opportunity for health education at the time when the individual should be most receptive to it. The patient who is examined and found to be free of detectable evidence of cancer might be told diplomatically by his physician that he is in a poor state of physical fitness. His performance of a functional capacity test and the information that he fell below standard might be his first introduction to the concept of physical fitness. The proper information at this time might awaken an interest which would be very important for his future welfare.

One of the most important concepts which the examiner must explain is that "normal" implies a range of values. In addition, what is "normal" at one age might be abnormal in another. That physical and physiological differences, other than the obvious ones, exist between the sexes is a surprise to many people. To report a finding to a subject without explaining its meaning may lead to confusion and misunderstanding which vitiate in part the purpose of the examination.

When it comes to reporting the results of functional testing to the subject, great care must be exercised by the examiner. The serious nature of very poor performance should not be understated, but the possibilities for improvement, if they exist, should be stressed. Functional capacities should be interpreted in terms of the needs of the particular individual and not on any arbitrary basis.

Finally, if the results of the examination lead to the conclusion that the subject has failed to meet the requirements or desired level of health and performance, the interpretation should include not only the specific reasons why this is the case but also recommendations concerning factors which are conceivably correctable. The interpretation may be difficult to a subject who considers himself healthy, but has a poor functional capacity, or to a person with a good functional capacity who has a specific disqualifying physical defect.

III. Qualifications of Individuals for Exercise Activity

Prevention of injury and illness in any program of physical activity must begin with the examination of the person or persons who will participate in this activity. There is a moral obligation on the part of the sports director not to allow the participation of one who because of some defect in his health or because of the unsuitability of his condition might become more seriously ill or might more easily suffer an injury. The individual has an obligation to himself and his family, if individual participation is concerned.

In the case of schools, colleges, voluntary sports associations, and professional teams, there is also a responsibility which has been increasingly recognized by the number of civil actions for damages which have been brought against them in recent years because of permanent disability or death sustained in supervised sports activity. Although this has been recognized in the past by having the participant (if of age) or the parents sign a release for responsibility in the event of injury, these releases have little effect under the law. In any event, it must be recognized that a parent cannot waive the rights of a minor, and that in the event of a permanent disability, the minor may bring action after reaching his majority, and that the limitations set by statute for such civil action do not become operative until that date has been reached.

Further, it is unquestionable that the ability of an individual to participate effectively and with enjoyment depends on his physical capacity to participate. In team sports the highest measure of those values which are thought to accrue from participation will be reached if the competitors are well suited to the activity by virtue of their physical qualifications, equalization of capacities is obtained, and neither team is handicapped by preventable disability.

These ideals can be realized only by requiring physical examinations before supervised sports activities and recommending it strongly for those participating in individual recreational sports. The dynamic physical examination is then combined with a thorough knowledge of the particular requirements of sports activities in general to determine what activity is suitable for the individual and which individuals must be disqualified from certain activities.

A. SELECTION OF SUITABLE ACTIVITY

Every type of physical activity requires a certain type or types of physical or performance capacities to ensure successful and safe participation. It has a certain characteristic environment or setting which may pose problems for the individual. There are certain hazards of injury or illness inherent in every type of sports activity. All of these factors must be considered in selecting the sport or other physical activity suitable for the particular individual.

An exhaustive survey of the somatotypes which favor certain types of sports activities or of desirable performance capacities is not within the scope of this work. A few examples will illustrate the principles involved.

The relatively short, squat, squarish individual makes the best weight-lifter. When well muscled he will not only be more efficient but less prone to muscle strain because of his short lever arms. There is little need for the weight-lifter to demonstrate cardiovascular endurance since his action occurs in short, explosive bursts.

The sprinter has the capacity to perform efficiently under essentially anaerobic conditions of work. His physique tends to be taller, more muscular, with a heavier skeleton than the long-distance runner who is typically shorter, lighter, and with more slender muscles. These types naturally lean toward the more suitable activity.

The athlete participating in contact sports should be well developed from a muscular standpoint whatever his height. This development should be maximal in the thighs in order to provide as much protection as possible to the knees which are exposed to serious hazards in these activities.

A person who lacks mental as well as physical toughness, or who lacks cardiorespiratory endurance, or is easily fatigued by hard physical work, should never select mountain climbing as a sport.

As far as the environment of the sports activity is concerned, the particular factors which are important are temperature, humidity, altitude, and whether the activity takes place on or under the water, on land, or in the air. Some persons by virtue of their constitution and by their previous experiences are well suited to physical activity in environments which manifest extremes of cold or heat. Acclimatization is more easily reached and maintained by some persons than by others. An individual with marked arteriosclerosis would be a poor candidate for outdoor winter sports if the period of exposure would be prolonged since there would be not only danger of frostbite to the extremities but of provoking a coronary attack if a severe wind chill occurred. A person with a congenital condition of the skin which impaired normal sweating would be a poor candidate for any strenuous physical outdoor effort in hot weather because of the danger of heat stroke.

In like manner, the problems raised by exercise under conditions where high humidity might be a factor would make the situation unsuitable for some persons at any time, and for all persons if extreme conditions are approached. It is possible to modify the individual's reaction in this instance, however, by means other than acclimatization through the administration of extra amounts of salt and water before and during exercise. This possibility must be considered in determining the suitability of the particular activity for the person concerned.

Where high altitudes will be attained during some sports activity, as in mountain climbing or sports parachuting, persons having circulatory or pulmonary problems will have to be ruled out in many instances. The critical factor for performance at high altitudes is the maintenance of adequate oxygen intake and consumption. Even though this behavior may be modified by the use of self-contained oxygen breathing apparatus, the modification itself may have an unfavorable effect on the person's functional defect, as in asthma.

Man is only beginning to learn how to adapt himself to an underwater environment. Individuals who are qualified physically and by training for underwater sports activity may become temporarily or permanently unsuitable if they develop disease in the sinuses or middle ear.

Each sport has a number of hazards associated with its practice opening the door to possible illness or injury. These will actually vary within the area of that sport according to the degree of expertise of those participating. For example, the beginning skier is in the greatest danger of breaking a leg because of his inability to control his skis and to fall correctly. The expert downhill racer is in less danger of this, but faced with the threat of serious if not fatal injury to his head or neck due to the great acceleration he achieves, which would be impossible for the beginner.

The fact that hazards of injury and death are present in most sports is not in itself a sufficient reason to ban or legislate against them. The so-called "blood" sports, such as bullfighting, are barred in many countries. Boxing has been banned in some jurisdictions from time to time and is under attack at present. Factors other than the hazards involved are operative in these cases, however. If danger of death were the only issue, then professional automobile racing should have been abandoned many years ago. On the other hand, the sports physician should advise the prospective participant of the hazards involved as well as the protective measures which can be undertaken.

It has been contended that certain sports and exercise activities are unsuitable for girls and women. The basis of these objections seems to be largely aesthetic and traditional since there is hardly any sport in which women have not participated at one time or another, sometimes on an equal basis with men. It does seem inadvisable for women, with their lighter bone structure, to participate in football where there could, at least theoretically, be a greater possibility for fractures to occur.

B. Basis for Disqualification from Certain Activities

Acute medical conditions from which complete recovery can be expected and the convalescent stage following surgery or injury are only temporarily disqualifying from sports and other strenuous physical activities. It is important to remember that reexamination should take place following recovery and before participation.

Congenital and chronic conditions may be disqualifying from certain types of sports and not from others. A useful guide in this regard has been issued by the American Medical Association and is reproduced in Table II.

It is important to have exact information before determining that a condition is disqualifying. The presence of a heart murmur, for example, is not significant unless other confirmatory evidence from the history, chest x-ray,

TABLE II

Disqualifying Conditions for Sports Participation

Conditions	Contact[a]	Noncontact endurance[b]	Other[c]
General			
Acute infections: respiratory, genitourinary, infectious mononucleosis, hepatitis, active rheumatic fever, acute tuberculosis, boils, furuncles, impetigo	×	×	×
Obvious physical immaturity in comparison with other competitors	×	×	
Obvious growth retardation	×	×	×
Hemorrhagic disease: hemophilia, purpura, and other bleeding tendencies	×		
Diabetes, inadequately controlled	×	×	×
Jaundice, whatever cause	×	×	×
Eyes			
Absence or loss of function of one eye	×		
Severe myopia, even if correctable	×		
Ears			
Significant impairment	×		
Respiratory			
Tuberculosis (active or under treatment)	×	×	×
Severe pulmonary insufficiency	×	×	×

TABLE II

DISQUALIFYING CONDITIONS FOR SPORTS PARTICIPATION

Conditions	Contact[a]	Noncontact endurance[b]	Other[c]
Cardiovascular			
Mitral stenosis, aortic stenosis, aortic insufficiency, coarctation of aorta, cyanotic heart disease, recent carditis of any etiology	×	×	×
Hypertension on organic basis	×	×	×
Previous heart surgery for congenital or acquired heart disease	×	×	
Liver			
Enlarged liver	×		
Spleen			
Enlarged spleen	×		
Hernia			
Inguinal or femoral hernia	×	×	
Musculoskeletal			
Symptomatic abnormalities or inflammations	×	×	×
Functional inadequacy of the musculoskeletal system, congenital or acquired, incompatible with the contact or skill demands of the sport	×	×	
Neurological			
History or symptoms of previous or serious head trauma or repeated concussions	×		
Convulsive disorder not completely controlled by medication	×	×	
Previous surgery on head or spine	×	×	×
Renal			
Absence of one kidney	×		
Renal disease	×	×	×
Genitalia			
Absence of one testicle	×		
Undescended testicle	×		

[a] Lacrosse, baseball, soccer, basketball, football, wrestling, hockey, Rugby, etc.
[b] Cross country, track, tennis, crew, swimming, etc.
[c] Bowling, golf, archery, field events, etc.

electrocardiogram, and functional testing indicates that it is a sign of organic heart disease. The same principle applies to a single finding of elevated blood pressure or of albuminuria.

Where a disqualifying condition is correctable by surgery or other means, reevaluation may permit participation after recovery. Hernia and hydrocele are examples of such defects. On the basis of experience it does not appear to be reasonable to allow full participation in vigorous sports for persons who have had surgery for the correction of congenital or acquired cardiac conditions, with the exception of uncomplicated persistent ductus arteriosus.

Continued participation in sports for a person with diabetes should depend on continued control. It is recognized that physical activity may reduce temporarily the need for insulin and that dextrose should be kept readily available for the treatment of hypoglycemic reactions. The chance to participate in sports often provides the best motivation for a juvenile diabetic to make a serious effort to control his disease.

Participation in sports activities by persons who suffer from a convulsive disorder must be closely supervised even if the condition appears to be under satisfactory control by medication. Physical effort and emotional excitement may upset the balance between subcortical and cortical areas of the brain so that an attack is precipitated. Sports situations which expose the individual to the "flicker-fusion" phenomenon should be avoided.

The situation resulting from certain injuries, even when healing has occurred, with or without surgical intervention, may cause an absolute contraindication to participation in certain sports. Fractures in the upper cervical vertebrae are an example of such injuries. Since solid healing does not always take place, and there is no absolute method of determining this by x-ray or other means, the danger of cord injury is too great to allow participation in contact sports.

No consideration other than what is best for the health of the prospective participant should determine the question of participation. The physician's authority in this matter must be paramount. It is the duty of all those concerned with the direction of athletes to support and reinforce the physician in these decisions.

IV. Principles of Safety in Physical Activity and Sports

Every type of sport or physical activity has the potential for the occurrence of an accident and, therefore, also an injury. Accidents may occur as a result of events which are entirely beyond human control. The great majority, however, occur as the result of human failure in one respect or another. This implies that in the case of such accidents at least, there are preventable factors.

It has been said that 300 unsafe acts that could cause an accident take place before one does cause an accidental injury. Only one in thirty injuries is disabling, that is, causes loss of time from work, sport, or other normal activity. One hundred disabling injuries occur on the average for each accidental death. It can be seen from these figures that the problem of preventing one accidental death might involve preventing as many as 900,000 unsafe acts, and that of preventing a disabling injury, 9000 such acts.

Since sports are characterized by acts that are unsafe by their nature it can easily be seen the risk of injury may be very high. This is especially true as the speed of the performer increases, as the performers come in contact with each other, or in deliberate combative sports, since the margin of safety is proportionately reduced in each instance. Injury prevention in sports, then, is often a matter of assisting the performer to carry out intrinsically unsafe acts in as safe a manner as possible, or of minimizing the effects of injuries which are almost inevitable in their occurrence. This can be accomplished chiefly by carrying out a program of conditioning and training, teaching and coaching correct skills in sports, using proper protective equipment, insisting on learning and following the rules, and providing good officials, and making suitable emergency care readily available.

A. ROLE OF CONDITIONING

Injury, broadly construed in the area of sports and physical activity, includes illness and disease states which may occur as the results of such activities as well as trauma. In discussing prevention by means of training and conditioning, it is necessary to consider the roles which may be played by nutrition, acclimatization, and rest, as well as by muscular exercise and the improvement of function in the pulmonary and cardiovascular systems. These subjects involve material sufficient to fill one or several books, but only the main principles involved can be included here.

A diet so deficient in quantity or quality of its composition that it fails to maintain normal weight in a person regularly participating in some physical activity over a period of time may result in the occurrence of disease due to a lessening of general resistance. Dietary supplements are not necessary for persons with normal metabolism or who are eating a well-balanced diet (see Chapter 5). When excessive fasting and dehydration are practiced for the purpose of rapid weight reduction, as by wrestlers and boxers, loss of muscle strength occurs, and other profound physiological disturbances, including convulsions, may result. Attempts to restore weight lost in this fashion very rapidly by consuming large quantities of food may cause severe digestive difficulties, including acute pancreatitis.

Overeating in the athlete, a practice which is common among football players today, if accompanied by overweight, may militate against safety by hampering the ability of the athlete to move quickly and efficiently for his own protection. A greater strain is also put on the cardiovascular system. In order to determine whether an athlete is obese or simply above average weight due to the development of muscle it may be necessary to determine his body density. This may be done by weighing him underwater, or more simply by taking four skin-fold measurements and relating them to a formula which gives the body density with an accuracy sufficient for clinical purposes (see Chapters 12 and 13).

Acclimatization is important in physical activities in relation to heat, cold, and altitude. These subjects are fully covered in other chapters. Since they can become very important practical considerations in the management of individual athletes and athletic teams, the sports physician must be thoroughly familiar with the mechanisms which can lead to illness and injury and the appropriate preventive measures.

Heat exhaustion and heat stroke are of major concern during the first month of practice for American football which takes place in September each year. The combination of hot, humid days, heavy equipment, insufficient salt and water replacement, and lack of acclimatization produce fatalities every year which are entirely preventable.

Problems relating to performance at altitudes considerably above sea level are of less serious importance to health except when one gets into the higher mountains. The average athletic team is at a moderate disadvantage when traveling up to play a team which is acclimatized to a lower atmospheric pressure. The individual performer in long-distance running or swimming events must accept a considerable decrement in performance as far as finishing time is concerned. Practical considerations prevent spending the time at altitude necessary to become acclimatized except in unusual circumstances.

To speak about the importance of rest when discussing training and conditioning seems paradoxical, but consideration of this subject is vital from three standpoints. Athletes should get enough rest each day, heavy practice and competition should be properly spaced out, and no period of training should be carried on indefinitely without a long break.

The intensive training schedules in many sports today which are prescribed by coaches or are self-imposed by athletes leave relatively little time for other activities and at the same time increase fatigue, so that adequate rest and sleep are even more important. Sleep requirements vary among individuals, but, in general, the young athlete in training requires at least 8 hr per night. If he is spending 6 hr per day training, and has either an academic program or a job to maintain, there is very little time to do anything else except eat his meals. Consistent failure to get adequate amounts of sleep will inevitably be reflected in a deterioration of performance.

The ancient Greek boxers and wrestlers at one time worked in a 4-day cycle of training. On the first day the athlete took exercises featuring light quick movements, on the second his powers of endurance were tested, on the third he relaxed with only very gentle movements, and on the fourth he practiced only movements of defense. This was similar to the system of training advocated by the Swedish physical educator, Ling, who advocated gradual increase and gradual diminution of work. Modern systems of training are very apt to continue 7 days a week before competition starts, reaching several peaks during the week. When competition starts, the day following is often devoted to complete rest and usually only light work is undertaken on the day before competition.

Due to the improvements in international communications and ease of travel, there is no longer any time of the year for many sports in which the opportunity for competition is not available somewhere in the world. The top-class athletes find it a matter of necessity to keep themselves in condition and available for competition the year around. This is especially true in track and field, swimming, tennis, and golf. If they wish to remain active continuously, they run the risk of "going stale" or reaching a state of "overtraining."

Although the signs and symptoms of overtraining are well defined and readily recognized, the exact mechanisms through which these phenomena occur are not understood in spite of all that has been written on the subject. The athlete, himself, is usually puzzled at first when he finds his performance falling off when he seems to be trying as hard or harder than ever. Finally, everything becomes an effort, and a feeling of lassitude and depression appears to accompany the symptoms of weakness, rapid heart beat, and easy fatigue. Not all athletes are affected by this condition even if they work through the year. Most seek to avoid it by·taking one month in which they stop intensive training and may not take any special exercise at all (see Chapter 14).

The athlete who does not get enough daily rest, rest between competitions, or who is overtrained is more susceptible to injury as well as to intermittent illness. Fatigue is an important factor in the production of injury as exemplified by the fact that the greatest number of accidents in skiing occur during the last hours of daylight when some have been on the hills almost continuously for hours.

Conditioning the muscles by exercise plays an important role in safety in sports for two principal reasons. The more powerful muscles are more able to resist the severe stresses which may occur without tearing. The greatest protection to the ligaments and joints is afforded by the strength of the muscles which cross them or whose tendons insert on or around the capsules. In addition, attention to a correct order of procedure during training and practice may prevent injury to the muscles themselves.

There is no proof that muscles with a large cross section are more resistant to strains than smaller ones, but as a matter of practical experience this seems to be so. However, they do not appear to be any more resistant to the effect of contusions. There is no real evidence to indicate that rapid increase in muscle mass due to overloading makes such a muscle more susceptible to injury.

The knee joint is particularly vulnerable to injury in many types of sports because of its complex mode of action, the unusual stresses to which it may be subject, and the fact that it is a weight-bearing joint. It seems apparent from a number of studies which have been done that when muscle strength in the thighs is increased the volume of serious knees injuries in football is less. The same situation seems to prevail in the shoulder.

It is generally believed that proper "warming-up" before exercise reduces the danger of muscle strains. This has never been demonstrated convincingly in any clinical study. It is apparent, however, that overstretching a muscle immediately before subjecting it to a maximum stress does decrease the danger of muscle strain or rupture.

Adequate conditioning of the pulmonary and cardiovascular systems is an important factor in safety mainly from two standpoints. If an athlete becomes excessively fatigued or exhausted during practice or competition he is more liable to suffer an injury. This is particularly true in a contact sport where a defensive attitude exposes an athlete to a greater danger of injury than an offensive one. In the second instance, if a person undertakes very strenuous physical activity over a prolonged period of time without any or very little conditioning for the cardiovascular system, damage to the heart or its coronary circulation may result. If such damage already exists, but has not been recognized previously, a serious heart attack or a fatality may occur.

B. IMPORTANCE OF CORRECT COACHING AND TEACHING

Since we are dealing in sports with many activities and types of movement which are essentially unsafe, it is natural that in order for them to be made as safe as possible, great care must be taken in teaching and learning these activities. Pole-vaulting is an excellent example of an unsafe activity which can be made safer by good coaching. The speed must reach a maximum on the runway, but the planting of the pole must be controlled so that it goes straight up and not to the side, or the performer will hit the standard or land out of the pit. The turn of the body in mid-air and push-off from the pole must be accomplished in such a way that the back and shoulder muscles are not strained. The fall should be controlled so that the vaulter lands sitting down or on his back and not on his head or neck.

If there are several ways of accomplishing the same objective in sports, the safer way should be taught by preference. There is sometimes, in sports such as football, a tendency for some coaches to teach a technique which may be effective but which may be fraught with danger for the user. Spearing the opponent with the helmet is an example of such a technique. Even though the major portion of the shock may be diverted from the head by the helmet, it is transmitted to the neck which has no protection other than the strength of its muscles and is poorly designed from a mechanical standpoint to resist such stress. Serious injuries and even fatalities have resulted from this practice.

Awkward or incorrect movements may result in chronic as well as acute injury. The baseball pitcher who throws the ball incorrectly or off balance may suffer a chronic strain in his pitching arm. Failure to hit the forehand or backhand drive with the correct motion in tennis may result in the development of a chronic inflammation at the tendonous attachments to the internal or external epicondyle, the so-called "tennis elbow."

A very special example of the teaching of a skill correctly but to a person who is not physically prepared to adopt it safely occurs in the baseball programs for boys 9–12 years of age. The use of the twisting motion of the arm and elbow which is necessary to make a baseball curve is capable of producing acute and chronic damage to the ununited epiphysis of the lower end of the humerus.

C. THE USE OF PROTECTIVE EQUIPMENT

One of the most important aspects of safety in sports is the use of appropriate protective devices and equipment. The requirements for sports vary according to the hazards involved but usage may follow custom rather than indicated needs. Where equipment is used, advantage should be taken of modern materials to afford the best and most lasting protection. Proper fit of personal protective equipment is essential to effective function. The use of worn-out or defective equipment is a false economy. Levels of protection offered in practice should be equivalent to those supplied for competition. Athletes must be carefully instructed in the proper use and care of the protective devices which are provided. They should not be overloaded with equipment which hampers effective participation. Protective devices may in themselves offer some hazard to athletes.

The protective devices used in sports may be placed on the athlete or may be placed in such a way as to protect him. A helmet is a characteristic device placed on him, and a wrestling mat, one which is provided for his protection. A third type is a device attached to some equipment used by the athlete, such as the rubber or plastic tip applied to the sharp rear end of the ice hockey skate. Protective devices may be substantial and may be reused repeatedly, as a shoulder pad for football, or they may be especially constructed for single use and be disposable, as in the protective strapping of an ankle with adhesive tape. In some instances, the safety device may be almost a duplication of regular equipment used as part of the sport, as the reserve parachute used in sports parachuting.

The sports which feature body contact, in general, employ the greatest weight and variety of protective equipment. American football and ice hockey lead the list in this regard. Soccer, however, does not ordinarily use any devices other than shin guards and not all players wear these. Participants in Rugby and football under Gaelic and Australian rules wear very little if any protective equipment by tradition. The types and character of protective equipment which may be used are sometimes specified in the rules laid down by the governing body for the sport.

The development of closed-cell plastic foam materials for use in protective sports equipment has made it possible to offer superior protection and comfort as well as to lighten the weight which the athlete has to carry. These materials are shock absorbent but have a slow recovery period. This material is used as a liner but may also be applied with tape as a protective pad cut to fit over an injured part. High-impact plastics have permitted the development of superior helmets and other types of equipment which are still moderately light in weight.

The finest protective equipment available will not do its job right if it is not fitted to the person who is going to wear it. This is particularly true of helmets which should fit snugly so that they cannot be turned on the head or easily dislodged. Hip pads for football players should be held in place so that they reach above the iliac crest to protect this sensitive area. Many young athletes if not watched closely have a tendency to allow the trousers and underlying pads to drop down over the hips.

When protective equipment becomes worn-out, broken, or loses its natural fit, it should be replaced before an injury occurs as the result of inadequate protection. It is often difficult to persuade the athlete to part with it since it has become "comfortable" for him. It is a mistake to pass it on to be used by a team of lesser rank, such as junior varsity or freshman, since there is little likelihood that it will fit properly and since they have an equal if not greater need for superior protection. Neither should inferior or worn-out equipment be used for practice since injuries of comparable severity may occur then as well as in games.

It is not difficult to have an athlete fitted with a mouth guard, but it may be very difficult to get him to wear it consistently. Athletes, like other people, tend to reject things which they do not understand or in which they do not believe. A little positive selling has to go along with the introduction of any new piece of protective equipment. The athlete must also be instructed in the proper care of protective equipment for which he will be personally responsible. The contact lens is a good example of such a situation. Improper storage and application of these aids to vision may result in eye infections or abrasions, and carelessness resulting in loss can create a financial problem since they are expensive.

When adding protective equipment to the costume or person of the athlete, careful consideration must be given as to how movement and effective participation may be hampered. Compromises must be accepted for certain purposes. The face guard on the football helmet causes some loss of vision in the lower half of the visual field.

Although the development of high-impact plastic has improved protective devices, this material is so hard that its contact with another player's anatomy may cause serious contusions. This problem cannot be settled by the use of padding on the outside of the plastic since the padding tends to focus the blow which might otherwise be harmlessly deflected.

The role of wrapping and taping in prevention of injury and reinjury is well established in practice, but has some aspects which are controversial. There does not seem to be any doubt that the wrapping of a previously uninjured ankle and taping of a previously sprained ankle offer some degree of protection to this joint. The effectiveness of this protection is gradually dissipated due to stretching once activity begins. Some persons are inclined to believe that tight strapping of the ankles predisposes to the development of knee injuries since the force which might otherwise twist the ankle is transmitted upwards to damage the knee. There is no substantial investigative evidence to indicate that this is actually so.

Protective strapping of unstable knees may help to stabilize them without substantially impairing efficiency in running and turning. The use of various types of knee braces including metal bars, springs, and other substances offers very little in the way of protection and may handicap the player considerably. Shoulder harness and other restraints are generally ineffective in preventing redislocations of the shoulder and should not be relied on for this purpose in contact sports.

D. FOLLOWING THE RULES

The rules of sports and games are codified primarily to make competition possible, to prevent unfair advantages, allow the establishment of records, establish reasonable numbers of players, and set boundaries of time and space for competitions. Many rules are written especially to eliminate hazards and prevent injuries. Others have this as a secondary object. The rules are enforced by the competitors themselves in practice and informal competition. In formal competition a varying number of officials with different titles may be employed to enforce these rules. One of the most important functions of the official is to enforce strictly those rules which help to prevent injury.

In American football the rules against blocking with one forearm and against blocking the legs from the rear (clipping) have as their sole purpose the prevention of injury. In wrestling certain holds, such as the full-nelson, are barred for this reason. In automobile racing, all competitors are required to slow down if track conditions are dangerous due to rain or oil. The wearing of certain types of protective equipment, such as a mouthguard, may become mandatory for safety reasons in some sports.

The rule against charging the goalkeeper in soccer and penetrating the area in front of the goal in hockey are designed partly to prevent an unfair advantage but also to protect the defender from injury. The rule against running into the kicker in American football is there primarily to prevent injury, but also helps to preserve an important and interesting part of the game by encouraging the use of the punt as an offensive as well as a defensive weapon.

Games officials as a rule are very safety conscious. They are quick to vary the interpretation of a rule if they are able to sense instantly that an element of danger to a contestant is involved. They will stop actions on the part of contestants which may be within the letter of the rules but might be dangerous to other contestants. They will put out of a game a player or players guilty of deliberate or repeated fouls or fighting. They will stop a contest immediately to allow aid to be given to an injured player. Because of their close proximity to the athletes they may be able to detect signs of injury before the coach, trainer, or physician. In the extremity, if a game gets out of hand because of rough behavior, they may call it off altogether.

Since their duties require them in many instances to be on the field or floor with the contestants, and even in the midst of the play itself, game officials are exposed to injury themselves. Few wear very much in the way of protective equipment, the umpire behind the catcher in baseball being a principal exception. Their principal protection lies in their sense of anticipation and ability to get out of the way quickly. Unfortunately, since the crowd tends to align itself with the contestants and against the officials, the referee who is struck with a hockey puck or mowed down by an errant blocker can·expect more derision than sympathy.

E. AVAILABILITY OF EMERGENCY CARE

In any sport where the danger of injury is common, where serious injuries are apt to occur, or where the number of contestants multiplies the possibility of injury, emergency care should be immediately available. This care may be supplied as first-aid by the coach, trainer, or the physician. Supplies and equipment are necessary and the existence of some type of facility is desirable. More definitive care must be provided by the physician who may be present or available nearby. This may require the use of an office, clinic, or hospital.

Provisions for suitable transportation should be made available in advance or on call on an emergency basis. These may all be made available by a sponsoring body, but in the case of individual sports, under certain conditions, it is up to the individual to provide his own emergency care.

The danger of injury is common in the so-called "contact" sports among which may be listed football, soccer, basketball, wrestling, judo, ice hockey, field handball, lacrosse, and baseball. It is important to have someone skilled in first-aid immediately available at practice and competitions. Most of the time during practice sessions the coach must fulfill this role but he may have the services of a trainer available. It is highly desirable to have a physician present at competitions in these sports. One who is familiar with the team and sports injuries should also be easily available during practice sessions.

Although injuries are numerically less common in the motor sports, the very serious nature of injuries which may occur usually makes the attendance of a physician mandatory at contests in these events. A physician's attendance at a dual meet in track or swimming would not ordinarily be expected but in a conference championship meet involving many teams this might be very necessary.

A first-aid room, training room, or a medical office at the scene of sports activity may provide the base for emergency care of the injured athlete. It should be well stocked with the types of bandages, dressings, splints, and other disposable and reusable supplies which may be required. Preferably it should be close to the locker rooms but separated in such a way that quiet and privacy can be secured. Severe injuries may require emergency care which cannot be rendered in such a facility. In this case a local physician's office, clinic, or hospital emergency room may be the appropriate site. It is unwise to schedule sports events with serious hazards far away from any facility where complete emergency care may be rendered.

Transportation equipment to take the player off the field or court should always be readily available in a contact sport. Provisions for other transportation to a medical facility by ambulance or other means should be made in advance and should be immediately available or on a standby basis. Equipment for resuscitation should be available in ambulances used for this purpose as well as at the site of activity, and personnel should be trained in its use.

An outstanding example of the application of emergency care to a difficult sports situation is the establishment of teams to assist injured skiers by the National Ski Patrol and the International First-Aid and Rescue Organization. Volunteers, trained in first-aid with particular application to the winter sports, not only bring first-aid to the skier at the site but arrange his transportation to a facility where definitive medical care may be provided.

V. Management of Illness and Injury Sustained in Exercise Activities

The role of the physician is a key one in the recognition and management of illness and injury in sports and games. As has already been indicated, this has led to the development of a specialty of sports medicine. The physician who only devotes part of his time to this field must learn to think in the same terms as the specialist in order to provide the best care, since there are important differences between the care of athletes and sportsmen and of others, even for the same conditions.

In playing his part the physician must utilize the services of other persons, especially the coach and trainer, but also the physiotherapist, psychologist, and perhaps other medical consultants. He must be the leader of the team and the coordinator of all efforts made in behalf of the athlete. He begins with a prompt diagnosis, carries out or supervises the first-aid procedure or emergency care, follows through with or brings the athlete to definitive medical care, and then plans and helps to carry out the procedures of rehabilitation.

One of the physician's principal functions in the team which carries out the total treatment of the athlete is to enlist and maintain the active cooperation of the sportsman himself. He will do this most successfully when he knows his patient before the event, when he understands the sport and demonstrates empathy with the athlete. He must be willing to identify himself with the latter's aims and aspirations as well as with the more general ideals of sport and all individual exercise activities.

A. PROMPT DIAGNOSIS

Early recognition of a problem makes possible its early correction. In sports injuries there is an almost unique opportunity to make a very early diagnosis since it is seldom, except by accident, that a physician can be on hand to witness the event of injury in most situations. The prompt institution of countermeasures may greatly shorten disability which is of great importance to the athlete. In the case of serious injuries a prompt diagnosis may be life-saving.

When an injury occurs there may be a few golden moments before the body's reaction to injury expressed in terms of pain, swelling, and muscle spasm begins to obscure the evidence of the damage which has taken place. This is particularly true in the case of injuries to the joints and especially the knee joint. Immediately following the tearing of lateral collateral ligaments of the knee it may be possible to determine abnormal lateral mobility which will require x-ray examination under anesthesia only a short time later.

Early diagnosis also makes it possible to institute rational and effective treatment in time to prevent or minimize complications. The immediate application of cold to the injured part greatly reduces swelling due to internal bleeding and often relieves pain significantly. Dislocations, particularly recurrent ones, can often be reduced without anesthesia during the first few minutes following injury. If a diagnosis of a fractured ankle can be made at once the victim would not be allowed to risk further injury by attempting to bear weight on it.

The prime example of a serious injury which may threaten life or result in severe permanent disability, if not suspected at the time, is a fracture of the cervical spine. The diagnosis can usually be made or surmised by a physician at the scene of the accident. This will lead to all suspected cases of neck fracture being handled in such a way that injury to the spinal cord, if it has not already occurred, may be prevented.

In the situation of illness in the sportsman prompt diagnosis of an infectious disease may prevent the spread to other members of the team or to opponents. The occurrence of herpes simplex infections on the skin of wrestlers is an example. The isolation and prompt treatment of the infected individual will stop future spread of the disease.

When symptoms of cramps, exhaustion, and collapse due to heat stress occur, prompt and accurate diagnosis can be life-saving. Once heat stroke occurs, the time in which the affected individual's life can be saved can be measured in minutes. In the acute pulmonary edema sometimes encountered in mountain climbers, prompt diagnosis is necessary to ensure the correct treatment which will yield almost universally favorable results.

B. First-Aid Procedures

There is essentially no difference in the type of first-aid which should be given sports injuries from that given for injuries due to other causes. The main differences are in the patient himself and the setting in which he is found. Everyone engaged in the supervision of athletes should have a knowledge of first-aid equivalent to that achieved in the advanced course taught by the American Red Cross. Appropriate equipment should be available for their use whenever sports are being practiced.

When contusions and other bruising and crushing injuries occur, the most important first-aid measures are applications of cold, support, and elevation. Cold and elevation minimize the swelling which results from the local outpouring of serum and blood into the wound. Support, provided by lifting, propping up, and elastic bandaging, relieves discomfort, prevents further injury, and promotes dependent drainage.

In the first-aid treatment of abrasions and lacerations, cleanliness is important both in dressing the wound and preventing further contamination.

Control of bleeding may be established by local application of pressure, elevation, or the use of tourniquets.

When injuries to the extremities occur, sprains, strains, fractures, or dislocations may result. The first principle of treatment is similar to that used in the treatment of bruises, the application of cold. Support is next in importance. Bandaging or splinting must not be too tight in order not to embarrass circulation.

Head injuries which result in even a momentary loss of consciousness require close observation. The victim may regain consciousness only to lapse off again, a most serious prognostic sign which usually indicates intracranial bleeding. If the victim is unconscious when first reached, care should be taken to see that his airway is clear, that artificial respiration is established if necessary, and that he is allowed to recover consciousness naturally without artificial stimulation. Every unconscious athlete who has been injured must be assumed to have suffered a neck injury until it can be proved otherwise.

All persons with suspected neck or back injuries should be carried flat on a board with the head supported in the midline and transported directly to the nearest hospital for definitive care. Mouth-to-mouth breathing may be necessary to maintain respiration. A diver with a suspected neck injury can be kept afloat on his back easily until a board can be floated under him for transportation.

Acute injuries to the chest in sports, exclusive of the shoulders, usually result at worst in broken ribs. The immediate treatment is support in the form of strapping or bandaging the ribs. It is important to remember that in a steering wheel injury there may be a rupture of the aorta which may cause the victim to go rapidly into shock and die.

Injuries to the abdomen in sports sometimes cause damage to the kidneys or the spleen. If there is reason to expect either, the victim should be transported immediately to a hospital on a stretcher. The most common injury is the so-called "solar plexus blow" which causes a momentary cessation of breathing. There is no better restorative than allowing the victim to lie flat on his back until respiration returns spontaneously.

Medical conditions, known and unsuspected, may cause problems in sports requiring first-aid. Diabetic acidosis leading to coma will respond to the administration of insulin. Insulin shock is treated by the administration of glucose, preferably in orange juice. Epilepsy may cause convulsions in which the victim must be protected from biting his tongue and from injury due to the violent clonic contractures which accompany the seizure.

The most serious nontraumatic condition which may occur in sportsmen is heat stroke. When it is suspected, the affected individual should immediately be put at rest in the shade, undressed, wrapped in cold towels with fans blowing over him, or placed in a cold shower or tub filled with ice water.

Water with salt dissolved in a quantity of one teaspoonful to a gallon should be given by mouth. Cooling procedures should be stopped when the rectal temperature reaches 99.0°F.

In drowning and near-drowning it is important to remember that the emergency treatment of the accidents in fresh and salt water must be different. The freshwater victim requires immediate mouth-to-mouth respiration and closed-chest cardiac massage. As soon as breathing and heart action are restored, he should be transported directly to the hospital to correct the disturbed fluid and salt balance in the blood. The saltwater victim requires the administration of oxygen under pressure since the lungs are flooded with water and every effort should be made to evacuate this water. On revival he should also be brought to the hospital for restoration of depleted blood volume and oxygen therapy.

C. Definitive Medical Care

It is not the purpose of this chapter to discuss the definitive care of sports injuries in detail but to indicate the principles which are involved in their management as they differ from that of injuries in general. The principal differences reside in the fact that the sportsman is usually a young and otherwise superbly healthy individual, that he is ordinarily highly motivated to recovery and that he must be returned to his sport as rapidly as possible with the closest return to normal function as possible.

The early phases of medical treatment for sports injuries are a continuation of the first-aid and emergency measures already described. Diagnosis already made or suspected is confirmed or disproved by x-ray examinations. If no surgery is contemplated, support is maintained for as short a time as necessary in order to keep swelling at a minimum and allow healing to begin. Efforts are made to maintain a good state of conditioning in the rest of the body by exercises and early ambulation.

There has been a profound change in attitude toward the management of severe injuries to the joints in recent years. This resulted from a reevaluation of the poor results which had been obtained by nonoperative treatment, particularly of knee injuries. At the present time most orthopedic surgeons are in agreement that the definite diagnosis of a laceration of the semilunar cartilage or a complete tear of the collateral ligament of the knee is an indication for surgical exploration and repair of the joint. A similar attitude is now assumed toward severe ligamentous injuries to the ankle and recurrent dislocation of the shoulder.

In other respects treatment of sports injuries is conventional except for the fact that rehabilitation begins almost at the start of treatment in intensive fashion and is carried out continuously through return to sports activity.

Every attempt is made to restore the injured athlete to contact with his team or the environment of his sport during his convalescence.

Definitive medical care for illnesses sustained in the course of sport and exercise activities is conventional. The principal difference is an attempt to maintain a state of physical conditioning in so far as is consistent with the degree of rest necessary for recovery. The administration of tetanus toxoid to those who have been previously immunized and of tetanus antitoxin (preferably prepared from human serum) to those who have not is of proven value in the prevention of tetanus in those who have suffered puncture wounds, abrasions, lacerations, or burns. The prophylactic administration of antibiotics has not been proven of value except in those cases where severe contamination and much destruction of tissue have taken place.

D. Rehabilitation Procedures

A certain amount of rest is required in the acute phase of injury to allow a reversal of the process of inflammation which accompanies it. Active restoration of function may begin as quickly as 24 hr after the injury occurs. In this effort, teamwork of the sportsman, physician, trainer, coach, and other therapists is extremely important to secure a successful result. A variety of methods may be employed but the means are conventional except for the intensity with which they may be utilized by the athlete. The goal is complete restoration of normal function.

In the rehabilitation of the injured athlete, the process begins with motion. This may at first be passive but becomes active assisted and then active as quickly as possible. When healing has progressed to the point where it is safe, resistive motions are practiced. In the meantime all noninjured parts of the body are kept in condition by active and resistive motions.

Isometric and isotonic exercises are introduced as early as possible into the program. Muscle strength and volume are lost very quickly following injury during immobilization. Where little or no motion is possible, isometric exercises may be very helpful. They are also easier for the bedfast patient since they do not require the use of any apparatus and can be done without having to seek any assistance. Isotonic exercises are done against resistance supplied by the therapist, the patient himself, a weight, or some other medium.

Work against resistance with progressive overloading is the most effective method of restoring muscle strength following injury. There is some cross transfer of strength in the extremities by exercising the normal side alone. The use of pulley weights, dumbbells, and barbells is practiced according to the particular requirements and capabilities of the individual. No additional contribution to strength is made by the administration of anabolic steroids and there are considerable dangers in their continued use.

The local application of heat is a mainstay in rehabilitation following injury. The principal modalities employed are moist hot pads, lamps, paraffin baths, electric pads, whirlpool baths, various forms of diathermy, and ultrasound. Since the purpose is to stimulate circulation in the affected part there is some value in delivering the heat as deeply as possible into the affected area. The ability to penetrate is the chief advantage which diathermy has over hot pads, packs, and lamps. The infrared spectrum is the effective portion of radiation from a lamp or from the sun. Ultraviolet light has no known therapeutic effect in trauma.

Ultrasound produces heat at interfaces of tissue such as the junction of bone and muscle. In spite of its wide usage in recent years there is a complete lack of significant evidence that it exerts any therapeutic effect in the treatment of trauma. There are some possible dangers connected with its use.

The whirlpool bath combines the effect of heat with the gentle massage provided by the passage of a current of air through the water. It is especially helpful in the reduction of swelling. The support which the water offers the affected limb also aids in active motions which can be carried out during the treatment.

Electrotherapy has no apparent value in rehabilitation except to stimulate muscle which has temporarily lost its effective innervation until this can be restored. It will probably never lose its appeal since it causes a contraction which can be felt by the patient and seen by the therapist.

The use of various enzymes reputed to have anti-inflammatory properties has been a great disappointment in the management of trauma. On the other hand, the use of some chemical agents with such supposed properties has been moderately encouraging, especially in the chronic state following injury. Local injections of the synthetic adrenogenic hormones have been helpful many times in the chronic state of inflammation in and around joints. The local injection of an anesthetic such as procaine for any purpose other than to relieve pain for diagnostic purposes, or to allow rest, is mentioned only to be condemned.

Massage and stretching exercises are of great value in stimulating circulation, reducing swelling, and restoring motion. They should be practiced only by persons experienced in physical therapy to avoid possible harm from their improper use.

In the first stages of rehabilitation of the sportsman, the physician, nurse, and physical therapist carry the burden of the patient's care. When the athlete is able to get back to the training area the trainer and then the coach become involved. Through their efforts in cooperating with the physician, the athlete is able to gradually widen his activities until he returns to a regular training schedule. In the meantime he remains under the supervision of the physician who is alert for any signs of failure to progress or for a deterioration of his condition below the levels already achieved during therapy. The attitude of the athlete himself is most important during this period.

Practice and, indeed, even competition may be resumed in many situations before complete restoration of function takes place. It should be remembered that not only the return to activity but as near normal restoration of function are the goals of rehabilitation. Active therapy may be continued during this phase. The goal of rehabilitation in an extremity has often been stated to be to make the injured side as strong or stronger than the uninjured one. This may be in some cases a practical impossibility but it is an excellent objective.

REFERENCES

Ackernecht, E. H. (1955). "A Short History of Medicine." Ronald Press, New York.
Aldrovandri, V. (1616). "De Quadrupedibus." Bologna.
Andry, N. (1741). "L'orthopédie, ou l'art de prévenir et corriger dans les enfants les déformités du corps." Paris.
Balke, B. (1960). *In* "Exercise and Fitness," pp. 73–81. Athletic Inst., Chicago, Illinois.
Brock, A. J. (1916). "Galen: On the Natural Faculties." Heineman, London.
Brock, A. J. (1939). "Greek Medicine." J. M. Dent, London.
Burette, J. (1748). "Dissertazione del Disco." Venice.
Byles, J. B., and Osborn, S. (1898). *In* "Encyclopedia of Sport," p. 394. Putnam, New York.
Cagnatus, M. (1602). "De Sanitate Tuenda." Padua.
Cardano, G. (1562). "De Subtilitate et de Rerum Varietate." Venice.
D'Acquapendente (1614). "De Motu Animalium." Venice.
Deusing, A. (1656). "Exercitations de Motu Animalium." Amsterdam.
Duchesne, G. (1855). "De l'électrisation localisée." Baillière et fils, Paris.
Duchesne, J. (1648). "Ars Medica Dogmatica Hermetica." Frankfort.
Duckworth, W. L. H. (1962). "Galen on Anatomical Procedures," Books X-XV. Cambridge Univ. Press, London and New York.
Einthoven, W. (1903). *Arch. Ges. Physiol.* **99**, 472.
Falls, H. B., Ismail, A. H., MacLeod, D. F., Wiebers, J. E., Christian, J. E., and Kessler, W. V. (1965). *J. Sports Med.* **5**, 185.
Fleishmann, E. A. (1964). "The Structure and Measurement of Physical Fitness." Prentice-Hall, Englewood Cliffs, New Jersey.
Green, R. M. (1955). "Asclepiades, His Life and Writing." Yale Univ. Press, New Haven, Connecticut.
Greene, H. C. (1927). "An Introduction to the Study of Experimental Medicine by C. Bernard, 1965" (Transl.). Macmillan, New York.
Guerra, F. (1960). "Book of Bodily Exercise" (Transl.). Elizabeth Licht, New Haven, Connecticut.
Heald, C. B. (1931). "Injuries and Sport." Oxford Univ. Press, London and New York.
Hyman, A. S. (1962). *J. Sports Med.* **2**, 86.
Ismail, A. H., Falls, H. B., and MacLeod, D. F. (1965). *J. Appl. Physiol.* **20**, 991.
Jackson, J. H. (1932). *In* "Selected Writings of John Hughlings Jackson" (J. Taylor, ed.), p. 103. Hodder & Stoughton Ltd., London.

Joubert, L. (1582). "Opera." Lugdoni.

Kruger, H. C. (1962). "Avicenna's Poem on Medicine" (Transl.). Thomas, Springfield, Illinois.

Littre, E. (1839–1861). "Oeuvres complètes D'Hippocrate." Paris.

McCormick, P. J. (1943, 1944). Two Medieval Catholic Educators (Vittorino da Feltre). *Catholic Univ. Bull., Wash.* **12** and **13**.

McKenzie, R. T. (1909). "Exercise in Education and Medicine." Saunders, Philadelphia, Pennsylvania.

McKenzie, R. T. (1916). *Proc. Roy. Soc. Med.* **9**, 31–70.

Mercuriale, G. (1569). "De Arte Gymnastica." Venice.

Pare, A. (1582). "Opera Ambrosii Parei Regis Primarii et Parisenis Chirurgi." Jacques Du Puys, Paris.

Perrault, C. (1680). "Mécanique des animaux." Paris.

Santorio, S. (1614). "De Medicina Statio Aphroismi." Venice.

Singer, C. (1956). "Galen on Anatomical Procedures," Books I-VIII, and 5 chapters of Book IX. Oxford Univ. Press, London and New York.

Vegius, M. (1613). "De Educatione Librorum." Lodi.

Weissbein, S. (1910). "Hygiene des Sports," Grethlein, Leipzig.

White, P. D. (1958). *J. Am. Med. Assoc.* **167**, 711.

Wright, W. C. (1940). "De Morbis Artificiorum: Latin Text of 1713 by B. Ramazzini" (Transl.). Univ. of Chicago Press, Chicago, Illinois.

12

PHYSIQUE AND EXERCISE

Albert R. Behnke

I. Introduction

The remarkable improvement in performance and the continual lowering of world records is due in part to the increased number of competitors, improved training methods, application of scientific principles underlying physiological mechanisms, and to increase in size, strength, speed, and agility of the athletes. More men are available with particular physical aptitudes that make for superior performance in specific events. The present shot-put record exceeds by 12 ft the world record of 1948, referred to at the time as "phenomenal."

The striking secular improvement, e.g., in putting and throwing events, may well serve to emphasize the importance of physique in terms of greater size and muscular development of the participating athletes. However, this conclusion is tempered by the fact that, in the hammer throw, the same athlete may increase his world record performance by 20 ft during a period of 9 years during which his size presumably remains the same.

In the evaluation of physique, the body can be described systematically, measured accurately, and quantified as to its gross components by physical and biochemical techniques. Thus, the classic description of body form has consisted of subjective evaluation, chiefly from photographs, of 3 structural components: fat, muscle, and bone. Extensive anthropometric measurements have been made on military personnel in connection with human engineering requirements. It is possible not only to follow standardized procedures in the course of linear and girth measurement but one has recourse to data on varied and sizeable populations (Hertzberg *et al.*, 1963). With reference to biochemical techniques, investigations during the past 3 decades have supported the concept that the human body is an entity amenable to structural analysis of its gross components. It is now possible to determine in the living person total amounts of blood, water, potassium, and other electrolytes (Brožek and Henschel, 1961) that previously were deduced from analysis of animal carcasses. One may conclude that definitive procedures for assessment of body build are available for application in the field of exercise physiology. In this chapter the size, shape, and proportions of the body (both external and internal) relative to bone, muscle, and fat, will be outlined chiefly in relation to athletic performance.

II. Concepts

A. ANTHROPOMETRIC RELATIONSHIPS

1. Perimetric Size and Body Weight

From measurements on several thousand persons it has been established (Behnke, 1961; Behnke and Royce, 1966) that selected circumferences (S) can be converted (S/K) into a value (D) which is interchangeable with $3F$, where F is the square root of weight divided by stature. For example, perimetric size S as described by 11 girths (some 6 m or more in extended length) and stature (h) are numerically equivalent to and can be substituted for body weight ($r = 0.99$). This remarkable equivalence in the absence of a correction factor for density is due in part to the fact that with the air normally present in the lungs, the density of the body as a whole is approximately unity. There are changes in shape also toward rotundity as fat accumulates which serve to render perimetric size (in contrast to body volume) numerically equivalent to body weight.

It is not the calculation of body weight, however, in which we are interested but the ability to convert each of the 11 circumferences or combinations of these girths into d quotients (girth/k). The k values represent the mean body proportions of any group selected for reference. The shape of any person may then be outlined on the "somatogram" (Fig. 1) as the percentage deviations of *d* quotients from *D* or from the factor (*F*). The somatogram is, therefore, a quantitative representation of body shape. If the girth proportions of an individual conform to group symmetry, then all of the *d* quotients are equal to *D* and body shape would appear as a vertical line (Fig. 1). Deviations from group symmetry are, however, characteristic of body build, chiefly because of accumulation of fat in adult life and the variation in phenotype of skeletal dimensions and muscle mass.

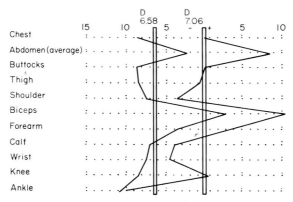

Fig. 1. Somatogram based on data in Table II showing the effect of weight reduction on body proportions. The *D* axis has shifted 6.8% to the left following a weight loss of 12.3 kg. Each circumference has been converted to a *d* quotient and the percentage deviations from each *D* axis, respectively, are shown before (*D* = 7.06) and after (*D* = 6.58) weight reduction. Initial weight was 100.0 kg.

2. Skeletal (Transimetric) Size, Reference Weight, Lean Body Weight, Minimal Weight

Selected anthropometric diameters and stature may be employed for the estimation of reference weight (Ref. *W*), and with a lower scaling factor applied, of lean body weight (*LBW*). The relationship that makes this projection possible is the nearly constant ratio between mean values of transimetric size and perimetric size (diameters/girths approach constancy) throughout the growth period beginning at about age four and continuing to maturity. One may calculate from "frame" (diameters and stature) size what any person should weigh relative to his skeletal build.

LBW is body weight minus excess fat (Behnke, 1961). In any male group the weights (minimal) of the leanest individuals approach *LBW*. The specific gravity of the body as a whole of such persons will approximate 1.100, a value identified generally with fat-free, adult, mammalian tissue. In the female, minimal weight computed from diameters and stature, in the same manner as for the male, will be several kilograms higher (e.g., 48 kg) compared with *LBW* (42 kg) derived from specific gravity, total body water, or potassium determinations.

B. RADIOGRAPHIC RELATIONSHIPS

The tape measure and anthropometer provide reliable data as to size and shape of the body but we can only make a guess as to the contents within the cutaneous wrapper. The x-ray technique employed by Tanner (1964) and his associates to visualize muscle, bone, and subcutaneous fat constitutes an essential procedure for delineation and width measurement especially of bone. From the diameters of the long bones in the arm and lower extremity as measured on the radiogram, one may derive a valid approximation of bone weight, notably in the Negro whose generally heavier skeletal mass (Seale, 1959) is, in our experience, not associated with increased anthropometric skeletal widths.

Tanner's advanced statistical treatment of anthropometric and radiographic data penetrates the "ratio" barrier into the more sophisticated (and perhaps more accurate) covariant and canonical analysis. However, in this chapter we shall use elementary conversions of measurements of bone, muscle, and fat in the effort to maintain close contact with the raw data at all times.

III. Methodology

A. SUBJECTIVE APPRAISALS AND PHOTOGRAPHY

1. Sheldon's Classification

This widely used procedure, described and evaluated by Dupertuis (1963) and Tanner (1964), is a system of rating on a 7-point scale each of 3 dominant components designated by Sheldon as follows:

(a) Endomorphy is relative predominance of soft roundness throughout the various regions of the body
(b) Mesomorphy is relative predominance of muscle, bone and connective tissue
(c) Ectomorphy is relative predominance of linearity and fragility of body build

Apart from recourse to the inverse of the ponderal index (height divided by the cube root of weight) the evaluation is subjective and requires consultation with a coterie for proper grading and interpretation of photographs. It is most helpful to have the somatotype evaluation. It should be pointed out that ratings of fatness, muscularity, and skeletal prominence, which may be discerned from Sheldon's classification, can be made objective as will be shown subsequently in the analysis of data from anthropometric and radiographic techniques.

2. Non-Sheldonian Appraisal

Without attempting to downgrade or compromise Sheldon's formal system we employ a simple rating scale: 1, 2, 3, 4, 5, 6, with values above 3 to designate corpulence-obesity, and values below 3 to denote leanness. A zero (0) added on the lean side would apply to any healthy person who appeared to be grossly underweight. Good muscular development is indicated by a STAR (∗). If the prime development is largely over the upper part of the body, as frequently observed in male Negroes, a "u" is placed in the upper right quadrant of the STAR (∗^{u}). If the lower extremities are muscular but the arms relatively undeveloped, as in distance runners, an "l" is placed in the lower segment of the STAR (∗$_l$). Individuals having been classified as to sex, age, or age group (adults), are then rated on a numerical "fat" scale accompanied, if appropriate, by a STAR subject to modification by a "u" or "l."

B. OBJECTIVE PROCEDURES

1. Anthropometric Evaluation

Krogman (1955) has provided guidelines based on his extensive experience and Hertzberg et al. (1963) have compiled standard, illustrated procedures in their exemplary survey of military personnel in Turkey, Greece, and Italy. Some essential points based on the author's experience (Behnke, 1961, 1963) follow. An examiner, a recorder (unless automated techniques have been established), and in the case of adolescents, a monitor, are required. The role of the recorder who is also an observer is most important in preventing error. The measurements are made with dispatch consistent with accuracy and with the least inconvenience to subject and examiner. A linen tape measure (a metal tape gives rise to error as a result of "bowing" around large ovoid girths) is applied in light contact with skin surface. An anthropometer with wide blades ($\frac{3}{4}$ inch) permits pressure to be applied in measurement of skeletal widths excepting the chest.

The scope of the examination (Table I) is determined by requirements; generally measurements have been too few. In the case of athletes, lengths and proportions of extremities (Cureton, 1951; Tanner, 1964) are informative. Technical detail is presented by Hertzberg et al. (1963) and Behnke (1961). It should be noted that an average is taken of homologous girths, the biceps are

TABLE I

DIMENSIONS AND CONVERSION CONSTANTS FOR A REFERENCE MAN AND WOMAN

Age group (years):	20–24	20–24
Stature (dm):	17.40 (68.5 inches)	16.38 (64.5 inches)
Weight (kg):	70.0 (154 lb)	56.8 (125 lb)
uS-W:	100	100
Ref. W (kg):	69.6	56.2
$3F$:	6.00	5.56
D:	6.00	5.56
Lean body weight (kg):	61.8	48.4
$3F$ (LBW):	5.656	5.157 ($3F$, minimal W)

Circumferences	cm	k	cm	k
Head	57.0	9.5	54.6	9.78
Arm extended	29.1	4.85	25.3	4.55
Abdomen (1) waist	77.0	12.84	65.6	11.83
Abdomen (2) omphalion	79.8	13.30	77.8	13.93
Chest	91.8	15.30	82.5	14.85
Abdomen (average)	78.4	13.07	71.7	12.90
Buttocks	93.4	15.57	94.2	16.93
Thigh	54.8	9.13	55.8	10.03
Shoulder	110.8	18.47	96.4	17.33
Biceps	31.7	5.29	26.7	4.80
Forearm	26.9	4.47	24.1	4.33
Calf	35.8	5.97	34.1	6.13
Wrist	17.3	2.88	15.2	2.73
Knee	36.6	6.10	34.9	6.27
Ankle	22.5	3.75	20.6	3.70
	S 600	K 100	S 556	K 100

Diameters	cm	k(Ref. W)	$k(LBW)$	cm	k(Ref. W)	k(minimal W)
Bideltoid	45.24	7.54	—	40.4	7.27	—
Biacromial	40.6	6.77	7.18	35.0	6.29	6.79
Chest width	30.0	5.00	5.31	25.5	4.59	4.94
Bi-iliac	28.6	4.77	5.06	28.6	5.14	5.55
Bitrochanteric	32.8	5.47	5.79	32.0	5.75	6.20
Wrists	11.1	1.85	1.96	9.6	1.73	1.86
Ankles	13.9	2.32	2.46	12.7	2.28	2.46
Knees	18.5	3.08	3.27	17.7	3.18	3.43
Elbows	13.9	2.32	2.46	11.9	2.14	2.31
S(8 diameters)	189.4	31.6[a]	33.5[b]	117.0	31.1[a]	33.5[b]

[a] K(reference weight).
[b] $K(LBW)$, male; K(minimal weight), female.

fully flexed, the knee diameter is measured at the tibiale (not the bicondylar width of the femur); ancillary measurements include circumferences of the head, the midarm (extended), and the bideltoid diameter. The time required for the examination is about 5 min. Standard error is $\pm 1\%$ of the girth or width measured.

2. Estimate of Body Volume by Underwater Weighing

The simple procedure of underwater weighing can be carried out in a small tank (1.5 m^3). The subject, suitably weighted, sits on a canvas sling, and while underwater assumes a "jacknife" position which facilitates full expiration. The temperature of the water is maintained between $31°$ and $34°$C (skin temperature, not deep body temperature). Weighing is performed (subject underwater) by means of a 15-kg scale calibrated to record to 10 gm. A comparison of hydrometric and spirometric vital capacities serves to monitor the procedure (Behnke *et al.*, 1942). Residual air volume is determined at any convenient time, not necessarily at the time of weighing. More important is preparation of the subject so that gas in the stomach and large bowel is minimal, to ensure normal hydration (applies chiefly to women), and to assure constancy of residual air volume. The range of error in replicate determinations should not exceed 0.003 density units. Technical details are discussed by Goldman and Buskirk (1961). Luft and Kim (1961) have improved the technique which can be applied clinically.

The helium dilution technique (Siri, 1956), which has been made available to us on many occasions, is highly reliable if the rigid controls exercised by Dr. Siri are established.

3. Measurement of Total Body Potassium

The 4π liquid scintillation counter, and γ-spectrometer (NaI crystal) housed in a shielded room ("human counter"), are becoming available for determination of total body potassium (Anderson, 1963; Miller and Remenchik, 1963). Because of its high intracellular concentration, potassium can provide an estimate of cell mass (Moore *et al.*, 1963) and specifically with the help of creatinine, an approximation of muscular development. Continual monitoring and calibration of apparatus are required in the effort to achieve reliable results. The S.E. of measurement (4π counter) is ± 5 gm of potassium out of a total of 150 gm.

4. Appraisal of Skinfold Thickness

One may obtain a crude estimate of the thickness of subcutaneous fat by means of calipers (White, 1963) but the assessment is too gross for anytning more than corroborative support of visual impression. Radiographic measurements of subcutaneous fat are quantitative but the conversion to estimates of total fat is tenuous. Garn (1961) gives an authoritative analysis of the problem.

5. Body Water and Electrolytes (Exchangeable Na, K)

The use of radioisotopes and meticulous technique as employed by Boling (1963) combined with whole body specific gravity provide the best estimate of LBW. The narrow range of variation in the concentration of Na_e and K_e per liter of total body water (tritiated water technique) serve as reference standards for calibration purposes.

C. Symbols and Definitions

W	weight in kilograms unless otherwise designated
h	stature in centimeters unless otherwise designated
$F\sqrt{W/h}$	F is properly derived as the average of the $\sqrt{W/h}$ quotients on each individual of a group. F may be derived from mean values of W/h without appreciable errors in groups that do not differ widely in weight.
$F_h{}^{0.7}\ \sqrt{W/h^{0.7}}$	This factor applies specifically to children and adolescents in whom head size (not included in the 11 girths) is disproportionate during the growth period to body size. In adults, F and $F_h{}^{0.7}$ are interchangeable
S	sum of 11 circumferences (cm)
$S(n)$	sum of n circumferences
Unit size-weight ($uS\text{-}W$)	$\sqrt{W}$ divided by stature (h)
Unit size-perimetric ($uS\text{-}P$) and $uS\text{-}W$	are equivalent and provide an estimate of perimetric size independent of stature
$uS\text{-}W$	reference man or woman (Table I) $= 100$
D	derived from S/K, where $K = 100 =$ sum of 11 k values
$K(n)$	sum of (n) k values
$K(\text{Ref. } W)$	sum of $k(\text{Ref. } W)$ values
$K(LBW)$	sum of $k(LBW)$ values
$K(\text{minimal } W)$	sum of $k(\text{minimal } W)$ values for the female
k	a proportionality constant expressed as a percentage, specific in Table I for each circumference, e.g., $k(\text{biceps})$ is 5.29% of the sum of the 11 girths
cm	any circumference measured in centimeters, e.g., cm (biceps)
d	the quotient (cm/k). An approximation of body weight may be obtained from single d values, as $d(\text{buttocks})$. The error in this type of calculation is proportional to the deviation of d from D

Circumferences May Be Allocated into Regional Categories

A	reflects fat accumulation in the obese and comprises the girths of abdomen, average; buttocks; and chest

A reflects fat accumulation in the obese and comprises the girths of abdomen, average; buttocks; and chest

A' is *A* minus cm (chest) and is used chiefly in connection with athletes whose chest size may be increased by muscular hypertrophy as in weight lifters

B reflects muscular development and comprises girths of the shoulder, biceps, forearm, and calf

WFCA comprises girths of wrist, forearm, calf, and ankle and is used in the estimation of optimal weight

d(A), *d(A')*, *d(B)*, *d(WFCA)* sum of respective *d* quotients for each group

Diameters

C comprises skeletal diameters from which Ref. *W* is calculated

$D(C)$ C/K(Ref. *W*), K(Ref. *W*) = 31.6 (male), 31.1 (female), 8 diameters

$D(LBW)$ $C/K(LBW)$, $K(LBW)$ = 33.5 (8 diam.), male and female (K, minimal *W*)

D. Formulas

To Adults Only: The Following Formula Applies

(1) $D^2 \times h \times 0.11i$ = Weight D(Ref. *W*) and $D(LBW)$ may be substituted in place of D in the calculation of Ref. *W* and *LBW*, respectively. Likewise $d(A) \ldots d(WFCA)$ may be substituted for D in the calculation of relative weights for the respective categories

All Ages from 4 Years Upward: The Following Formulas Apply

(2) $D^2 \times h^{0.7} \times 0.263$ = weight (male)
(3) $D^2 \times h^{0.7} \times 0.255$ = weight (female)

All of the substitutions that were made in (1) as $d(A) \ldots d(WFCA)$ can also be made in (2) and (3)

(4)   mean $LBW = 0.204h^2$ (male)
(5)   mean (minimal W) $= 0.18h^2$ (female)
  $uS\text{-}W = 208\sqrt{W}/h$ (male), $217.3\sqrt{W}/h$ (female)
  $uS\text{-}P = 0.695S/h^{0.5}$ (male), $0.728S/h^{0.5}$ (female)

E. Derivation of Proportionality Constants (k Values) for a Reference Man and Woman from Military Data

1. k Values from Circumferences

The proportions of any designated group may be employed for reference (Table I). Initially on a Navy group (Behnke *et al.*, 1959; Behnke, 1961) the factor (F) was computed for each of 31 men differing widely in stature and weight. The mean value of F was 2.087 and the mean value for the sum (S) of the 11 girths was 626 cm ($S/F = 300$, $D = 6.26 = 3F$).

The mean values for the dimensions of the "reference man" were divided by $3F$ ($= 6.00$) to give the proportionality constants for each circumference. The sum of the k values (for 11 girths) $= 100$; for 12 circumferences (S + head girth), $K(12) = 109.5$ (male).

2. k(Ref. W) Values

Each mean value for the 8 diameters was divided by $3F$ (as well as the bideltoid width), to derive the quotients under the heading (Table I) k(Ref.W). Transimetric size as measured by the 8 diameters is 31.6% of perimetric size for the male, and 31.1% for the female.

3. k(LBW) Male and k(minimal W) Female

From Eq. (4) mean *LBW* (male) $= 61.8$ kg and $3F(LBW) = 5.656$
From Eq. (5) mean minimal weight (female) $= 48.4$ kg, $3F$(minimal W) $= 5.157$

The values for $k(LBW)$ and k(minimal W) are the quotients derived for each diameter divided by $3F(LBW)$ and $3F$(minimal W), respectively.

IV. Physique and Fatness

Excess Fat Load Carried by Many Adults

The amount of fat in the body may well be our first consideration in evaluation of physique. The excessive fat burden on many adults would not be credible were it not for unequivocal data that cluster around such low values of *LBW* as 62 kg (136.4 lb) in the male (h, 17.40 dm), and 42 kg (92.4 lb) in the female (h, 16.38 dm). Both men and women frequently support a fat load of more than 20 kg ($+44$ kg) which may constitute from 50 to 75% of the musculoskeletal framework. The difficulty of assessing the amount of work performed on a treadmill, e.g., is obvious. The problem of quantifying the amount of fat in the body is rendered difficult, e.g., by exceptionally good muscular development of former athletes, who acquire excess fat during the sedentary period of middle life, if not earlier.

1. Quantification of Body Fat in a Moderately Obese Man

In Table II are data pertaining to a 52-year-old man who in earlier life was accustomed to heavy manual work, 60 hr per week. After the age of 25, when sustained physical activity was greatly curtailed, he gained 25 kg (55 lb). The anthropometric data indicate that before weight reduction there is both excess fat and increased muscularity, notably in the arms [*d*(abdominal average) is 8.7% greater than *D*; *d*(biceps) is 10.6% greater than *D*]. The percentage of fat, based on density and total body water, was 28.3% (28.3 kg of excess fat, body *W*, 100 kg).

If the *d* quotients are grouped in the *A* and *B* categories, *d*(*A*) and *d*(*B*) are both higher than *D* and, by contrast, *D*(*C*) from diameters is low (8.2% less than *D*). The *WFCA* (optimal weight) component is also low (4.4% less than *D*). On inspection the examinee was rated 5 STAR, and in a formal manner by somatotype (5, 6.5, 1.5). Reference weight (*W*, *C*), Table II, is 83.4 kg (about 11% fat) and this was the examinee's weight at age 30. If 20% of body weight for fat is a reasonable estimate for an older man, then reference weight would be about 90 kg. This is the weight projected from the *WFCA* component.

2. Effect of Weight Reduction

Following a regimen of increased exercise and dietary restriction over a period of 3 months, body weight loss amounted to 12.3 kg, the percentage of body fat was reduced to 22.8%, and body density increased from 1.035 to 1.047. From these values it was deduced that weight loss consisted of 8.3 kg of fat and 4.0 kg of lean tissue. An independent estimate of the amount of lean tissue lost is obtained from total body water which decreased by 1 liter— equivalent to 1.25 kg lean tissue.

Analysis of regional weight losses (Table II and Fig. 1) shows that the decrement of *W*(*A*), relative weight computed from the *A* component, is more than twice (18.4 kg) that of *W*(*B*). An average of *W*(*A*) and *W*(*B*) weight losses is equal to 14.0 kg compared with a scale weight loss of 12.3 kg. Of interest is the 2 to 1 ratio of weight loss from *W*(*A*) to *W*(*B*). This ratio may approach unity reflecting a greater loss of lean tissue in persons reducing on inadequate diets. The objective anthropometric rating gives numerical values for the decrease in *A* and the relative increase in the *B* as well as in *C* components. The somatotype rating following weight reduction is in accord with these changes. The decrease in *LBW*(anthropometric) of 3.8 kg and *LBW* (density) of 4.0 kg is coincidental; the one being accounted for by loss of subcutaneous fat, the other is attributed to loss of lean tissue from the whole body.

It is generally agreed, and it has long been our experience, that exercise in later life is essential for body economy, specifically to limit fat accumulation, and what is less often emphasized, to preserve muscular tissue and bone architecture. Attention is invited to the pertinent paper by Jokl (1963)

TABLE II

ANTHROPOMETRIC DIMENSIONS OF A 52-YEAR-OLD MALE[a]

		Preweight loss			Postweight loss		
Stature (dm):		17.88 (70.4 inches)			17.88		
Weight (kg):		100 (220 lb)			87.7 (193 lb)		
3F:		7.09			6.64		
uS-W:		116.3			109.0		
D:		7.06			6.58		
uS-P:		116.0			108.2		

	Circumferences	cm	d	% Dev.	cm	d	% Dev.
A	Chest	108.0	7.06	0	98.8	6.46	−1.8
	ABD. (avg)	100.3	7.67	8.7	89.7	6.86	4.3
	Buttocks	108.0	7.06	0	100.4	6.45	−1.9
	Thigh	64.2	7.03	−0.4	59.0	6.46	−1.8
	Shoulder	125.7	6.80	−3.5	120.4	6.52	−0.9
B	Biceps	41.3	7.81	10.6	38.2	7.22	9.7
	Forearm	31.9	7.14	.1.1	30.2	6.80	3.4
	Calf	40.4	6.77	−4.1	39.2	6.57	−0.1
	Wrist	19.4	6.74	−4.5	18.9	6.56	−0.3
	Knee	43.3	7.10	0.6	39.5	6.48	−1.5
	Ankle	23.8	6.35	−10.0	23.6	6.29	−4.4
		706					

	C 8 Diameters	cm	D(Ref. W)	$D(LBW)$	cm	D(Ref. W)	$D(LBW)$
		204.9	6.48	6.12	199.7	6.32	5.96

	Change in D and in d categories				Change in relative weights			
	D	$d(A)$	$d(B)$	$D(C)$	$d(WFCA)$	$W(A)$	$W(B)$	$W(C)$[b]	$W(WFCA)$[c]
Before	7.06	7.26	7.13	6.48	6.75	104.6	100.9	83.4	90.4
After	6.58	6.59	6.78	6.32	6.56	86.2	91.2	79.3	85.4
						18.4	9.7	4.1	5.0

	Physique ratings: somatotype			Anthropometric rating			
	Inspection	End.	Mes.	Ect.	(% deviation d quotients from D)			
Before	5*	5	6.5	1.5	$d(A)$ 2.8	$d(B)$ 1.0	$D(C)$ −8.2	$d(WFCA)$ −4.4
After	3*	2.5	6.5	2.0	0.2	3.0	−4.0	−0.3

[a] Anthropometric dimensions converted to d quotients and the percentage deviation of d from D before and after weight reduction, also the effect of weight reduction on group categories (A, B, C, and $WFCA$) and on physique ratings.

[b] $W(C)$ is reference weight, age group 20–24 years.

[c] $W(WFCA)$ is a first approximation to optimal weight.

dealing with physical activity and body composition and to his earlier classic experiments concerning the effects of exercise and rest on the carbohydrate content of the body (Jokl, 1933).

V. Physique of the Athlete

A. GENERAL COMMENTS

The physique best suited to the requirements of the ultimate in physical performance emerges from the pioneer investigation of Kohlrausch (described by Cureton and Tanner) of Olympic competitors in the 1928 Amsterdam games; from the comprehensive analysis of Cureton (1951) dealing with physique, performance, and organic efficiency of champion athletes; and from the outstanding treatise of Tanner (1964) covering Olympic athletes in Rome, 1960. Tanner and his associates have examined not only a large number of athletes (137 tri-racial track and field participants from 23 countries) but the technical excellence of their measurements, notably the radiographic data obtained despite considerable handicap, and the statistical treatment of results serve as a model in future studies.

From the exposition of these investigators one is aware of striking differences in physique of athletes pre-eminent in competition. For the most part body build is revealed essentially as a lean mass free from the blanket of fat that frequently adds difficulty to the assessment of skeletal size and muscle as pointed out previously. The distribution of athletes based on photoscopic rating is restricted entirely to about one-half of the somatotype field dominated by mesomorphy and ectomorphy. Some characteristics of these athletes may be summarized from Cureton and Tanner who are substantially in agreement.

Briefly, sprinters were found to be more muscular than other runners, but their legs are shorter than 400-m and 1500-m men. Tanner states, "High hurdlers, however, though as muscular as sprinters, have legs as long as middle-distance men and are thus a sort of cross between 100-m and 400-m runners. Since an Olympic class hurdler must on the one hand be capable of very fast sprinting times and on the other must have a long stride and a high stepping action over hurdles, his physical specification is obvious enough. Since Negroes have longer legs than Whites relative to their trunk length, they should dominate this event, and so they do, to the extent that they comprised four out of six Olympic finalists in Rome, and won all three medals."

Tanner's measurements show a clear gradient of build in athletes running 400 m to the marathon. "The 400 m men are large, long-legged, broad-shouldered in relation to their hips, and fairly heavily muscled. Long distance runners are small, short-legged, narrow-shouldered and relatively lacking in muscle. There is no overlap between 400 m and marathon distributions in height or weight or muscle width in arm, calf, and thigh." In the putting and throwing events (shot, discus, and javelin) the athletes are not only tall, heavy, and muscular but have long arms relative to their limb bones. The remarkable increase in size of current champion athletes in the shot put compared with the 1948 champion will be presented in subsequent tables. It is an adage in the prize ring that a good, little man cannot beat a good, big man. Hence the advantage of size in events that demand strength as well as agility.

There is an interesting and rather striking parallel between physique of horses relative to performance and the different body builds of athletes. To quote or abstract from Marguerite Henry's classic descriptions (1962), comparable to the field men in the throwing and shot put events, are "The Big Four of the Draft World," Belgians, Percherons, Shires, and Clydesdales. "These four drafters are much alike. They are all enormous, blocky horses, each weighing about a ton. The feet are big; their shoulders, thighs, and legs bulge with muscle; they are the very picture of power." The American quarter horse is comparable to the sprinters. To continue the quotation, "For a quarter of a mile he can burn up the track. He can beat a thoroughbred. He can even outdash a motocycle. From a standing start he can reach top speed in two leaps." This breed of horse is well muscled, blocky, but quick and nimble on his feet. However, after the first quarter of a mile the slender, long-legged thoroughbred is the winner.

B. ANALYSIS OF DATA

The systematic analysis and mature presentation of data concerning the physique of champions and of Olympic athletes cannot be taken out of context but requires study of the original texts prepared by Cureton and Tanner. However, the anthropometric and radiographic measurements fit in well with the type of analysis represented by the data in Tables I and II. Although the anthropometric data on the exceptional athletes are unduly restricted in number, it is possible to record major physical differences in competitors in different events in the light of the elementary analysis woven into this chapter.

1. Gymnasts and Swimmers (from Cureton, 1951)

Cureton's data (Table III) present the opportunity to derive a set of k values for each of two groups of athletes, Danish gymnasts and American swimmers. The k values of the Reference Man (Table I) are not applicable because the anatomical sites of measurement apparently differ and because of the unique physical characteristics of the two groups of athletes, who are nevertheless remarkably similar except for stature.

a. Table III. Factor (F) is the average of square root of weight divided by stature for each athlete in the two groups respectively. Since only 6 girths were measured, the value for $K(6)$ is the sum of the 6 individual k values equal to 50.8 for the gymnasts and 51.9 for the swimmers compared with

TABLE III

Derivation of Proportionality Constants (k Values) from the Mean Dimensions of Danish Gymnasts and American Swimmers[a]

	Danish gymnasts ($n = 10$)		American swimmers ($n = 10$)	
Stature (dm):	16.76		18.39	
Weight (kg):	74.1		75.6	
$3F$:	6.24		6.08	
uS-W:	104.4		98.3	
Circumferences	cm	k[b]	cm	k[b]
Biceps	33.5	5.38	33.3	5.48
Thigh	55.3	8.86	54.3	8.94
Calf	36.5	5.85	35.8	5.89
Ankle	22.1	3.55	21.9	3.60
Waist	77.2	12.38	77.1	12.29
Buttocks	92.1	14.77	93.0	15.29
	$S(6)$ 316.7	K 50.8	$S(6)$ 315.4	K 51.9
Diameters	cm	k(Ref. W)	cm	k(Ref. W)
Biacromial	39.9	6.39	41.0	6.74
Chest width	31.0	4.97	30.8	5.07
Bi-iliac	28.6	4.58	29.6	4.87
S(3 diameters)	99.5		101.4	
K(Ref. W) = S(3 diameters)/$3F$	15.94		16.68	

[a]Analysis of Cureton's (1951) data.
[b] k = cm/$3F$.

52.6 for the reference man. With the exception of k(biceps) and k(Ref. W) for chest width, the k values are lower than those in Table I, notably for calf, buttock, and ankle girths which are usually amendable to uniformity in the matter of measurement.

b. Table IV. In Table IV the dimensions in centimeters for each athlete may be obtained from the product of d and the respective k values. In the case of the Danish gymnast, $S(6)$ divided by $K(6)$ is equal to D (6.31) which is identical to $3F$ derived from stature and weight. The 3 athletes have approximately the same perimetric size (uS-W or uS-P) per unit of stature, although the gymnast is short compared with the other 2 athletes. The quotient (q) is uS-P/D, and the product, dq, is the correction of each converted girth (d) for

TABLE IV

BODY PROPORTIONS OF THREE ATHLETES[a]

	Danish gymnast			Swimmer			Shot-put champion (1948)		
h (dm):	17.09			18.54			18.65		
W (kg):	75.5			86.4			89.3		
$3F$:	6.31			6.48			6.57		
uS-W:	105.8			104.3			105.4		
D:	6.31			6.41			6.43		
uS-P:	106.1			103.5			103.5		
q:	16.81			16.14			16.09		
	d^b	dq	%Dev.	d^b	dq	%Dev.	d^b	dq	%Dev.
Circumference									
Biceps	6.14	103.2	−2.7	6.40	103.3	−0.2	6.97[a]	112.2	8.4[d]
Thigh	6.39	107.4	1.3	6.40	103.3	−0.2	6.68	107.5	3.9
Calf	6.21	104.4	−1.6	6.26	101.0	−2.4	6.68	107.5	3.9
Ankle	6.51	109.5	3.2	6.43	103.7	0.2	6.14	98.8	−4.5
Waist	6.26	105.2	−0.8	6.44	104.0	0.5	6.30	101.4	−2.0
Buttocks	6.36	106.9	0.8	6.44	104.0	0.5	6.44	103.7	0.2
Diameter									
Biacromial	6.28	105.6	−0.5	6.52	105.2	1.7	5.80	93.4	−9.8
Chest	6.18	103.9	−2.0	6.16	99.5	−3.9	6.31	101.6	−1.9
Bi-iliac	6.60	110.9	4.6	6.52	105.2	1.7	6.49[c]	104.5	1.0

[a] Analysis of data from Cureton (1951) pertaining to champion athletes.
[b] d = cm/k, k values from Table III for gymnast and for American athletes, respectively.
[c] k (bi-iliac) for Negro athletes derived from Tanner's (1964) data (= 4.50).
[d] k (biceps) derived for the arm extended from Tanner's (1964) data (= 4.85).

difference in stature. Thus dq for the thigh of the gymnast is equal to dq for the shot-put champion. The raw data converted to d quotients and corrected for stature can therefore be compared across the board.

The proportions of the swimmer are nearly identical with those of his group and the striking symmetry is shown by the narrow range in variation of percent deviation of d from D. The shot-put champion (1948 Olympics) has ample arm size for this event (if the arm were measured extended and not in the same manner as for the swimmers). The 6 circumferences, however, are probably not representative of his actual size since D is significantly less than $3F$ (>2 S.E.). The lower k (Ref. W), 4.50, derived from Tanner's data and other sources, compared with 4.87 (swimmers) reflects the relatively small pelvic size which is a characteristic of body build in the Negro.

2. Olympic Athletes, 1960 (Analysis of Tanner's Data, 1964)

a. Derivation and Comparison of k Values of Negro, Asian, and Caucasian Athletes. Mean values (Table V) representing 8 events from Tanner's Table V (1964) were treated as individual measurements in the derivation of the $(3F)$ factors. Since the range of body weights is restricted in each particular event, the error in utilizing mean stature and weight data is not significant for group and racial comparisons. Perimetric size per unit of stature as inferred from uS-W (Table V) is approximately the same for the three groups of athletes and reference man. The anthropometric k values are remarkably similar for the three races with the exception of the small bi-iliac width ($k = 4.50$) previously referred to in the Negro. The k values (Ref. Man) are in close agreement with those of the Caucasian athlete with the exception of knee width. The larger knee width (level of femoral condyles) of the athlete is probably related to the site of measurement; for the reference man the diameter is transtibial.

Obviously, the advantage of the radiographic technique lies in the delineation of muscle, bone, and fat widths in the extremities. Surprisingly, the Caucasian athlete has relatively less muscle than his Negro and Asian peers. It is in the measurement of bone width and a better estimate of actual skeletal size (and probably weight) that the radiogram is essential. The larger bone width of the Negro ($k = 1.52$) is in accord with data on cadavers (Seale, 1959) that the skeleton of the Negro is heavier than the skeleton of the Caucasian, although greater ponderosity is not associated with greater "frame" size as recorded by 8 diameters. The heavier bone structure of the Negro would also contribute to a higher body density which tends to exclude Negroes from competitive swimming.

b. Physical Characteristics of Two Shot-Put Champions, 1960. Conversion of anthropometric and radiographic measurements to d and dq equivalents (Table VI) facilitates comparison of physical characteristics associated with exceptional build. Per unit of stature (uS-W) their body size is about 15% (about 2 σ) greater than that of the reference Caucasian athlete. The enlargement of arm size is the feature (apart from massive structure) of their build. The agreement of radiographic and perimetric conversions indicates not only technical accuracy but constancy of the ratio of transmetric (x-ray) to girth dimensions.

TABLE V

Derivation of Conversion Constants (k Values) for a Caucasian, Negro, and Asian Reference Athlete from Mean Values of Anthropometric and Radiographic Data Representing Eight Group Events[ab]

	Caucasian		Negro	Asian	Reference man (military)
Stature (dm):	17.86		18.10	17.44	17.40
Weight (kg):	74.3		74.4	70.6	70.0
3F:	6.11		6.07	6.00	6.00
uS-W:	101		99	100	100
	cm	k^c	k^c	k^c	k
Diameters					
Anthropometric					
Biacromial	41.32	6.76	6.83	6.84	6.77
Bi-iliac	29.16	4.77	4.50	4.83	4.77
Elbow × 2	14.46	2.37	2.36	2.36	2.32
K (Ref. W, 3 diameters)		13.90	13.69	14.03	13.86
Knee × 2	19.91	3.26	3.25	3.25	3.03[d]
Radiographic					
(arm, calf, thigh)					
Muscle	31.75	5.20	5.35	5.31	—
Bone	8.73	1.43	1.52	1.43	—
Fat	2.29	0.375	0.309	0.335	—
(muscle + bone + fat)					
Arm	10.74	1.76	1.77	1.69	—
Calf	12.42	2.03	2.04	2.14	—
Thigh	19.61	3.21	3.36	3.25	—
Circumferences					
(tape)					
Arm	29.70	4.86	4.86	4.79	4.85
Calf	—	6.06[e]	—	—	5.97
Thigh	56.65	9.27	9.36	9.34	9.13

[a] Eight group events, Caucasian and Asian (400 m, marathon, 400-m hurdles, long jump, triple jump, hammer, weightlift, wrestling); Negro (100/200 m, 400 m, 5000 m, 110-m hurdles, steeplechase, high jump, long jump, weightlift).

[b] Pertinent k values for the reference man (Table I) have been introduced for comparison with Caucasian reference athlete (analysis of Tanner's (1964) data on Olympic Athletes).

[c] The cm divided by respective $3F$ factors.

[d] Intercondylar width of tibia; other groups, intercondylar width of femur.

[e] Estimated from calf/thigh (military) × 9.27.

TABLE VI

Conversion of Anthropometric and Radiographic Measurements into d and Unit Size (uS-P) Values for Two Olympic Champion Athletes (1960) in the Shot-Put Event[a]

	Athlete No. 1				Athlete No. 2				
h (dm):	19.27 (75.9 inches)				18.97 (74.7 inches)				
W (kg):	114.5 (252 lb)				108.2 (238 lb)				
$3F$:	7.31				7.17				
uS-W:	115.5				114.1				
q:	15.80				15.91				
	cm	d	dq	%Dev.	cm	d	dq	%Dev.	k
Diameters									
Biacromial	46.2	6.85	108.3	−6.3	47.1	6.99	111.2	−2.5	6.74
Bi-iliac	32.5	6.83	107.9	−6.6	32.9	6.91	109.9	−3.6	4.76
Elbow × 2	16.4	6.95	109.8	−4.7	16.2	6.86	109.2	−4.3	2.36
Knee × 2	21.8	6.71	106.0	−8.2	22.0	6.78	107.9	−5.4	3.25
Average	116.9	6.83	107.9	−6.6	118.2	6.91	109.9	−3.6	17.11
Radiographic (9 arm, calf, thigh)									
Muscle	37.65	7.27	114.9	−0.5	38.13	7.36	117.1	2.7	5.18
Bone	10.06	7.09	112.0	−3.0	10.06	7.09	112.8	−1.1	1.42
Fat	4.62	12.38	195.7	69.4	2.89	7.75	123.3	8.1	0.373
Radiographic									
Arm	14.98	8.56	135.3	17.1	13.71	7.83	124.6	9.2	1.75
Calf	13.53	6.67	105.4	−8.8	14.12	6.96	110.8	−2.9	2.03
Thigh	23.82	7.44	117.6	1.8	23.25	7.27	115.6	1.4	3.20
Perimetric (tape)									
Arm	41.3	8.52	134.6	16.6	38.1	7.86	125.0	9.6	4.85
Calf	42.3	7.00	110.6	−2.0	44.3	7.34	116.8	2.4	6.04
Thigh	69.7	7.54	119.2	3.2	66.9	7.24	114.9	1.0	9.24

[a] Analysis of Tanner's (1964) data.

The amount of fat (x-ray widths) appears to be considerably higher in one athlete compared with the other. How does one convert the shadow widths (which have reliability if not validity) to kilograms of fat? The ratio, $d(\text{fat})/D \times 10.2$, or $d(\text{fat})/D^2 \times 10.2$ where 10.2 is the mean percentage of body fat for the reference athlete computed from skeletal frame size, appeared promising. Individual estimates of fat were either too low (the simple proportion) or too high if squared values were substituted.

A more basic approach to the estimate of body fat by simple technique is the computation of *LBW* from anthropometric diameters. This calculation requires a value for $K(LBW)$ which we do not have in Table V. However, K (Ref. *W*) is the same for the reference Caucasian athlete and reference man if biacromial, bi-iliac, and elbow ($\times$ 2) diameters are used. Since *LBW* is calculated in the same manner as Ref. *W* but on a lower scale, it is reasonable to employ for $K(LBW)$ the value of 14.7 for the above selected diameters from Table I. Then $D(LBW)$, athlete No. 1, is 7.23 (diameter 14.7), and 7.30 for athlete No. 2. If the respective $D(LBW)$ conversions are substituted in Eq. (1), *LBW* (No. 1) = 89.5 kg and *LBW* (No. 2) = 90.2 kg. These weights represent mean values based on the average amount of lean tissue relative to skeletal frame size. In men with better than average musculature (and perhaps bone width although Tanner's data indicate little correlation between the two components), it is necessary to correct *LBW* for excess muscle (and bone?).

The radiographic muscle plus bone widths provide the data for this correction. Ref. *W* (athlete No. 1) computed from muscle + bone (K, Ref. *W*, muscle + bone = 6.6) is 111.8 kg which is less than body weight (114.5 kg); hence, no correction is required. Ref. *W* (athlete No. 2) computed from muscle + bone is 112.3 kg compared with body weight (108.2 kg). A correction of +4.1 kg will be added to *LBW* (anthropometric). The estimate of body fat in the 2 athletes, is as follows:

Corrected *LBW* (anthropometric), No. 1 = 89.5; body weight 89.5 = 25 kg fat (21.8% of weight)

Corrected *LBW* (anthropometric), No. 2 + 4.1 kg = 94.3 kg; fat = 13.9 kg (12.9% of weight)

3. Long Distance and Specifically English Channel Swimmers

We now turn to the most arduous type of endurance effort and it is reassuring to find older and even moderately obese men (endowed with adequate musculature) as firmly established competitors. A commentary on endurance swimming is the performance of adolescent girls and women who periodically excel the best male swimmers. The chief advantage conferred by added fat is increased buoyancy. A relatively lean swimmer (weight 80 kg; sp.gr., 1.080; 10% fat) has a net weight (weight corrected for the volume of air in the lungs) in fresh water of about 6 kg. A corpulent swimmer (weight 100 kg; sp. gr., 1.040; 30% fat) has a net weight of 3.8 kg in fresh water. Thus, an athlete who weighs 20 kg more in air may weigh 2.2 kg less than a lean swimmer in water. The 100-kg swimmer with an amount of air in the lungs normally present (expiratory reserve volume + tidal volume) enjoys neutral or even positive buoyancy; the lean swimmer has a negative buoyancy of about 2.2 kg.

Physique, therefore, plays a most important role in this type of competive effort. Not only must the swimmers have powerful muscles trained for sustained effort but also extra fat. In addition to improvement of buoyancy, fat provides insulation which reduces heat loss in cold water. The accumulation of fat alters the shape of the body in the direction of rotundity which in turn decreases the ratio of surface area to volume. A lean scientist (5% body fat), accustomed to the cold and hardship of Mt. Everest expeditions, was incapacitated after a short exposure in water (13° to 16°C). A moderately obese Channel swimmer, on the other hand, could remain immersed in the cold water for long periods without shivering despite minimal activity (Pugh and Edholm, 1955).

TABLE VII

BODY SIZE AND PERCENTAGE OF FAT OF ENGLISH CHANNEL SWIMMERS[a]

Swim-mer (No.)	Age (years)	Stature (dm)	Weight (kg)	$3F$	uS-W	Den-sity	%Fat[b]	Sp. gr.	%Fat[c]
1	58	16.40	91.2	7.08	121.2	1.032	29.6	1.037	31.5
2	37	17.45	82.6	6.53	108.4	1.038	26.9	1.043	28.5
3	37	18.26	102.9	7.12	115.6	1.040	26.0	1.045	27.5
4	26	17.86	85.6	6.57	107.8	1.075	10.5	1.080	10.0
5	31	17.32	81.9	6.53	108.8	1.068	14.1	1.073	13.5
6	31	17.13	98.7	7.20	120.7	1.036	27.7	1.041	29.5
7	34	16.02	76.5	6.56	113.4	1.049	21.8	1.054	23.0
8	26	17.78	72.6	6.06	99.7	1.065	14.8	1.070	15.0
9	27	17.02	87.3	6.79	114.2	1.022	34.3	1.027	36.5
10	18	18.55	103.2	7.08	114.0	1.047	22.8	1.052	24.0

[a] Based on data reported by Pugh *et al.* (1960) and Pugh (1965).
[b] From Siri (1956) equation. Percentages in original paper not used.
[c] % Fat = (1.100 − Sp. gr.)/0.002. Sp. gr. calculated from density + 0.005.

The physical characteristics with respect to the amount of body fat, chiefly, are presented in Table VII based on the studies of Pugh *et al.* (1960) and résumé (Pugh, 1965). The uS-W estimates of unit perimetric size vary from about 100 to 121 with an average of 112.4, somewhat less than the uS-W for shot-put champions. In the original data, the calculated percentages of fat appear to have been derived from a formula which incorporates a value of 0.873 for density (fat), much below an experimental value of 0.90 for the density of lipid extracted from adipose tissue and the overall estimate of 0.915 for the density of all body lipids (Brožek, 1963). The formulas of Siri (1956) (density) and of Rathbun and Pace (1945) based on specific gravity incorporate the higher values. Percent fat (density) = 495.0/density − 450.0;

% fat (sp. gr.) = 554.8/sp. gr. − 504.4. We have used the simple approximation: % fat = (1.100 − sp. gr)/0.002. The percentages of fat (Table VII) have been recalculated from density using Siri's formula and from specific gravity (sp. gr. = density + 0.005) water temperature (32°C approximately) by our thumb rule calculation. The average percentage body fat of the swimmers is about 23% so that an average weight of 88 kg incorporates some 20 kg of fat.

As a concluding note to these paragraphs, it is of interest that the estimated metabolic cost of swimming the English Channel (Pugh, 1965) is about 11,000 kcal. This cost is independent of the crossing time which is in the range of 9.5 to 27 hr over a direct distance of 22 mi. In view of the inordinate energy requirement, it is remarkable that a 15-year-old girl, and a man of 57 years, have succeeded in swimming the Channel. On the incredible side is the feat of Abertondu, the Argentinian who swam the Channel both ways in 43 hr.

4. Professional Football Players (circa, 1940)

In professional football, speed, agility, coordination, balance, and lean weight (muscle and bone) are prime factors. In a previous era (Welham and Behnke, 1942), it was impressive to find big men who had these qualifications and who did not carry an added burden of excess fat (Table VIII). Today these attributes are taken for granted; in addition, there is an increase in weight of backfield men and ends of 15 to 25 lb, and in linemen, up to 50 lb. With regard to increased lean weight, an estimate is made that backfield men average 190 lb (h, 70–74 inches), and the linemen about 220 lb (h, 75–79 inches).

Noteworthy in Table VIII is the uniformity of the 2 groups with respect to stature, lean body weight, and lung volumes. The range of residual air volume is restricted, 1.190 to 1.790 liters. The importance of lung volume and fractions of lung volume, which incorporate both morphological and functional parameters, is emphasized. It was anticipated at the time that a high correlation would be found between LBW and total lung volume. The correlation coefficient ($r = 0.67$) was too low to have much predictive value since CV of the fraction, lung volume/LBW, was $\pm 6.7\%$ which is about one-half the CV of each parameter.

Although a few anthropometric measurements were made at the time, it was found that the difference between average chest and waist girths for the entire group of 25 men was 6.9 inches (40.0 − 33.1) compared with 6.8 inches (36.5 − 29.7) for 38 lean Navy men who had about the same specific gravity. It would have been highly informative to have had not only the comprehensive type of examination outlined in Table I but linear dimensions of extremities and the radiograms as developed by Tanner. On the other hand, solidly grounded techniques in contrast to tenuous skinfold appraisal, such as

TABLE VIII

Mean Values for Lean Body Weights, Percentage of Fat, and Pulmonary Volumes of 25 Professional Football Players (circa 1940)[a]

	Group I	Group II
Age (years)	24.9	26.4
Stature (dm)	18.13	18.49
(inches)	71.4	72.8
Range (I and II) (inches)	(68.7–75.3)	
Weight (kg)	84.5	98.8
(lb)	186	217
Range (lb)	169–196	194–260
$3F$	6.48	6.94
uS-W	105.5	111.9
Specific gravity[b]	1.097–1.088	1.080–1.051
Fat %[c]	1.5–6.0	10.0–24.5
Lean body weight (kg)	81.6	81.9
Range	75–86	76–97
Total lung volume (ml)	7420	7130
Range	6040–8400	5890–8920
Vital capacity (ml)	5930	5700
Range	4630–6600	4500–7250
Residual air (ml)	1490	1430
Range	1340–1790	1190–1670

[a] Divided into two groups: (I) chiefly backfield men and ends, and (II) linemen (from Welham and Behnke, 1942).

[b] Density (approximately) = Sp. gr. − 0.005.

[c] % Fat = (1.100 − Sp. gr.)/0.002.

specific gravity and measurements of lung volumes, have not been exploited in recent years for evaluation of athletes.

5. A Professional Football Player, 1966 (Table IX and Fig. 2)

a. Anthropometric Data. Examination was made of an outstanding athlete who played guard position. In evaluation of his physique it is necessary to make an estimate both of excess fat and better than average musculature. Perimetric size per unit of stature, uS-P (Table IX), was 124.3 compared with uS-W (115) for the shot-put champions. Excess fat is indicated by the larger d (abdominal average) quotient compared with D, and excess muscle (including fat also) is reflected in the high d(biceps) and d(thigh) quotients relative to D. Weight calculated from D (by substitution in Eq. (2), $h^{0.7}$ = 7.91) was 127.6 kg compared with a scale weight of 127.5 kg. In exceptionally tall men, Eq. (2) may provide a closer estimate of body weight than Eq. (1); by substitution of D in either equation the difference is not large.

TABLE IX

Anthropometric Description and Somatolytic Analysis of a Professional Football Player, 1966

h (dm):	19.18 (75.5 inches)
W (kg):	127.5 (280.5 lb)
$3F$:	7.74
uS-W:	122.2
D:	7.83
uS-P:	124.3
q:	15.87

	Circumferences	cm	d	dq	% Dev.
	Chest	116.5	7.61	120.8	−2.8
A	Abdomen				
	(average)	110.6	8.46	134.3	8.1
	Buttocks	120.5	7.74	122.8	−1.2
	d(A)	7.94			1.4
	Thigh	76.1	8.34	132.4	6.5
	Shoulder	142.4	7.71	122.4	−1.5
	Biceps	44.3	8.37	132.8	6.9
B	Forearm	34.6	7.74	122.8	−1.2
	Calf	47.1	7.89	125.2	0.8
	d(B)	7.93			1.3
	Wrist	20.2	7.02	111.4	−10.4
	Knee	43.7	7.16	113.6	−8.8
	Ankle	27.1	7.23	114.7	−7.7
		S 783			
$WFCA$	d($WFCA$)	7.56			−3.5

Diameters	cm	d(Ref. W)		cm	d(Ref. W)
Bideltoid	56.3	7.47			
Biacromial	43.6	6.44	Wrists	11.9	6.43
Chest width	33.8	6.76	Ankles	14.8	6.38
Bi-iliac	30.0	6.29	Knees	21.6	7.01
Bitroch.	36.0	6.58	Elbows	15.0	6.47
Sum 8 diameters	206.7	K(Ref. W) = 31.6			% Dev.
C		$D(C)$ = 6.54			−16.5
$K(LBW)$ = 33.5		$D(LBW)$ = 6.17			

Inspection Rating: 4∗

Anthropometric rating			
A	B	C	$WFCA$
1.4	1.3	−16.5	−3.5

TABLE IX

Anthropometric Description and Somatolytic Analysis of a Professional Football Player, 1966

		Calculated weights (kg)		
$W(D)$	$W(A)$	$W(B)$	$W(C)$	$W(WFCA)$
127.6	131.2	130.9	89.0	118.9

Lean body weight (anthro.) 79.2 kg

Tissue	Somatolytic analysis		
	$\% LBW$	W(kg)	Potassium (mEq)
Bone Marrow Tendons Cartilage Nonmuscular	21	16.6	310
Lean	39	30.9	2100
Muscle	40	31.7	2760
		79.2	5170

"Excess" K = 2036 mEq, 7206–5170
"Excess" Muscle[b] = 23.4 kg

Corrected LBW
    79.2 + 23.4 = 102.6 K
Fat = 24.9 kg, (127.5–102.6)
% Fat = 19.5

[a] Total body potassium (40 K analysis) = 7206 mEq (281.8 gm).
[b] Excess muscle = excess K/87 based on 87 mEq K/kg of muscle.

The component analysis reveals that $d(A)$ and $d(B)$ are nearly identical but are much higher than $D(C)$ from which Ref. W is computed. LBW (anthropometric), calculated from 8 diameters and the 0.7 fractional power of stature, was 79.2 kg. Weights calculated from the d components emphasize the differences; $W(A)$ 131.2, $W(B)$ 130.9, $W(C)$ 89.0, and optimal weight, $W(WFCA)$ 118.9, weights in kilograms.

 b. Somatolytic Analysis Based Chiefly on Total Body Potassium. A startlingly high value of 281.8 gm (7206 mEq) compared with 150–160 gm (Ref. Man) was recorded in a run of 50 min duration in the 2π shielded chamber housing a NaI crystal spectrometer. Prior to the determination a satisfactory calibration test was carried out on a subject whose total body potassium (166 gm) was known both from radioisotopic (K_e) and chamber ^{40}K

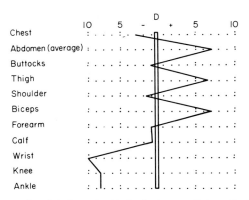

Fig. 2. Somatogram showing the percentage deviation of d quotients from the D axis based on data in Table IX. The relative enlargement with respect to body size of the abdomen, thigh, and biceps points to excess fat combined with heavy musculature. Professional football player 1966. Stature dm 19.18 (75.5 inches); weight kg, 127.5 (280.5 lb).

analysis. Nevertheless, without replication the high potassium figure is regarded as tentative but it will serve to illustrate the principle underlying our analysis. Potassium can be allocated to bone, nonmuscle lean tissue (n-m lean), and muscle. Bone weight was estimated from mineral, organic, water, and fat content (expanded to include all essential lipids in the body) as 16% of $LBW = 12.57$ kg, water content 3.56 liters and potassium in bone as 310 mEq (3.56 × 87). The n-m lean (skin, glands, viscera, fat-free adipose tissue) was estimated as 39% LBW (= 30.9 kg, 24.1 liters of water). Muscle normally present in LBW is 40% (= 31.7 kg, 23.8 liters water) and the potassium, 2760 mEq (23.8 × 116). Total potassium in LBW(anthropometric) = 5170 mEq. The "excess" muscle of the football player may be estimated from the difference, total K—5170 = 2036 mEq, weight of excess muscle = 2036/87 = 23.4 kg. Corrected LBW(anthropometric) = 79.2 + 23.4 = 102.6 kg; total weight of muscle = 55.1 kg. Body fat = weight − corrected LBW = 24.9 kg (19.5%). If the fat allowance is 15% of body weight, the reduced weight from 127.5 kg would be 121 kg and this is approximately equal to $W(WFCA)$, the "Optimal" weight (118.9 kg) computed from the anthropometric girths and stature.

VI. Summary

A system of analysis of body build drawing upon photography, anthropometry, radiography, determinations of specific gravity, and total body potassium, has been applied to evaluate the physique of gymnasts, swimmers (short and long distance), track and field athletes, and football players. Data have been utilized from several sources but in no instance was a comprehensive appraisal of body build possible. There should be no doubt from our exposition that body build can be examined systematically by the media of simple techniques, carefully executed, and with attention directed to the rigorous control of physiologic variables. Advanced methods are available in the laboratories of the biophysicist and biochemist.

The feasibility of ^{40}K monitoring to assess total body potassium is largely a matter of transportation to specially equipped and manned laboratories. Metabolic balance studies and analysis of urinary excretory products, as one endeavor to quantify the muscle mass as distinct from nonmuscular lean tissue, are routinely possible in medical centers. The yield from and contribution of radioisotope laboratories is meager relative to potential. Finally, with reference to the athlete, he should be studied systematically in "home" surroundings, well before he engages in national and international competition. The site of Olympic games is no place for the type of controlled examination, simple though it be, that we have outlined. The results of our studies must have daily return to the athlete himself. The groundwork for a new era in quantitative somatology has been prepared by such pioneers as Kohlrausch, Jokl, Cureton, and Tanner. Vital and imaginative administrative efforts primarily are required for accomplishment.

REFERENCES

Anderson, E. C. (1963). *In* "Body Composition" (H. E. Whipple and J. Brožek, eds.), Part I, pp. 189–212. N.Y. Acad. Sci., New York.

Behnke, A. R., Guttentag, O. E., and Brodsby, C. (1959). *Human Biol.* **31**, 295.

Behnke, A. R. (1961). *J. Appl. Physiol.* **16**, 1960.

Behnke, A. R. (1963). *In* "Body Composition" (H. E. Whipple and J. Brožek, eds.), Part II, pp. 450–464. N.Y. Acad. Sci., New York.

Behnke, A. R., and Royce, J. (1966). *J. Sports Med.* **6**, 75.

Behnke, A. R., Feen, B. G., and Welham, W. C. (1942). *J. Am. Med. Assoc.* **118**, 495.

Boling, E. A. (1963). *In* "Body Composition" (H. E. Whipple and J. Brožek, eds.), Part I, pp. 246–254. New York Acad. Sci., New York.

Brožek, J., Grande, F., Anderson, J. T., and Keys, A. (1963). *In* "Body Composition" (H. E. Whipple and J. Brožek, eds.), Part I, pp. 113–140. N.Y. Acad. Sci., New York.

Brožek, J., and Henschel, A., eds. (1961). "Techniques for Measuring Body Composition." Natl. Acad. Sci.—Natl. Res. Council, Washington, D.C.

Cureton, T. K., Jr. (1951). "Physical Fitness of Champion Athletes." Univ. of Illinois Press, Urbana, Illinois.

Dupertuis, C. W. (1963). *In* "Anthropometric Survey of Turkey, Greece, and Italy," pp. 35–65. Pergamon Press, Oxford.

Garn, S. M. (1961). *In* "Techniques for Measuring Body Composition" (J. Brožek and A. Henschel, eds.), pp. 36–58. Natl. Acad. Sci.—Natl. Res. Council, Washington, D.C.

Goldman, R. F., and Buskirk, E. R. (1961). *In* "Techniques for Measuring Body Composition" (J. Brozek and A. Henschel, eds.), pp. 78–106. Natl. Acad. Sci.—Natl. Res. Council, Washington, D.C.

Henry, M. (1962). "All About Horses." Random House, New York.

Hertzberg, H. T. E., Churchill, E., Dupertuis, C. W., White, R. M., and Damon, A. (1963). "Anthropometric Survey of Turkey, Greece, and Italy." Pergamon Press, Oxford.

Jokl, E. (1933). *Arch. Ges. Physiol.* **232**, 687.

Jokl, E. (1963). *In* "Body Composition" (H. E. Whipple and J. Brozek, eds.), Part II, pp. 778–793. N.Y. Acad. Sci., New York.

Krogman, W. M. (1955). *Monographs Soc. Res. Child Develop.* **20**, no. 60.

Luft, U.C., and Kim, T. P. K. (1961). *In* "Techniques for Measuring Body Composition" (J. Brozek and A. Henschel, eds.), p. 107. Natl. Acad. Sci.—Natl. Res. Council, Washington, D.C.

Miller, C. E., and Remenchik, A. P. (1963). *In* "Body Composition" (H. E. Whipple and J. Brozek, eds.), Part I, pp. 175–188. N.Y. Acad. Sci., New York.

Moore, F. D., Olesen, K. H., McMurrey, J. D., Parker, H. V., Ball, M. R., and Boyden, C. M. (1963). "The Body Cell Mass and its Supporting Environment." Saunders, Philadelphia, Pennsylvania.

Pugh, L. G. C. E. (1965). *In* "Physiology of Breath-Hold Diving and the AMA of Japan" (H. Rahn and T. Yokoyama, eds.), pp. 325–346. Publ. 1341, Natl. Acad. Sci.—Natl. Res. Council, Washington, D.C.

Pugh, L. G. C. E., and Edholm, O. G. (1955). *Lancet* **II**, 761.

Pugh, L. G. C. E., Edholm, O. G., Fox, R. H., Wolff, H. S., Hervey, G. R., Hammond, W. H., Tanner, J. M., and Whitehouse, R. N. (1960). *Clin. Sci.* **19**, 257.

Rathbun, E. N., and Pace, N. (1945). *J. Biol. Chem.* **158**, 667.

Seale, R. U. (1959). *Am. J. Phys. Anthropol.* **17**, 37.

Siri, W. E. (1956). *Advan. Biol. Med. Phys.* **4**, 239–272.

Tanner, J. M. (1964). "The Physique of the Olympic Athlete." Allen & Unwin, London.

Welham, W. C., and Behnke, A. R. (1942). *J. Am. Med. Assoc.* **118**, 498.

White, R. M. (1963). *In* "Anthropometric Survey of Turkey, Greece, and Italy," pp. 61–65. Pergamon Press, Oxford.

13

BODY COMPOSITION AND RELATIONSHIPS TO PHYSICAL ACTIVITY

A. H. Ismail

I. Influence of Physical Activity on Body Composition

Experience has shown that children and adults leading an active and vigorous life have firmer, stronger, and more supple muscles with sturdier physiques and less adipose tissue than those individuals who follow a sedentary existence. Hence, it is reasonable to believe that there are real differences between structural and functional measurements of active and nonactive individuals. The body responds to exercise in a dynamic fashion, and several mechanisms simultaneously affect fluid shifts during exercise. The mechanisms may be altered with the kind of exercise, the duration, and the conditions under which it is performed. Therefore, no single exercise state can reasonably serve as a reference for all types and duration of exercise.

Type of exercise may be classified as acute or chronic. By definition, acute exercise may be considered in terms of the effect of one single bout of exercise on body composition. Chronic exercise may be considered in terms of the effect of exercise on body composition when repeatedly undertaken for a length of time. This may involve a short-term physical conditioning program for a month or two or habitual exercise which is followed for years. Furthermore, exercise may be classified as to kind in terms of degree of severity into either light, moderate, or heavy.

A. Effect of Acute Exercise on Body Composition

The light or moderate exercise does not affect body composition. Although fat reduction may take place after heavy exercise, body composition will return to pre-exercise values gradually within a short time. Cureton (1958) pointed out that intermittent games, e.g., bowling, golf, and volleyball, will not change body composition. However, research studies have shown that the effect of acute exercise can differentiate between obese and nonobese subjects.

Auchincloss *et al.* (1963) found that when the increase in oxygen consumption from rest to exercise was related to body weight, a steeper slope was found for higher body weights indicating a reduction in mechanical efficiency. During the steady state, the obese subjects increased their ventilation in order to maintain normal alveolar carbon dioxide tensions.

Administering 12 physical performance tests to groups of mesomorphs, ectomorphs, and endomorphs, Sills and Everett (1953) concluded that excess body fat may be a handicap to physical performance.

There is an agreement among researchers pertaining to the relationships between various components of body composition and the maximal oxygen uptake. The relationships indicate that obesity limits the capacity for strenuous exertion by increasing the energy cost of exercise without a proportional increase in the maximal capacity for oxygen uptake. As substantiation for this statement, Balke and Ware (1959) tested more than 500 Air Force personnel on a work capacity test and found that overweight subjects scored lower than those classified as either normal or underweight.

In sedentary college men, Dempsey (1964b) found that the time taken for the heart rate to attain 180 beats/min in the Balke Test was significantly and negatively related to the fat per total body weight ratio. He concluded that the obese individual is under a substantial handicap in physical performance requiring exhausting work because of the load of fat which does not contribute to his performance and which he must carry with him.

It can be concluded that acute exercise may have a momentary effect, if any at all, on body composition. However, acute exercise, especially the heavy kind, can differentiate functionally among individuals with different body compositions.

B. Effect of Chronic Exercise on Body Composition

Chronic exercise affects the individual functionally and structurally. To bring about significant changes in body composition, the individual should adopt a regular workout regime. Body composition data from individuals who exercised habitually were compared with similar data from sedentary men (Buskirk *et al.*, 1955). The results showed that habitual exercise was associated with a greater lean body mass. These results were obtained from three groups of students who varied with respect to the type and amount of habitual physical activity. It was found that body fat was inversely related to the extent of participation in physical activity. For example, athletes averaged less fat than intramural participants who averaged less fat than sedentary students.

In two matched adult groups, Keys and Brožek (1953) found that the physically active group showed a lower estimated fat content of their body than the sedentary group. Furthermore, the physically active group had larger lean body mass and showed little of the "disease atrophy" characteristic of the "normal" aging. In contrast, some researchers (Christian et al., 1964a) maintain that change in body composition in adult populations is due to reduction of fat only and not due to increase in muscle mass. Such a claim is supported by the measurement of potassium K^{40} which has been found to be constant in adult individuals for a long period of time.

Pascale et al. (1955) studied body composition measurements before and after a physical training course. As a result, it was found that body fat decreased and fat-free body weight increased.

In several studies it was reported that body fat, particularly subcutaneous fat, could be altered by strenuous training and that body density usually increased even if no loss in weight occurred. Relative to this point, Kireilis and Cureton (1947) concluded that weight is not a good guide in fat loss because fat loss might be compensated for by increased muscle density due to exercise. This finding was supported by Leedy et al. (1965) when they concluded that physical exercise alone did not result in a significant loss of weight. They studied the effect of an organized program of physical fitness on a group of middle-aged males and found that the percent of lean body weight, rather than the amount of lean body weight, was the factor associated with the ability to score highly on physical performance items.

Christian et al. (1964b) and Ismail et al. (1963) studied preadolescent boys who were involved in a physical fitness program. They found that the percent of lean body weight was the most important item for measuring motor fitness. The same finding was achieved by Falls et al. (1965) when they studied adults. A series of studies by Wells et al. (1962a, b, c) showed that physical training caused a "proportional and absolute increase of lean tissue and a correspondingly opposite response of excess fat."

Evaluating the effect of a typical 6-week period of physical fitness for underwater trainees, Cureton (1963) found significant reduction in abdominal fat, total fat index, and abdominal girth. Among middle-aged men, Cureton and Phillips (1964) found significant reduction in abdominal girth, body weight, body surface area, and total fat due to a continuous conditioning program.

Studies utilizing the factor analysis techniques have shown that the heavier the man, the smaller the oxygen intake per kilogram of body weight (Cureton

and Sterling, 1964; Falls *et al.*, 1965). Negative correlations were obtained
between body weight and aerobic work capacity in heavy exercise.

The studies reviewed above indicate a general agreement among researchers
that regular exercise of certain duration and intensity brings about definite
changes involving a decrease in body fat and increase in muscular mass, especially among a young population (Dempsey, 1964a), with variations in
total body weight depending upon the proportional changes in these two
components. Meanwhile, acute or even intermittent activities have negligible
effect. Inactivity has the reverse effect.

II. Body Composition, Growth and Development, and Aging of the Organism

Profound changes take place with time, not only in the total bulk of the
human organism but also in the absolute and relative contribution of individual organs and tissue. A summary of the literature on changes in body
composition with age was made by Mickelsen (1959).

Friis-Hansen (1958) found that in the human fetus the total body water
expressed as a percentage of body weight decreases from 94% in the first to
82% in the eighth lunar month. The rapid decrease in water content continues
through the first year of life from about 78% in the newborn child to 60% in
the age group of one-half to 2 years. Further, Friis-Hansen's data were
supplemented by information on body water in adults with particular reference to sex differences. The total body water accounted for 54% and 49%
of body weight in males and females, respectively. This was supported by
determinations of the total exchangeable potassium. There is no significant
difference between males and females in terms of potassium concentration
(grams per kilogram of gross body weight) until approximately the age of
puberty. After this period the proportion of lean to total body weight in
females drops rapidly till 16 years of age. Beyond 16 years of age, there is a
gradual decline in potassium concentration with age paralleling the slope of
the male curve but 0.3 to 0.4 gm/kg lower concentration. Anderson and
Langham (1959) reported body potassium measurements in 1590 subjects in
both sexes ranging in age from less than one year to 79 years. The average
concentration of potassium per kilogram of gross body weight showed interesting correlations with age and sex; one of the permanent features was a
steady decline with increasing age for adults. The results have been confirmed
by other workers in the field (Schifferdecker *et al.*, 1964). Measurement of
adult females (20 years or more) at Purdue University showed 12 to 14% less
lean body mass on the average than males of the same age.

In the age range from 20 to 60 years, density decreases both in men and
women and reflects largely a tendency toward the accumulation of body fat.

The changes in body composition associated with aging involve the accumulation of certain body constituents, namely fat, and simultaneous decrement in other tissues especially muscles and some demineralization of bones. It could be concluded that the total body potassium content (K) is proportional to the body mass minus bone mineral, fat, and water (M_3).

During growth, body potassium and M_3 increase linearly with age. During maturity, changes in body composition are likely to be complex and nonlinear. In adulthood, M_3 and potassium appear to depend on both age and sex. The ratio of K/M_3 decreases with increasing age and is lower for females than for males (Seppanen *et al.*, 1963).

When dealing with the concept of aging, two kinds of interpretations present themselves—biological age and chronological age—and these are quite different. Until now, adequate definition of biological age has not been presented. However, many possibilities exist: (1) of two individuals of the same age, the one who outlives the other is biologically younger; (2) of two individuals of the same age, the one who can sustain effort best without exhaustion is biologically younger; and (3) of two individuals of the same age, the one with greater work capacity is biologically younger than the other. The difficulty in defining biological age is perhaps not a serious handicap since long-life expectancy, high resistance to stress, and greater work capacity tend to correlate in persons attaining an exceptionally great age (Jalavisto and Makkonen, 1963). Therefore, chronological age may be considered as a rough measure of aging.

In research pertaining to aging and longevity (Jalavisto and Makkonen, 1963) it was found that the absence of excessive obesity is one of many important factors influencing the organism. Other factors are familial longevity, active life, unfailing general health, and absence of heavy smoking. Jalavisto and Makkonen (1963) extracted a factor of overweight pertaining to aging. They indicated that overweight may be associated with hypertrophy of the heart. Hypertrophy of the heart is known to be connected with increased duration of systole which is indicative of heart failure. Further, cardiac involvement is more common among overweight persons and consequently insurance companies consider them to be higher risks.

The differences in the factorial structure of the male and female results concerning obesity, hypertension, and association of coronary sclerosis are in conformity with previous experience (Seppanen *et al.*, 1963). For example, in men, Moses (1963) noted a higher incidence of atherosclerotic coronary lesions in obese-hypertensive and normotensive individuals than in thin men. In women, a difference was noted between hypertensive obese and normotensive obese individuals. Obesity in old women seems to have very little pathogenetic connection with the development of hypertension, atherosclerosis, or heart disease in general.

As to the effect of physical activity on body composition and the aging of the organism it has been pointed out that long-term physical activity has a positive effect on body composition and the aging of the organism. In adolescence, obesity is frequently accompanied by marked delay in puberty, and exercise exerts a remedial influence upon developmental retardation (Wells *et al.*, 1962a). Using 14-year-old high school girls in an experiment geared toward studying the effect of physical activity programs on body composition, it was found that the lightest girls gained weight while the heaviest girls lost weight at the end of the training program. The increase of weight was due to increase of active tissue while the loss of weight was due to loss of excess fat (Wells *et al.*, 1962c).

REFERENCES

Anderson, E. C., and Langham, W. H. (1959). *Science* **130**, 713.
Auchincloss, J. H., Jr., Sipple, J., and Gilbert, R. (1963). *J. Appl. Physiol.* **18**, 19.
Balke, B., and Ware, R. W. (1959). *U.S. Armed Forces Med. J.* **10**, 675.
Buskirk, E., Taylor, H. L., and Simonson, E. (1955). *Intern. Z. Angew. Physiol.* **16**, 83.
Christian, J. E., Combs, L. W., and Kessler, W. V. (1964a). *Clin. Nutr.* **36**, 156.
Christian, J. E., Ismail, A. H., and Kessler, W. V. (1964b). *Intern. J. Appl. Radiation Isotopes* **15**, 441.
Cureton, T. K. (1958). "Professional Contributions," pp. 25–40. Am. Acad. Phys. Educ., Washington, D.C.
Cureton, T. K. (1963). *Res. Quart.* **34**, 440.
Cureton, T. K., and Phillips, E. E. (1964). *J. Sports Med.* **4**, 87.
Cureton, T. K., and Sterling, L. F. (1964). *J. Sports Med.* **4**, 1.
Dempsey, J. A. (1964a). *Res. Quart.* **35**, 275.
Dempsey, J. A. (1964b). *Res. Quart.* **35**, 288.
Falls, H. B., Ismail, A. H., MacLeod, D. F., Wiebers, J. E., Christian, J. E., and Kessler, W. V. (1965). *J. Sports Med.* **5**, 185.
Friis-Hansen, B. (1958). *Exita Paediat.* Suppl. 110.
Ismail, A. H., Christian, J. E., and Kessler, W. V. (1963). *Res. Quart.* **34**, 462.
Jalavisto, E., and Makkonen, T. (1963). *Ann. Acad. Sci. Fennicae: Ser. AV. Med.* **100**, 38.
Keys, A., and Brožek, J. (1953). *Physiol. Rev.* **33**, 245.
Kireilis, R. W., and Cureton, T. K. (1947). *Res. Quart.* **18**, 123.
Leedy, H. E., Ismail, A. H., Kessler, W. V., and Christian, J. E. (1965). *Res. Quart.* **36**, 158.
Mickelsen, O. (1959). *Public Health Rept. (U.S.)* **73**, 295.
Moses, C. (1963). "Atherosclerosis." Lea & Febiger, Philadelphia, Pennsylvania.
Pascale, L. R., Frankel, T., Grossman, M. I., Freeman, S., Faller, I. L., and Bond, E. E. (1955). *U.S. Army Med. Nutri. Lab., Denver, Rept.* **156**.
Schifferdecker, G. E., Kessler, W. V., and Christian, J. E. (1964). *J. Pharm. Sci.* **53**, 269.
Seppanen, A., Lindquist, C., and Jalavisto, E. (1963). *Ann. Acad. Sci. Fennicae. Ser. AV. Med.* **104**, 20.
Sills, F. D., and Everett, P. W. (1953). *Res. Quart.* **24**, 223.
Wells, J. B., Parizkova, J., and Jokl, E. (1962a). *J. Assoc. Phys. Mental Rehabil.* **16**, 3.
Wells, J. B., Parizkova, J., and Jokl, E. (1962b). *J. Assoc. Phys. Mental Rehabil.* **16**, 35.
Wells, J. B., Parizkova, J., and Jokl, E. (1962c). *J. Assoc. Phys. Mental Rehabil.* **16**, 69.

PART 3: **RUNNING AND WATER SPORTS**

14

TRAINING FOR COMPETITIVE RUNNING

Fred Wilt

I. Introduction

Competitive racing distances may be generally described as sprints (up to and including 440 yd or 400 m), middle distances (880 yd or 800 m to and including 6 mi or 10,000 m), and long distances (all races beyond 10,000 m, and including the marathon, which is 26 mi 385 yd or 42,195 m). The 440 yd race might be described as an endurance sprint, while the middle distances may properly be divided into short–middle distances (880 yd to 2 mi) and long–middle distances (3 mi to 6 mi). It is important that these distances be clearly identified when selecting the type of training to be used if optimum physical preparation for competition is to be achieved.

II. Training Terminology (Wilt, 1964)

Training, the series of physical activities executed for the purpose of increasing efficiency in running and racing, should be a continuum throughout an athletic lifetime. The specific physical fitness that permits an athlete to run a given distance in a faster time is acquired most efficiently through use of carefully planned training which is tailored to the length and anticipated speed of the racing distance. In order to identify the factors involved in our discussion of training, organize the material presented, and establish precision of meaning for the purpose of this chapter, certain terminology is reviewed hereafter in ultrasimplified form.

Each workout, the physical activities which occur during one session of training, should be preceded by a warmup and followed by a warmdown. The warmup refers to the preliminary exercise used as physical and mental preparation for strenuous exertion which is to follow immediately; the warmdown is simply exercise gradually diminishing in intensity following severe exertion, for the purpose of facilitating return of the circulatory system and bodily functions to the pre-exercise state. The same warmup should be used prior to both training and competition. A useful warmup for all racing distances is 1 mi of continuous running, at a speed of 3 min for the first 440 yd, $2\frac{1}{2}$ min for the second, 2 min for the third, and alternately sprinting 50 yd and jogging 50 yd throughout the final 440 yd. This should be followed by 5 min of calisthenics, after which the athlete is ready to go directly into the training session. The same warmup prior to competition may be followed by 10 min of rest before going directly into the race. The usual warmdown is merely 880 yd to 1 mi of jogging. Jogging refers to running at a speed of 2 to 3 min/ 440 yd, or 8 to 12 min/mi.

Sprinting means running at maximum speed. Cadence in good sprinting is $4\frac{1}{2}$ (occasionally 5) strides per second. It requires about 45 steps to run a 100 yd sprint race. Stride length, indicating the distance covered with one step, varies in length between 7 ft (84 inches) and $8\frac{1}{2}$ ft (102 inches) in sprinting. An athlete's optimum sprinting stride is usually 1.17 times his height, ± 4 inches. By contrast, stride length in middle distance running varies between 5 ft (60 inches) and 6 ft (72 inches). In sprinting, both feet are off the ground about 60% of the time, while in middle-distance running the body is out of contact with the ground about 50% of the time.

Striding is any running speed between jogging and sprinting.

From a training viewpoint, recovery implies restitution, restoration, or return to a relatively normal resting state following exercise.

Stress indicates any condition which places an unusual burden on the organism. It may be regarded as rate of wear and tear, or simply anything of which an individual experiences too much. Stress may be any infectious, painful, adverse, or deleterious force or various abnormal state that tends to disturb the body's normal physiological equilibrium (homeostasis).

Fatigue, by common usage, indicates a sensation of tiredness or a psychic state. It is a condition in which the performance of a certain amount of work meets with increased difficulties and is carried out with a decreasing effect. There is a subjective feeling of locomotor inhibition which eventually leads to complete muscular impotence. Biochemically, it indicates the accumulation of lactic acid in the muscles to the extent of seriously impeding muscular contractility.

Metabolism is the term applied generally to all chemical reactions which occur in living cells. This includes all of the chemical processes by which food is converted into either work or structure. This term is, however, often confined to oxidations which are the ultimate source of biological energy.

Aerobic means "with oxygen." Aerobic metabolism occurs in muscles when there is available an adequate supply of oxygen, and results in the complete utilization of the carbohydrate to produce carbon dioxide and heat. When starting work at a steady rate which can be prolonged over a considerable period of time, there is a 3- to 5-min period of increasing oxygen consumption preceding a steady state of oxygen consumption. This type of submaximal work, wherein oxygen intake tends to meet oxygen requirement, is known as aerobic work.

Anaerobic, the opposite of aerobic, means "without oxygen." With reference to utilization of carbohydrate in the muscle, anaerobic (without oxygen) metabolism may occur when there is an inadequate supply of oxygen. The performance of physical exercise wherein the oxygen cost per minute always exceeds the oxygen intake is known as anaerobic work. During severe exercise, oxygen intake is inadequate to supply the oxygen requirement for production of the energy demanded, and the energy for muscular contraction is derived anaerobically from a complex series of chemical reactions. This liberation of energy in the absence of oxygen is an anaerobic chemical reaction. During the course of this complex reaction, lactic acid ($C_3H_6O_3$) is formed as the end product of anaerobic metabolism of glucose or glycogen. Lactic acid is adverse to muscular economy. Even slight accumulations in the blood often result in muscular pain and contraction of the muscles ceases. Although lactic acid must eventually be oxidized, buffers in the blood (collectively known as the alkaline reserve) can neutralize great quantities of lactic acid during exercise. The accumulation of lactic acid in the muscles and blood is the most common limiting factor of muscular activity, as there is a limit to the amount each individual is willing to tolerate before decreasing his rate of work or ceasing the activity. For a variable period of time after exercise this anaerobically produced accumulation of lactic acid demands oxygen for oxidation. During the post-exercise period, the "oxygen debt" is paid in terms of oxygen intake for oxidation of the lactic acid accumulated during exercise.

Oxygen debt is the difference between the oxygen requirement during exercise and oxygen intake during the performance of the exercise (oxygen requirement minus oxygen intake). It is the amount of oxygen required during the post-exercise recovery period to reverse the anaerobic reactions of the exercise period.

The alkaline reserve is the amount of alkali (bases or buffers) in the blood, primarily sodium bicarbonate, available for neutralizing acids.

Adaptation in a training sense is the advantageous change in function or constitution of tissue, organ, system, or body to meet new conditions.

Speed may be considered the rapidity with which successive movements can be performed. It is largely dependent on inherited ability to contract muscle fibers rapidly and on efficient neuromuscular coordination. In terms of athletic performance, speed involves the coordinated effort of muscles and nerves and the ability of the central nervous system to eliminate all antagonistic braking movements not concerned with the performance of the desired motion. While nothing can be done about the inherited structure of the muscle fiber, speed can nevertheless be improved by continuous high speed repetitions of desired movements until all components form a more rational pattern of overall action and internal muscular viscosity is reduced (Jarver, 1964).

Strength is the capacity to exert muscular force against resistance. It is determined by the size and number of muscles activated, number of muscle fibers involved, muscle group coordination, muscle condition, and lever action involved. Increased strength results from training so as to increase the diameter of the muscle fibers involved (hypertrophy). Increased strength (hypertrophy) results from working the muscle against resistance greater than that to which it is accustomed, or "overloading" the muscle in terms of the demand made upon it. The stimulus for muscular hypertrophy is overload (Morgan and Adamson, 1961).

Power is rate of work, or work per unit of time. It implies a combination of speed and strength to develop fast, explosive movements against resistance. Power suggests the ability to apply maximum force in the shortest length of time. The ability to propel one's own body rapidly over the ground as observed in sprinting requires tremendous power (Morgan and Adamson, 1961).

The overload principle specifies that increases in muscular hypertrophy, strength, and endurance result from an increase in intensity of work performed in a given unit of time. Work may be intensified by raising the cadence as experienced in running faster, or by increasing the resistance against which the muscles contract as experienced in lifting heavier weights. This principle provides the rationale for all progressive resistance exercise programs.

Progressive resistance exercise (progressive loading) specifies that the total work done by muscles in a given time in regular exercise periods must be increased progressively. This may be done either by increasing the resistance which the muscles are required to overcome, or increasing the number of repetitions against the same resistance in work periods of equal duration.

Endurance is the ability to withstand fatigue, or the ability of the body to withstand the stresses set up by a prolonged activity which produces fatigue. The term includes aerobic endurance (general endurance), anaerobic endurance, and muscular endurance (which may be subdivided into aerobic muscular endurance and anaerobic muscular endurance). These types of endurance are closely related within the unity of the human organism. The effectiveness of each to some extent is dependent upon the others, and the development of each type complements the effectiveness of the others. The identification and development of the various types of endurance become important in accordance with the competitive racing distance for which the athlete seeks to prepare himself. In terms of running a given distance in the fastest possible time, it would be most ineffective for the sprinter to concentrate primarily on the development of aerobic endurance, or for the long-distance runner to concentrate mainly on the development of anaerobic endurance.

Aerobic endurance, also known as general endurance or stamina, is the general ability to withstand fatigue of the entire organism in the presence of a sufficient supply of oxygen over a prolonged period. It involves the ability to resist fatigue under conditions where oxygen intake and oxygen requirement for the activity are kept at a steady and equal level. This quality, sometimes called cardiovascular endurance and circulorespiratory endurance, is most evident in work of medium intensity involving the entire organism (Nett, 1965).

Anaerobic endurance is endurance in the absence of oxygen. It is the general ability to withstand fatigue of the entire organism when oxygen is in insufficient supply. In running, this type of endurance is of special importance in the short–middle distance events, and to an appreciable extent in the long–middle distance events. Anaerobic endurance may be termed speed-endurance (Nett, 1965).

Muscular endurance is local endurance which may be either aerobic or anaerobic. Aerobic muscular endurance is the ability of the muscles to withstand fatigue of the locally active muscle groups in the presence of a sufficient oxygen supply. Anaerobic muscular endurance is the ability to withstand fatigue in locally active muscles or muscle groups in the absence of an adequate supply of oxygen. Efficiency of the blood supply in the muscles involved, muscle tissue viscosity, and strength are among the qualities upon which muscular endurance is dependent (Nett, 1965).

A well-trained athlete can absorb approximately 6 liters of oxygen per minute during severe exercise, and can tolerate a total oxygen debt of approximately 15 to 20 liters.

Weight training is simply lifting of weights to develop strength. Numerous repetitions of lifting light weights appears to develop endurance in the muscles involved, while the lifting of progressively heavier weights, necessitating fewer repetitions, develops greater strength. Essential features of weight training for strength development are lifting heavy weights, using a near maximum number of repetitions of which the athlete is capable at the moment, and the gradual increase of the poundage lifted as strength of the athlete increases. Weight training for runners might be opposed on grounds that it could increase body weight. The best advice on this issue is to include heavy weight lifting as part of the runner's training, but discontinue it when and if a significant increase in body weight is noted.

III. Selected Methods of Training

A. Sprint Training

Sprint training involves the repetition of short sprints as a means of preparation for competitive running. Since sprinting means running at absolute maximum speed, there can be no such phenomenon as an "easy sprint." The faster the running speed, the longer the stride. A runner therefore takes his longest stride when sprinting. When starting from a static position, it requires about 6 sec to accelerate to maximum speed. Sprinters should therefore run at least 60 yd on each training sprint, so as to produce the experience of moving at maximum speed. Top sprint speed is about 36 ft/sec. The maximum strength exertion required in sprinting will cause the heart to beat in excess of 200 beats/min. At this rate the heart does not fill maximally during diastole. For this reason, a heart-expansion stimulus does not occur during sprinting. Sprint training therefore does not produce an increased stroke volume of the heart, although it strongly stimulates metabolism in the muscles. Thus sprinters have relatively small hearts, hardly different from the hearts of nonathletes. Because sprinting muscles contract with great speed against high resistance, they become thicker, faster, and stronger. The effect of sprinting as a means of training is the development of speed and muscular strength.

B. Continuous Slow-Running Training

Continuous slow-running training refers to running long distances at relatively slow speeds. The distances covered in this type of training should be related to the racing event. For example, a miler might run 3 to 5 times his racing distance or more. A 3 miler might run 6 to 12 mi, and a 6 miler might run 12 to 18 mi continuously at slow speeds. The heart beats approximately 150 beats/min during this type of training, and the speed depends upon the ability of the athlete (Nett, 1960a). For example, 8 min/mi or 120 sec/440 yd might be sufficiently fast for a relatively inexperienced high school miler, while 6 min/mi or 90 sec/440 yd might be the appropriate speed for an international class 5000 m runner to bring the heart rate to 150 beats/min. This type of training has maximum effect in terms of producing aerobic endurance. It is the superior method of increasing the stroke–volume of the heart, capillarization of the musculature, and facilitation of the circulatory ability of the organism. This training represents the first step in gradually adapting the organism to tolerating the stresses of running and the ability to withstand fatigue. It is not limited to any particular racing distance and forms the basis upon which later to apply faster training more nearly related to the specific racing speed and distance. This type of training should not be timed, and for psychological reasons it is usually done on crosscountry, golf courses, or roads, but may take place on the running track.

C. Continuous Fast-Running Training

Continuous fast-running training differs from slow continuous running in terms of speed. Because the pace is faster, fatigue is encountered sooner. The distances covered are often in excess of racing distance, but not usually so long as those used in slow, continuous running. An 880 yd runner might run $\frac{3}{4}$ mi to $1\frac{1}{2}$ mi, and repeat the distance 1 to 4 times, recovering by alternately walking and jogging 5 min after each run. A 6 miler might run 8 to 10 mi at a steady, fast, continuous pace, or perhaps run 4 to 5 mi on 2 to 3 occasions, alternately walking and jogging for 5 min after each during one workout. Although varying with individual differences, the pace is sufficiently fast to cause the heart to beat well in excess of 150 times/min, perhaps approaching 180 beats/min during the latter stages of the distance covered. This training develops aerobic endurance. It represents a more intense form of effort than slow, continuous running, and seeks gradually to condition the organism to tolerating the stresses encountered in running at faster and faster speeds.

D. Interval Training

Interval training (interval running) is a form of training for competitive running involving a formal pattern of alternately running fast and slow. Briefly, it is fast–slow running. Five variables are found in interval training: the distance of the fast runs, the interval of rest or recovery between fast runs, the number of repetitions of the fast run, the time of the fast run, and the type of activity during the recovery or rest between fast runs. Note that the first four of these variables can be remembered by the code word, D-I-R-T. The fifth variable, activity between fast runs, is usually either walking or jogging. Interval training involves repeatedly running a specific distance at a predetermined speed, resting a specific interval following each fast run, recovering through use of a specific activity (walking or jogging) during the interval between fast runs. This type of training usually takes place on the track, with the fast runs being carefully timed with a stopwatch. However, this need not always be the case, and in areas where winds are high and snow covers the ground a major portion of the winter, carefully clothed athletes can be seen doing interval-training workouts on the roads with the wind at their backs, recovering while returning by jogging to the starting point against the wind, often without the benefit of stopwatch timing. The quality of work is much higher in interval running than in continuous running. Both 10×110 yd in 14 sec, with 110 yds recovery jogging after each, and 10×660 yd in 2:00 min, with 220 yd recovery jogging after each, would be examples of interval training. However, their effects would be entirely different in terms of which develops aerobic endurance and which benefits anaerobic endurance. For this reason, a careful distinction should be made between slow and fast interval training.

1. Slow Interval Training

Slow interval training is thought to develop aerobic endurance. The speed is faster than in continuous fast-running training, thus adapting the athlete to running at a more intense effort. In this type of formal fast–slow running, the heart beats at the rate of approximately 180 beats/min during the "effort" or fast phase. Slow interval training is usually confined to distances up to 880 yd. These include repetitions of 110, 220, 440, and 880 yd. The speed of the effort phase may be empirically determined in the following ways:

(a) Add 4 or more seconds to the athlete's best 110 yd time with a running start. As an example, if the athlete's best 110 yd is 12 sec. his time for repetitions of 110 yd in slow interval training would be $12 + 4 = 16$ sec. For this athlete, 20 to 40×110 yd in 16 to 20 sec, jogging 110 yd in 45 sec after each fast 110 yd, would be a slow interval-training workout. This workout might take the form of 2 to $4 \times (10 \times 110$ yd, jog 110 yd after each fast 110. Walk 2 to 4 min after each series of 10×110.)

(b) Add 6 or more sec to the athlete's best 220 yd with a running start. For example, if the athlete's best 220 yd is 26 sec, his time for repetitions of 220 yd would be $26 + 6 = 32$ sec. For this athlete, 10 to 20×220 yd in 32 to 36 sec, jogging 220 yd in 90 sec after each fast 220 yd, would be a slow interval-training workout.

(c) Ascertain the best average speed an athlete can maintain for 440 yd in the middle-distance race in which he expects to compete, and add 4 or more sec. As an example, a 6 miler whose best mark is 30:00 min will average 75 sec/440 yd. Thus his 440 yd pace for slow interval training might be 75 + 4 = 79 sec (or even slower if he so desires). For this athlete, an example of a slow interval-training workout might be 4 to 5 × (10 × 440 yd in 80 sec each, jogging 110 to 220 yd each. Walk 3 to 5 min after each set of 10 × 440 yd.)

A 9:20 ability 2 miler averages 70 sec per 440 yd. His pace in slow interval training would be 70 + 4 = 74 (or possibly slower) sec per 440 yd. For this athlete, 3 × (10 × 440 yd in 74 sec, jog 220 yd in 90 sec after each. Walk 5 min after each set of 10 × 440) would represent a slow interval-training workout.

A 4:12 ability miler averages 63 sec/440 yd in this race. His 440 yd pace in slow interval training would be 63 + 4 = 67 (or more) sec. For this miler, 3 × (5 × 440 yd in 67 sec, jog 220 yd in 90 sec after each. Walk 5 min after each set of 5 × 440) would represent a slow interval-training workout.

A 1:48 ability half miler would average 54 sec/440 yd. His 440 yd pace in slow interval training would be 54 + 4 = 58 or more sec. For this 880 yd runner, 3 × (3 × 440 yd in 58 to 60 sec, jog 440 yd after each. Walk 5 min after each 3 × 440) would represent a slow interval-training workout.

2. Fast Interval Training

Fast interval training is thought to develop anaerobic endurance or "speed endurance". It is used after a background of aerobic or general endurance has been established. The heart should beat in excess of 180 beats per minute during the "effort" or fast phase in this type of interval training. It develops the ability of the runner to withstand fatigue in the absence of an adequate oxygen supply. Although it has not been proved that fast interval training increases the alkaline reserve, the result is nevertheless an apparent increased ability of the organism to tolerate the acid products of fatigue. As a practical matter, experienced runners have empirically discovered this training develops a "specific" endurance necessary to run a given middle-distance race at a faster pace. Fast interval training is considerably more intense in terms of speed than continuous slow running, continuous fast running, or slow interval training, and therefore results in a more powerful stimulus to muscle metabolism. It is ordinarily confined to repetitions of 110, 220, and 440 yd, although this need not be the case.

The speed during the effort phase of fast interval training may be empirically determined in the following ways:

(a) For 110 yd repetitions, add $1\frac{1}{2}$ to $2\frac{1}{2}$ sec to the athlete's best time for that distance with a running start. If an athlete's best 110 yd is 12 sec, his time for repetitions of this distance in fast interval training would be $12 + 1\frac{1}{2}$ to $2\frac{1}{2} = 13\frac{1}{2}$ to $14\frac{1}{2}$ sec. For this athlete, 2 to 3 × (10 × 110 yd in $13\frac{1}{2}$ to $14\frac{1}{2}$ sec, jog 110 to 220 yd after each. Walk 5 min after each set of 10 × 110 yd) would represent a fast interval-training workout.

(b) For 220 yd repetitions, add 3 to 5 sec to the athlete's best time for that distance using a running start. If an athlete's best 220 yd is 25.0 sec, his time for repetitions of this distance would be 25 + 3 to 5 = 28 to 30 sec. For this athlete, 3 to 5 × (5 × 220 yd in 28 to 30 sec, jog 220 yd after each. Walk 3 to 5 min after each set of 5 × 220 yd) would represent a fast interval-training workout.

(c) For 440 yd repetitions, ascertain the best average speed an athlete can maintain for 440 yd in the middle-distance race in which he expects to compete. Subtract 1 to 4 sec from this figure. If an athlete's best mile time is 4:40 (averaging 70 sec/440 yd), his time for repetitions of 440 yd might be 70 − 1 to 4 = 66 to 69 sec. A 4:00-min miler (averaging 60 sec/440 yd) might subtract 1 to 4 from 60 and run repetitions of 440 yd in 56 to 59 sec during fast interval training. For the 4-min miler, such workouts as 2 × (5 × 440 yd in 58–59 sec, jog 440 yd after each. Walk 5 min after each set of 5 × 440 yd), 3 × (3 × 440 yd in 57 sec, jog 440 yd after each. Walk 5 min after each set of 3 × 440), and 5 × (2 × 440 in 56 sec, jog 440 yd after each. Walk 2 to 4 min after each set of 2 × 440), would be examples of fast interval training.

(d) Because the pace is slower in longer middle-distance races, the length of training repetitions may be extended to cover 880 yd during fast interval training for athletes competing at these distances. In this case, the speed is determined merely by subtracting 4 sec from the average pace the athlete can maintain for 880 yd over the full longer middle-distance event. For example, the 15:00 min 3 miler and 30:00 6 miler will average 2:30 per 880 yd. For these athletes, the pace for repetitions of 880 yd would be 2:30 − 4 = 2:26. A workout of 6 to 12 × 880 yd in 2:26, jog 440 to 880 yd after each, would represent fast interval training for such athletes.

In the case of longer middle-distance runners, it has not been positively established whether more thorough adaptation to running stress results from fast interval-training repetitions of 880 yd, or the use of this and longer training distances performed as repetition running (described hereafter). Short middle-distance performers usually prefer repetitions of 880 yd and longer distances in the form of repetition running.

E. REPETITION RUNNING

Repetition running differs from interval training in terms of the length of the fast run and the degree of recovery following each fast effort. It involves repetitions of comparatively longer distances with relatively complete recovery (usually by walking) after each. Interval training includes repetitions of shorter distances (ordinarily 110 to 440 yd) with less than complete recovery after each by jogging a distance equal to the fast run in a time period 2 to 3 times as long as required to complete the fast run. Repetition running is usually concerned with repetitions of distances such as 880 yd to 2 mi with relatively complete recovery between, during which time the heart rate reduces well below 120 beats/min. Such repetitions at reasonably fast pace in accordance with individual competitive objectives over distances approximating the athlete's competitive event tend to duplicate the duration of stress encountered under racing conditions. The speed in this type of training determines whether a training benefit accrues in terms of aerobic or anaerobic endurance. Repetitions at a pace considerably slower than racing speed tend to develop aerobic endurance. At a pace approaching racing speed, repetition running appears more likely to enhance anaerobic endurance. Repetitions of running beyond racing distance should be significantly slower than racing speed. When repetition running reaches racing speed, the length of the fast runs should not exceed half the competitive distance for which the athlete is training. Because of the higher speed involved, repetition running tends to be more exhausting than continuous slow-running training, continuous fast-running training, and slow interval training.

It would be unwise to specify rigid training times in repetition running due to the role played by individual differences among athletes. However, the following suggestions may serve as a rough guide in terms of speed when using this type of training.

(a) The half-miler may run 2 to 4 × 660 yd at average racing pace plus 2 to 3 sec for the 660 yd or 1 to 3 × $\frac{3}{4}$ mi at average racing pace plus 10 sec/440 yd. Thus a 2:00 min half-miler, averaging 60 sec/440 yd or 1:30 for 660 yd in competition, might run 2 to 4 × 660 yd in 1:32 to 1:33 during one workout. A 1:54 half miler, averaging 57 sec per 440 yd in competition, might run 1 to 3 × $\frac{3}{4}$ mi in 57 + 10 = 67 sec/440 yd or 3:21 each.

(b) A miler may run 2 to 4 × $\frac{3}{4}$ mi in average racing pace plus 3 to 4 sec/440 yd, or 1 to 3 × $1\frac{1}{4}$ mi at average racing pace plus 5 to 6 sec/440 yd. Thus a 4:16 miler, averaging 64 sec/440 yd, might run 2 to 4 × $\frac{3}{4}$ mi in 64 + 3 to 4 = 67 to 68 sec/440 yd, or 3:21 to 3:24. A 4:20 miler, averaging 65 sec/440 yd, might run 1 to 3 × $1\frac{1}{4}$ mi in 65 + 5 to 6 = 70 to 71 sec/440 yd, or 5:50 to 5:55.

(c) A 2 miler might run 4 to 6 × $\frac{3}{4}$ mi, 3 to 4 × 1 mi, 2 to 4 × $1\frac{1}{4}$ mi, or 2 to 3 × $1\frac{1}{2}$ mi at a pace of average racing speed plus 3 sec/440 yd.

(d) A 3 miler might run 5 to 8 × $\frac{3}{4}$ mi, 4 to 6 × 1 mi, or 2 to 4 × $1\frac{1}{2}$ mi at average racing speed plus 3 sec/440 yd. He might also use repetition running workouts such as 2 to 4 × 2 mi at average racing speed plus 5 sec/440 yd.

(e) A 6 miler might run 8 to 10 × $\frac{3}{4}$ mi, 6 to 8 × 1 mi, 5 to 8 × $1\frac{1}{4}$ mi, or 4 to 5 × $1\frac{1}{2}$ mi at average racing speed plus 3 sec/440 yd. He might also use repetition-running workouts such as 3 to 5 × 2 mi, 2 to 3 × 3 mi, or 1 to 2 × 4 or 5 mi at average racing speed plus 5 sec/440 yd.

F. Speed Play

Speed play is a form of training featuring informal fast–slow running, as opposed to the formal fast–slow running found in interval training. It means running at alternate fast–slow pace, preferably (though not necessarily) over natural surfaces such as golf courses, grass, or woods, with a basic emphasis on fast running. Fast and slow interval running, repetition running, sprinting, walking, and continuous fast-running training are informally combined in speed-play training over unmarked surfaces not unlike the crosscountry course. This psychologically stimulating form of training, when properly executed, should develop both aerobic and anaerobic endurance, in addition to muscular hypertrophy. Speed-play training, formerly known as "fartlek" (a Swedish word meaning speed-play) when originally developed in Sweden during the 1930's, has the disadvantage of lack of control by the coach. Unless the athlete is alert, responsible, conscientious, and devoid of laziness, speed-play training is apt to degenerate to nothing more than a long, slow jog in the country, thus depriving the runner of most of the training benefits which accrue when this form of training is properly executed (Wilt, 1959).

The various forms of training previously described may be combined in almost innumerable ways as speed-play training. The following is an example of one speed-play workout which might be used by an experienced miler. The distances and speeds specified are approximate.

(a) Jog 10 min as a warmup

(b) 5 min brisk calisthenics

(c) 1 to 2 × $\frac{3}{4}$ to $1\frac{1}{4}$ mi at a fast, steady pace which might be described as $\frac{3}{4}$ full speed. Walk 5 min after each

(d) 4 to 6 × 150 yd acceleration sprints (jog 50 yd, stride 50 yd, and sprint 50 yd, and walk 50 yd after each)

(e) 4 to 6 × 440 yd at slightly faster than racing effort. Jog 440 yd after each.

(f) Walk 10 min

(g) 2 mi continuous slow run

(h) Walk 5 min

(i) 8 to 12 × 110 yd at $1\frac{1}{2}$ to $2\frac{1}{2}$ sec slower than best effort, jogging 110 yd after each. Walk 5 min

(j) 4 to 6 × 60 yd sprints uphill, and walk back after each

(k) Jog 1 mi as a warmdown

G. Interval Sprinting

Interval sprinting is a method of training whereby an athlete alternately sprints 50 yd and jogs 60 yd for distances up to 3 mi. In this type of training, the athlete sprints 4 × 50 yd/440 yd, jogging 60 yd after each. This training is believed to develop aerobic endurance.

After the first few sprints, fatigue tends to inhibit the athlete from running at his absolute top sprint speed. Similarly, fatigue causes the athlete to slow his recovery jogging to a speed perhaps as slow as walking. For this reason, the training effect of interval sprints is quite unlike that of sheer sprinting followed by adequate recovery (Berben, 1965).

H. Acceleration Sprinting

Acceleration sprinting is the gradual acceleration from jogging to striding, followed by sprinting. For example, an athlete may do repetitions of jog 50 yd, stride 50 yd, and sprint 50 yd, followed by walking 50 yd and repeating. Other examples of acceleration sprints include jog 60, stride 60, sprint 60, and walk 60 yd; and jog 110, stride 110, sprint 110, and walk 110 yd. It is important that the athlete walk for recovery after each acceleration sprint, so as to be sufficiently recovered to run at maximum speed during the next effort. This type of training primarily develops speed and strength. Acceleration sprints are especially valuable when sprinting outdoors in cold weather, since the athlete gradually reaches top speed and thereby avoids the risk of muscle injury which might occur when suddenly reaching top speed in low atmospheric temperatures.

TABLE I

DEVELOPMENT OF TRAINING FACTORS ACCORDING TO TYPES OF TRAINING[a]

Type of training	Speed	Aerobic endurance	Anaerobic endurance
Repetitions of sprints	90	4	6
Continuous slow running	2	93	5
Continuous fast running	2	90	8
Slow interval	10	60	30
Fast interval	30	20	50
Repetition running	10	40	50
Speed play	20	40	40
Interval sprinting	20	70	10
Acceleration sprinting	90	5	5
Hollow sprints	85	5	10

[a] Figures in table are percentages.

I. Hollow Sprints

Hollow sprints are two sprints, joined by a "hollow" period of recovery jogging. Examples include sprint 50, jog 50, sprint 50, and walk 50 yd for recovery prior to the next repetition; sprint 110, jog 110, sprint 110, and walk 110 yd before the next repetition; and sprint 220, jog 220, sprint 220, and walk 220 yd before repeating. If sufficient recovery occurs during the walking following each hollow sprint, this type of training should develop muscular strength and speed.

It seems logical to suspect that each of these types of training has at least some effect upon speed, aerobic endurance, and anaerobic endurance. Nevertheless, it is known that some forms of training accrue a greater training benefit to certain of these factors than others. Table I illustrates the approximate percentage of development of each of these factors which possibly results from various types of training. It is admitted without hesitation that these figures are influenced by the empirical observations of this author, although they are based to some extent upon research results of others (Roskamm *et al.*, 1962).

IV. Recovery during Training

Recommendations for the duration of recovery between fast training runs and the nature of activity during such recovery are made on an empirical basis.

In middle distance training at repetitions of running which cause the heart to beat approximately 180 times per minute, recovery need be no more than walking until the heart slows to two-thirds this rate, or 120 beats per minute (20 beats in 10 sec), before starting the next repetition. When recovery is by walking, runners may check their heart rate after fast repetitions by placing one hand directly over the heart and counting the beat for 10 sec with a stopwatch. Simply multiply the 10-sec count by 6 for the rate per minute (Wilt, 1964).

If recovery is by jogging, the athlete is usually advised to jog a distance equal to that of the preceding fast run in a time period equal to 2 to 3 times the number of seconds required to negotiate the fast run. This, however, is subject to certain refinements, as the speed used during the fast run will influence the duration of recovery jogging.

As an athlete improves in physical condition and ability, recovery jogging during slow interval training may be gradually reduced. For example, superior athletes might jog only 110 yards after slow intervals of 220 and 440 yd, even though athletes of lesser ability might require a full 440 yd jog for recovery.

During fast interval training, the speed of the fast efforts is of sufficient intensity to justify recovery by jogging a distance equal to that of the fast run, and sometimes a longer distance. As an example, a runner using fast repetitions of 110 yd might jog 220 yd for recovery after each.

In both slow and fast interval training, recoveries are intentionally kept incomplete so as to start each repetition with some fatigue products in the blood and muscles. The recovery should be sufficiently long to allow the next repetition to be run at the same speed as the previous effort, but a longer recovery should be avoided if optimum training benefit is to result.

At the present time most superior middle-distance runners recover during interval training by jogging. It is unknown as to whether jogging or walking is preferable or more desirable from a training viewpoint in either slow or fast interval training. One minute of walking usually results in as much or more recovery as two minutes of jogging, on the basis of decrease in heart rate. In jogging, contact is broken with the ground and there is a period of "double float" wherein both feet are off the ground during the course of each step, thus the energy requirement is higher than for recovery walking. Since jogging requires more energy than walking and is therefore more fatiguing, it is generally assumed that jogging has a more beneficial training effect. The physical motions used in jogging have little, if any, more relationship to the movements used in running at racing speed than do the movements used in walking. It might be argued that a greater number of fast repetitions could be run within a given workout during the time saved by walking for recovery, thus producing a more beneficial total training effect.

During fast continuous-running training, repetitions of $\frac{3}{4}$ mi, 1-mi, $1\frac{1}{4}$-mi, etc., may be followed by recovery walking until the heart rate slows to 120 beats per minute.

Walking is recommended for recovery during repetition running. The high speed and longer distances used in this type of training demand that the recovery be more complete than in slow- and fast-interval training. The heart may be permitted to reduce in rate well below 120 beats per minute during recovery walking, so as to permit the next repetition to be run at the desired speed.

As in repetition running, walking is also recommended for recovery between repetitions of sprinting. If recovery is insufficient, then what might be intended for sprinting becomes slower than maximum speed, and the net training effect is quite different from that expected of sprint training, namely the development of sheer speed.

V. TRAINING VOLUME

The total volume of training, exclusive of warmup, warmdown, and recovery walking and jogging, which an athlete may reasonably use in a single workout in an effort to achieve optimum training benefit must be determined with due regard to numerous factors, not the least of which is individual differences. Youths and novices are advised to err on the side of too little rather than too much running in the beginning and early stages of their training. More experienced athletes in reasonable physical condition usually have no need to fear too much running, and indeed one of the problems in the past has been failure to use enough total running volume to achieve best competitive results. A total of 10 to 20 sprints with walk recovery following each is not unreasonable during one workout for the sprinter. Middle-distance runners may cover $1\frac{1}{2}$ to 2 times racing distance during a fast interval-training workout. For example, a miler might run 12 to 16 × 220 yd, jog 220 yd after each, during a fast interval-training workout. The middle-distance runner may cover a total of 2 to 3 times racing distance during the course of a slow interval-training session. For example, a 2 miler might run 16 to 24 × 440 yd during slow interval training. Olympic and world-record caliber

TABLE II

ROLES OF OXYGEN UPTAKE (INVOLVING AEROBIC ENDURANCE) AND
OXYGEN DEBT (INVOLVING ANAEROBIC ENDURANCE) IN SUPPLYING THE
TOTAL OXYGEN REQUIREMENTS FOR RACES OF VARIOUS DISTANCES[a]

Event	Total O_2 requirement (liters)	Liters from oxygen uptake	Liters from oxygen debt
Marathon in	763.0	745.0	18.0
2 hr 15 min		97.5%	2.5%
10,000 m,	178.0	160.0	18.0
29:00.0 min		90%	10%
5000 m	90.0	72.0	18.0
		80%	20%
2 mi,	40.0	22.0	18.0
9:00.0 min		55%	45%
1500 m,	38.0	20.0	18.0
3:40.0 min		52.5%	47.5%
800 m,	27.6	9.6	18.0
1:45.0 min		35%	65%
800 m,	27	9.0	18.0
2:00		33.3%	66.6%
400 m,	22.1	4.1	18.0
45.0 sec		18.5%	81.5%
200 m	20.0	1–2	18–19
		5–10%	90–95%
100 m	8–10	0	8–10
		0%	100%

[a] Nett (1959a, b); Robinson (1956); Nett (1960b).

runners frequently far exceed the above training volumes, but there is always a question as to the point of diminishing returns in excessive training volumes. This question cannot be answered on the basis of present knowledge (Wilt, 1964).

VI. Training Emphasis According to Racing Distances

From Table II it is apparent that after an athlete has undergone a basic conditioning period and acquired a foundation of general endurance which has produced gradual adaptation of the entire organism to the stresses of running, his training during the speeding-up period for competition, and during the actual racing season, might logically receive specific training emphasis in accordance with the speed, aerobic, and anaerobic requirements of his racing distance. It is the opinion of this author that in the case of the

TABLE III

RECOMMENDATIONS FOR TRAINING EMPHASIS
ACCORDING TO RACING DISTANCE

Event	Speed	Aerobic endurance	Anaerobic endurance
Marathon	5[a]	90	5
6 mi	5	80	15
3 mi	10	70	20
2 mi	20	40	40
1 mi	20	25	55
880 yd	30	5	65
440 yd	80	5	15
220 yd	95	3	2
100 yd	95	2	3

[a] Percentage of emphasis.

middle- and long-distance runner, regardless of the aerobic and anaerobic requirements of his race, he should include at least some sprinting during most training sessions. Table III, reflecting the author's personal recommendations, may serve as a rough guide to the percentage of speed, aerobic, and anaerobic training to utilize.

VII. Annual Training Plan

When utilized as a continuum throughout an athletic lifetime, training may be divided on a yearly basis into the basic conditioning period, speeding-up period, racing season, and the season of active rest. These four periods are different in length, do not sharply change from one to another, and should tend to overlap as the training is gradually intensified.

The period of active rest immediately follows the racing season. Rest is only relative during this period. General physical condition is maintained through games and activities such as basketball and swimming. Some running may be done, but the training load should be considerably reduced. The level of physical condition previously achieved should not be permitted to completely deteriorate, thus active rest rather than complete rest is recommended. This period should occupy approximately four weeks.

The basic conditioning period is used to develop aerobic endurance and strength, while gradually adapting the organism to tolerating increasingly more intense efforts of running. This phase may occupy three months, with the fourth month gradually overlapping the first month of the speeding-up period.

During the speeding-up phase, major emphasis is placed upon the development of speed and anaerobic endurance. The first month of this phase overlaps the fourth month of basic conditioning, while the fourth month of speeding-up overlaps the first month of the racing season. The principle of progressive loading is evident here, as the overload principle is used in applying training efforts more intense in terms of speed and greater in terms of total volume (distance) than can be anticipated during actual competition. The repetitions of running are faster than racing speed (though by necessity much shorter than racing distance), and their total when added is far in excess of the actual competitive objective.

The first month of the racing season overlaps the fourth month of the speeding-up period, and may cover approximately 5 months. Training is adjusted to maintain and increase previously developed aerobic and anaerobic endurance and speed, while simultaneously introducing sufficient rest to permit best competitive efforts. Longer recovery periods prior to competition may be recommended, and the total number of workouts per week may be reduced. The more severe workouts are taken a reasonable number of days prior to competition, and in some cases the intensity of training may be curtailed. A certain volume and speed of training, depending upon individual differences, must nevertheless be maintained during racing season as it is well known that insufficient training, even when racing frequently, can result in an athlete losing his previously acquired preparation for fast competitive efforts.

Table IV will serve to illustrate the approximate duration of training phases on a yearly basis.

For specific examples of training programs for sprinting and short, middle, and long distances the reader is referred to Wilt (1959, 1964).

TABLE IV

ANNUAL TRAINING PLAN[a]

Type of training	Months	Training periods
Aerobic endurance	1	Basic conditioning
	2	
	3	
Anaerobic endurance and speed	4	Speeding up
	5	
	6	
	7	
Maintain and increase previously ac-	8	Racing
quired speed and aerobic and	9	
anaerobic endurance. Introduce	10	
sufficient rest to produce best com-	11	
petitive efforts		
Informal general physical activity	12	Active rest

[a] It should be recognized that there is considerable overlap between adjacent segments of the table.

VIII. The Status of Training for Running

Although running is among the oldest of competitive sports, its history in terms of measurement is relatively short. The attempted application of scientific knowledge to training is an even more recent development, and has a parallel not unlike the history of scientific thought.

The ancient practitioners of the pseudoscience of alchemy sought to transform base metals into silver and gold. Thanks to the efforts of research and scientific thought, we now know the futility of this endeavor. This is not to say that alchemy has vanished, as the hope of great wealth through conversion of cheap materials into precious metals did not die gladly. Though they have sunk to the level of the witch doctor, alchemists may exist even today.

In a sense, the training advocated by coaches in the past has resembled the alchemists' search for the philosopher's stone, alias world records. Gradually the application of scientific knowledge has been introduced, and modern coaches now tend to seek a scientific foundation upon which to base their methods. Nevertheless, it is still possible to hear of training methods being advocated with reckless disregard for scientific foundation, promising magical results.

This superficial survey of training for running is much less than all inclusive. The problems of how far, how fast, and how often to run in training for optimum competitive results still remain largely unsolved. Progressive coaches today are by no means comfortable and secure in their knowledge of training. There can be no doubt that considerably more physiological research in a number of directions is urgently needed if the art of training is to be placed on a more scientific basis.

REFERENCES

Berben, D. (1965). *Die Lehre der Leichtathletik.* **40**, 1231.
Jarver, J. (1964). "The How and Why of Physical Conditioning for Sport." Rigby Ltd., Adelaide, Australia.
Morgan, R. E., and Adamson, G. T. (1961). "Circuit Training." Bell, London.
Nett, T. (1959a). *Die Lehre der Leichtathletik.* **46**, 1091.
Nett, T. (1959b). *Die Lehre der Leichtathletik.* **47**, 115.
Nett, T. (1960a). *Die Lehre der Leichtathletik.* **2**, 35.
Nett, T. (1960b). "Der Lauf." Bartels & Wernitz, Berlin.
Nett, T. (1965). *Die Lehre der Leichtathletik.* **34**, 1023.
Robinson, S. (1956). *Intern. Track Field Dig.* p. 219.
Roskamm, H., Reindell, H., and Keul, J. (1962). *Die Lehre der Leichtathletik.* **28**, 659.
Wilt, F. (1959). "How They Train." Track and Field News, Los Altos.
Wilt, F. (1964). "Run, Run, Run." Track and Field News, Los Altos.

15

PHYSIOLOGY OF SWIMMING AND DIVING

John A. Faulkner

I. Surface Swimming

The inaccessibility of aquatic environments, and the difficulty of monitoring most parameters on or under the water, apparently deterred early investigators from undertaking physiological studies of swimmers. However, during the past 40 years improved instrumentation, increased availability of pools and experimental tanks, and field studies in lakes and oceans have provided data on competitive swimming (Åstrand *et al.*, 1963; Karpovich and Pestrecov, 1939; Karpovich and LeMaistre, 1940; Karpovich and Millman, 1944), channel swimming (Pugh and Edholm, 1955; Pugh *et al.*, 1960), underwater swimming (Hong *et al.*, 1963; Scholander, 1962; Scholander *et al.*, 1962; Teruoka, 1932), skin and SCUBA diving (Duffner and Lanphier, 1960), deep sea diving (Miles, 1962), and swimming for survival (Molnar, 1946). Different aspects of the research on swimming have been reviewed by

Cureton (1940), Swegan and Thompson (1959), and Faulkner (1966). Goff (1955) and Lambertsen and Greenbaum (1963) have both edited Symposia on Underwater Physiology.

Although considerable data are now available on limited aspects of aquatics, conflicting results and gaps in knowledge have resulted from the diversity of groups involved in aquatic research. Investigators from different disciplines tend to approach a problem with differences in design, instrumentation, procedures, and controls. Consequently, with the exception of underwater physiology (Goff, 1955; Lambertsen and Greenbaum, 1963), a coherent, well-organized body of knowledge has not been developed.

Throughout this chapter, "swimming" will refer to the four competitive strokes: the front crawl, back crawl, butterfly, and breaststroke. "Diving" may be applied to any method of getting under water. The Conference for National Cooperation in Aquatics (1962) has defined a diver as "under water, bare or in a flexible suit, and thus exposed to increased surrounding pressure." Two types of diving may be designated—breath-hold diving and compressed-air diving. In breath-hold diving, the diver simply holds his breath throughout the period of submersion. All other divers remain submerged longer than a breath-hold period and must be supplied with an appropriate gas mixture. The skin diver is supplied with gas through a hose or "snorkel" and a self-contained underwater breathing apparatus delivers an appropriate mixture to the "SCUBA" diver. Both skin and SCUBA divers are usually "finned" for added mobility. The conventional "booted" diver operates in a flexible suit and rigid helmet into which compressed gas is pumped from the surface.

A. BODY COMPOSITION OF SWIMMERS

Swimmers are taller and heavier, and have less fat than other individuals of the same sex and age (Table I). Using a modified somatotyping technique Cureton (1951) observed that sprint swimmers were relatively higher on mesomorphy and middle-distance swimmers relatively higher on endomorphy. Based on empirical measures of floating position and buoyancy, the distance swimmers floated closer to a horizontal position and had greater buoyancy.

Although there was considerable overlap in the two distributions, middle-distance swimmers tended to have greater subcutaneous fat depots* and lower specific gravity (Bloomfield and Sigerseth, 1965) than did sprint swimmers. The mean specific gravities were 1.0729 for the distance swimmers and 1.0786 for the sprint swimmers. Unfortunately, the data necessary to convert the

* Unpublished data, University of Michigan (this entry applies to all following data referred to by an asterisk).

TABLE I

MEAN BODY BUILD DATA FOR MALE AND FEMALE SWIMMERS COMPARED TO MEANS FOR THE SAME AGE AND SEX

Sample	Age (years)	Height (cm)	Weight (kg)	Skinfolds[a] 4 sites (mm)	Body fat[b] (%)
College men[c]	20	176	72	56	14
(N = 158)[d]	(0.28)[e]	(9.9)	(9.8)	(23.0)	—
College swimmers[c]	20	182	77	31	10
(N = 22)	(0.32)	(5.7)	(7.7)	(11.7)	—
American girls[f]	14	159	53.1	—	—
(N = 170)	(0.50)	(6.3)	(11.4)	—	—
American girl swimmers[c]	14	164	55.1	45	—
(N = 24)	(0.51)	(1.5)	(9.5)	(22.6)	—
Swedish girl swimmers[g]	14	165	54.2	—	—
(N = 30)	(1.3)	(6.5)	(7.2)	—	—

[a] Sites for skinfold measures were triceps, infrascapular, supra-iliac, and umbilical.
[b] Percent of the body weight fat = 5.783 + (0.153 × sum of 4 fat measures).
[c] Unpublished data, University of Michigan.
[d] N = number of participants in sample.
[e] Numerals in parentheses are standard deviations.
[f] Montoye et al., 1965.
[g] Åstrand et al., 1963.

specific gravity to body density were not presented (for discussion, see Keys and Brožek, 1953).

The lower skinfold measurements yet greater body weight of girl swimmers compared to their age mates is probably due partly to a greater muscular development and partly to a greater body size. There was no significant change in the weight–height ratio (Åstrand et al., 1963).

Pugh and others (1960) somatotyped 12 channel swimmers. Although the majority were found to be extremely high on endomorphy, the winners and runners-up in the channel swims tended to be less fat than the slower swimmers (Pugh et al., 1960).

Data on the body build of underwater swimmers and divers apparently have not been published. The body surface area of "booted" divers in Donald and Davidson's study (1954) ranged from 1.59 to 2.10 m². The subjects were described as "fit" and of "tough" physique, probably indicative of predominantly mesomorphic somatotypes.

B. PHYSIOLOGICAL RESPONSE TO WATER IMMERSION

Swimmers at rest have the low heart rates (Bloomfield and Sigerseth, 1965), large heart size (Åstrand et al., 1963; Deutsch and Kauf, 1927), high total body hemoglobin (Åstrand *et al.*, 1963), and large vital capacities (Åstrand *et al.*, 1963; Bloomfield and Sigerseth, 1965; Carey *et al.*, 1956; Newman *et al.*, 1961) of highly trained endurance athletes. Compared to most other activities the physiological response to swimming is complicated by the physiological response to immersion, to a horizontal body position, to restricted ventilation, and to predominantly arm work.

1. Heart Rate Response

The heart rate is normally reduced on immersion in water of swimming pool temperature (18° to 30°C) (Wells, 1932; Tuttle and Coreleaux, 1935; Tuttle and Templin, 1942). The decrease in heart rate varies directly with the resting heart rate (Table II). Variability in the response to immersion is attributed to psychological and physiological adjustments. An increased heart rate may result from fear of immersion. When emotional factors were controlled, a failure to respond normally has been credited to a "sensitivity to water" (Tuttle and Templin, 1942) or a "hypersensitivity to cold" (Horton and Gabrielson, 1940).

Immersion in warm water (35° to 37°C) resulted in a rise of heart rate (Keatinge and Evans, 1961) and in extensive vasodilatation (Herrington, 1949). Keatinge and Evans (1961) observed an increase in heart rate, hyperventilation, a fall in end tidal P_{CO_2}, and a constricted peripheral vascular field associated with immersion in cold water (15°C). Between 26° and 38°C, Goff and others (1956a) have concluded that "The heart rate is more directly influenced by average skin temperature than by immersion per se."

Three of seven subjects who had increased heart rates on their initial immersion in 18° to 30°C water displayed a "normal" decrease in heart rate after approximately 6 class hr of swimming instruction (Tuttle and Templin, 1942). In a study by Keatinge and Evans (1961), the initial tachycardia and

TABLE II

RELATION BETWEEN RESTING HEART RATE TO THE DECREASE IN RATE CAUSED BY IMMERSION IN WATER OF SWIMMING POOL[a,b]

Resting heart rate (per min)	Drop due to immersion
70–79	5
80–89	11
90–99	14
100–109	16

[a] From Tuttle and Templin, 1942.
[b] Temperature from 18° to 30°C.

overbreathing observed in 12 subjects on immersion in water of 15°C was reduced or abolished after 8 immersions. The changes were attributed to central nervous system conditioning rather than peripheral factors.

2. Metabolic Response

With the subjects in a supine position on a slatted duck board, immersion in water of 29° to 33°C had little effect on resting oxygen consumption (Goff et al., 1956a). Shivering was encountered in all but one subject after 20 min of immersion in water below 29.5°C. Above 33°C a slight though variable increase in resting oxygen consumption of approximately 1 liter/m²/hr was observed. Submerged at a depth of 3.66 m in an open tank at a water temperature of 21°C, 13 "booted" divers wearing a suit of strong rubberized gabardine had a mean sitting oxygen uptake of 250 ml/min and a standing uptake of 270 ml/min compared to 240 ml/min under basal conditions (Donald and Davidson, 1954). Seven men had sitting uptakes less than basal. The remarkably low sitting and standing uptakes were attributed to the neutral buoyancy.

3. Respiratory Response

Ventilation seldom limits maximum performance at sea level on land (Riley, 1954). In swimming and in diving, ventilation often becomes inadequate, particularly for untrained swimmers, even at modest work loads. Increased water pressure may impair respiration by restricting the airways, increasing the resistance in the breathing apparatus, or increasing the density of the breathing mixture. Although the work rate must be reduced at depth, the artificial atmosphere may be modified to provide the maximum performance capacity and comfort possible.

Many investigators have commented on the large vital capacities of swimmers. For male swimmers, Bloomfield and Sigerseth (1965) report a mean vital capacity of 5.32 liters, Magel and Faulkner (1967) 6.08 liters, Newman et al. (1961) 5.90 liters, and Cureton (1951) 6.28 liters. For female swimmers, Åstrand et al. (1963) report 4.00 liters and Newman et al. (1961) 4.55 liters. The values range from 6 to 13% over predicted vital capacity for age, height, and sex (Kory et al., 1961; Åstrand et al., 1963). The one-second forced expiratory volume of swimmers (Newman et al., 1961; Åstrand et al., 1963) is greater than that of normals and 8–15% over predicted values.

Immersion to the neck in water reduces the vital capacity approximately 9% and is equivalent to negative pressure breathing of −20.5 cm H_2O (Agostoni et al., 1966). During immersion, the hydrostatic pressure impedes the respiratory muscles and displaces blood into the thorax. The counteraction of the force of the respiratory muscles accounts for 6% of the reduction and the shift of blood into the thorax accounts for 3%.

In swimming, the vital capacity is reduced by both the horizontal body position and the hydrostatic pressure. The average water pressure on the chest is greatest in the breaststroke and least in the backstroke. Karpovich (1933) estimates a depth of from 12 to 22 cm in the front crawl. The excess energy required for respiration in swimming is 1.3 to 2.8 ml of oxygen for each liter of gas inhaled (Karpovich, 1939).

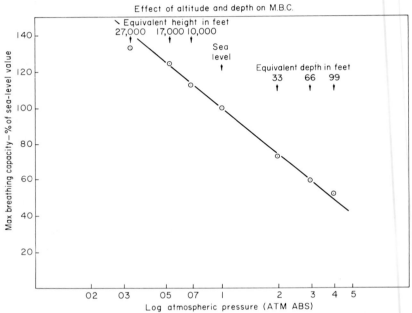

Fig. 1. The effect of altitude and depth on maximum breathing capacity. From Miles (1962).

Vital capacity decreases rapidly with increasing depth and very little air can be inspired through an open system at atmospheric pressure below a depth of 50 cm. The effective depth for a snorkel tube is much less. Since few snorkel tubes include a valve system to void expired gas, the amount of respiratory dead space is increased considerably. The dead space is a function of the total volume of the snorkel. The critical factor in resistance is the radius. The resistance is proportional to the length of the tube and inversely proportional to the fourth power of the radius.

Increases in maximum breathing capacity have been noted at high altitudes. Miles (1957) extended the series to increased barometric pressures. At 2, 3, and 4 atm the maximum breathing capacity was decreased to 72, 60, and 51% of the sea level value (Fig. 1). With other parameters constant, the maximum breathing capacity may be taken as inversely proportional to the square root of the density (MBC $\propto 1/D$).

The resistance to breathing is a function of the rate of flow, the diameter and length of the tubes, and the viscosity and density of the gas. The resistance is roughly proportional to the square root of the density (Miles, 1962). A 58% increase in flow resistance occurs with immersion to the neck. The increase has been attributed to the decreased lung volume by Agostoni *et al.* (1966).

Flow rates during respiration follow a sine curve (Miles, 1962). At a pulmonary ventilation of 30 liters/min the peak flow in inspiration and expiration is about 100 liters/min. Peak inspiratory and expiratory flow rates exceed 300 liters/min in maximum exercise. The peaks become flattened when respiratory resistance is increased. Peak flows rather than minute ventilation must be considered in developing specifications for mouthpieces, tubes, demand valves, and carbon dioxide-absorbing canisters.

The Korean diving women (amas), who undergo respiratory stress day after day in gathering food from the ocean floor, have vital capacities 25% higher than predicted (Song *et al.*, 1963). The increase is due entirely to a greater inspiratory capacity (Song *et al.*, 1963). Similarly, 16 instructors at an Escape Training Tank had a mean vital capacity of 5.68 liters (Carey *et al.*, 1956) which was 15% over the value predicted from body surface area. The tank instructors were engaged in daily underwater dives to and "free ascents" from 32-m depths. Significant increases observed after training (Carey *et al.*, 1956) suggest the large vital capacities were developed through aquatics rather than that large inherited vital capacities predispose persons to participation in aquatics.

C. Water Resistance and Propulsion

The propulsive force of swimmers is not known except during tethered swimming. Water resistance may be determined by towing (Karpovich, 1933; Karpovich and Pestrecov, 1939). Since, at constant velocity, propulsive force equals water resistance, the work done swimming may be calculated.

Investigations of ship models indicate that total water resistance is the summation of skin friction, eddy resistance, and wave-making resistance (Karpovich, 1933). The water resistance of human bodies has been determined for swimmers in the prone and supine position (Karpovich, 1933; Karpovich and Pestrecov, 1939) and for SCUBA divers (Goff *et al.*, 1957).

The great drag of the SCUBA diver is due to the bulky breathing apparatus and resultant change in body attitude (Fig. 2). Based on the exponential relationship between water resistance and velocity ($r = kv^2$), Karpovich (1933) determined the constants for the front and back crawl (Table III).

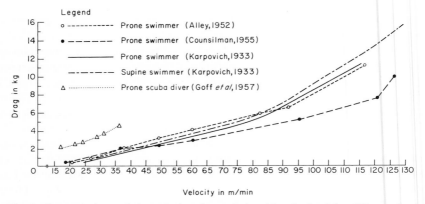

Fig. 2. A comparison of the velocity–drag relationship obtained by different investigators.

Alley (1952) and Counsilman (1955) measured resistance at different swimming velocities through the development of an instrument that released a tethered swimmer at a given speed and simultaneously measured the force he was exerting on the restraining device. The summation of the force exerted on the restraining device and the force equal to the water resistance at the velocity the swimmer was being let out by the restraining device was termed effective propulsive force (Alley, 1952). Theoretical estimates may also be made based on the principles of fluid mechanics (Karpovich and Pestrecov, 1939). The extrapolation of both types of data to a self-propelled human body moving through the water with intermittent accelerations and decelerations due to stroke mechanics appear hazardous. The greatest effective propulsive force, approximately 14 kg in the front crawl, is exerted at zero velocity (Alley, 1952; Counsilman, 1955).

TABLE III

CONSTANTS FOR THE ESTIMATION OF WATER RESISTANCE IN SWIMMING CRAWL AND BACK STROKE[a]

Sample	Skin surface area (m²)	Constant (k)[b] Prone glide	Back glide
Men	2.23–1.77	3.17	3.66
Men and women	1.77–1.53	2.68	2.93

[a] Data from Karpovich (1933).
[b] The constant k is kg-sec²/m².

Effective propulsive force declines steadily with increasing swimming velocity up to 48 m/min when it is about 75% of maximum. The reduced speed of the arms relative to the water and increased water turbulence are possible explanations. Water resistance is reduced by a hydroplaning action between 36 and 90 m/min and increased by the development of a bow wave at 120 m/min (Fig. 2).

Various data on water resistance are compared in Fig. 2. Counsilman's data are considerably lower than those of Karpovich (1933) and Alley (1952). Counsilman's data are likely the most valid due to his superior instrumentation and his use of Alley's procedure for releasing the swimmer.

Estimates of the force or work in swimming may be determined by Eqs. (1)–(3):

$$f = kv^2 \tag{1}$$

$$w = fs = rs \tag{2}$$

$$w = kv^2s = k\,(s/t)^2s \tag{3}$$

where

w = work in kgm; f = force in kg; r = resistance in kg; s = distance in meters; t = time in seconds; v = velocity in meters/second; k = constant (see Table III)

The use of the formulas requires the assumption that the swimmer maintains constant velocity with no starts, no turns, and no changes in hydroplaning, bow wave, water turbulence, or propulsive force. Although such assumptions can never be made, these formulas appear to provide reasonably

TABLE IV

MEAN PROPELLING FORCE (IN KG) DURING 20-SEC AND 60-SEC SWIMS[a]

Stroke	Sample[b]	20 Sec	60 Sec	Time (100-m race)
Front crawl	Males ($N = 2$)	14.4	10.6	0:58.0
	Females ($N = 2$)	10.6	8.8	1:03.6
Back crawl	Males ($N = 2$)	14.0	10.8	1:06.0
	Females ($N = 2$)	9.8	8.7	1:11.4
Butterfly stroke	Males ($N = 1$)	13.1	9.9	1:03.2
	Females ($N = 2$)	6.4	5.8	1:10.6
Breaststroke	Males ($N = 2$)	22.3	17.0	1:15.2
	Females ($N = 2$)	14.4	10.8	1:21.8

[a] From Mosterd and Jongbloed, 1964.
[b] N = number of participants in sample.

accurate estimates of force exerted and work done through the usual range of swimming velocities.

The propelling force at zero velocity has been assessed by swimmers pulling (Karpovich and Pestrecov, 1939; Mosterd and Jongbloed, 1964) or pushing (Cureton, 1930) on a measuring device. Mosterd and Jongbloed (1964) have made a comprehensive analysis of the 4 competitive strokes. The swimmer was attached by a harness and nonstretchable nylon cord to a dynamometer. Each stroke had a characteristic kymograph tracing due to the accelerations, decelerations, and magnitude of the forces exerted during the arm stroke and the kick. Within strokes, individual differences were observable in timing and stroke mechanics. Although the breaststroke has the slowest maximum velocity of all the strokes during free swimming, breaststroke swimmers exerted the greatest force at zero velocity (Table IV).

D. ENERGY EXPENDITURE IN SWIMMING

Most energy expenditure data are based on the physical activities of clothed humans in air (Passmore and Durnin, 1955). In addition to the reduction in heart rate due to immersion in water of swimming pool temperature, swimmers perform primarily arm work, in a prone or supine position, in a medium favorable to heat exchange, with much of their body weight supported by the water.

The unique aspects of training habitat, posture, and stroke mechanics of swimmers require that evaluation of oxygen uptake and physical work capacity be made during swimming (Faulkner, 1966) rather than during the traditional laboratory activities of bicycling or running (Åstrand et al., 1963; Rowell et al., 1964). Maximum oxygen uptake in swimming has been reported as 15% less than that obtained during running, cycling, or skiing (Åstrand et al., 1963; Åstrand and Saltin, 1961). Unfortunately, neither the stroke, the swimming velocity, nor the number of strokes per minute were indicated.

The determination of the maximum oxygen uptake of a subject requires that the test involve a large muscle mass and that the muscles have sufficient endurance to continue contractions until the circulatory system becomes the limiting factor. Swimming and running may each fulfill these criteria. Subjects untrained in a specific task reach local muscle fatigue before a maximum oxygen uptake is attained. Three laboratory technicians had a mean maximum oxygen uptake of 3.66 liters/min during treadmill running compared to 2.92 liters/min during tethered swimming—a 20% reduction.* Magel and Faulkner (1967) have found that trained college swimmers attain about the same maximum oxygen uptake swimming ($\bar{x} = 4.14$ liters/min) as they do running ($\bar{x} = 4.20$ liters/min). However, among a total population far greater variability in performance and energy expenditure is evidenced in swimming than in the more routine activities of running or bicycling. It is doubtful that other than highly trained swimmers can approximate their maximum oxygen uptakes swimming.

The mean and range for maximum oxygen uptake in liters/min is about the same for well-trained college swimmers and well-trained college runners (Table V). The swimmers, however, average 12 kg heavier than the runners.

TABLE V

THE MAXIMUM OXYGEN UPTAKE OF HIGHLY TRAINED COLLEGE RUNNERS AND SWIMMERS[a]

Sample[b]	Weight (kg)	$\dot{V}_{O_2}$ max (liters/min)	$\dot{V}_{O_2}$ max (ml/kg/min)
Distance runners	67.2	4.453	66.2
(N = 6)	(5.57)[c]	(0.52)	(0.52)
Middle distance swimmers	79.7	4.411	55.5
(N = 11)	(7.02)	(0.42)	(0.43)

[a] The maximum oxygen uptakes of the runners were determined during treadmill running at 14 mph and those of the swimmers during all-out 50 yd swims with 10-sec rest intervals.

[b] N = number of participants.

[c] Numerals in parentheses are standard deviations.

Consequently, when maximum oxygen uptake is represented as ml/kg/min male college swimmers average 55 ml/kg/min compared to 66 ml/kg/min for male college distance runners. Unlike running, the body weight is not supported by the swimmer and the energy expenditure swimming is not proportional to body weight. Since water resistance is only grossly related to body surface area (Karpovich, 1933) and buoyancy is an ameliorating factor, the expression of oxygen uptake in ml/kg/min does not appear an appropriate concept in aquatics. The greater body weight is not a serious handicap and a modest percentage of body weight in fat may even be an advantage. World-class distance swimmers (1500 m) approximate 12 to 13% of their body weight as fat compared to 6 to 7% for distance runners.

A variety of procedures have been used to determine the energy expenditure of swimming. Karpovich and Millman (1944) had the swimmers hold their breath during 50 yd swims. The expired gas of the swimmers was collected for 20 to 40 min after the completion of the swim. The energy cost of the swim was assumed to be equivalent to the raised metabolism. Energy expenditure has been measured during tethered swimming (Van Huss and Cureton, 1955; Magel and Faulkner, 1967) and during free swimming (Andersen, 1960; Åstrand et al., 1963; Pugh et al., 1960; Magel and Faulkner,

1967). However, the energy expenditure data are not complete for a reasonable range of swimming velocities in each of the four strokes.

The oxygen uptakes obtained during swimming (Andersen, 1960; Pugh *et al.*, 1960) appear to be a more linear function of swimming velocity than those estimated from recovery data (Karpovich and Millman, 1944). Metabolism may be raised for many hours after strenuous exertion (Margaria,

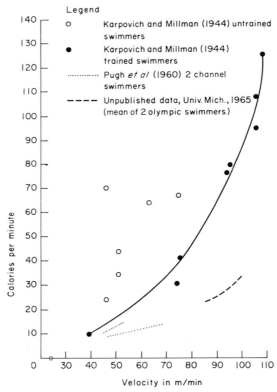

Fig. 3. A comparison of data on the caloric cost of swimming the front crawl stroke at different velocities.

1963). Since the collection period necessary to measure "true" oxygen debt has not been resolved any collection period is arbitrary. The discrepancy between the curvilinear oxygen uptake–swimming velocity relationship reported by Karpovich and Millman (1944), as opposed to the more linear relationship reported by Andersen (1960), Pugh and others (1960), and unpublished data from the University of Michigan,* is apparently due to the method used to estimate the energy expenditure of the swimmer (Fig. 3).

The strokes in order of increasing energy cost are front crawl, back crawl, breaststroke, and side stroke (Karpovich and Millman, 1944). This order is consistent for any given velocity between 37 m/min and maximum. The energy cost of the butterfly stroke relative to the other strokes varies greatly. For a given velocity, it requires the greatest energy expenditure below 54 m/min and above this velocity it requires less energy expenditure than the side or the breaststroke. Although the energy cost is less, swimmers tire quickly in the butterfly stroke because of local fatigue in the muscles of the shoulder girdle.

The individual variance in the energy cost of running is minimal and reasonable prediction of a runner's time for a distance event may be made from his maximum oxygen uptake (Balke, 1963). Among individuals the energy cost of swimming is widely variable as skilled swimmers perform at any specified velocity with a much lower energy cost than do less skilled swimmers (Fig. 3). Consequently, the maximum oxygen uptake of a swimmer provides little insight into his swimming ability.

E. SWIMMING EFFICIENCY

Efficiency is clearly defined in physics as the ratio of work input to work output converted to a percentage. In swimming, the term is much less precise, although it is quite feasible to compare relative efficiencies of different individuals swimming the same stroke or of individuals swimming different strokes. However, any attempt to precisely estimate the absolute efficiency of swimming appears hazardous (see comments on water resistance, Section I, C).

A rough estimate of efficiency of swimming may be calculated from Eq. (4):

$$\% \text{ efficiency} = kv^2s(0.0004686)100/O_2 \text{ uptake (liters)} \qquad (4)$$

where

k = constant (Table III); v = velocity in meters/second
s = distance in meters; 0.0004686 liters oxygen = 1 kgm

Note: s and O_2 uptake must be for the same time period.

Karpovich and Pestrecov (1939) found swimming efficiency varied from 0.5 to 2.2%, and in a more recent study from 1.71 to 3.99% (Karpovich et al., 1966). The average efficiency for eight channel swimmers tested by Pugh and others (1960) was 2.8%. The fastest male and female swimmers had efficiencies of 7.8% and 4.6%, respectively. The efficiency of man swimming appears very low compared to his efficiency of 25 to 30% running (Robinson, 1961). However, efficiencies in arm ergometry are approximately 6%[*] and the efficiency of motor boats is of about the same magnitude (Karpovich, 1933).

Karpovich *et al.* (1966) have compared the efficiencies of the leg kick, arm stroke, and whole stroke of the front crawl. The efficiency was highest for the arms alone, 0.56 to 6.92%, and lowest for the legs alone, 0.05 to 1.23%. These data support the present tendency of distance swimmers to emphasize the arm pull and de-emphasize the leg kick.

The biomechanics of swimming remain a relatively untouched field of research. The extreme differences in efficiency even among highly trained swimmers indicate the complexity of swimming skills. Although body form, buoyancy, body position, and the size and flexibility of the "paddles" contribute or detract from the economy of the stroke, world-class swimmers are of a variety of shapes and sizes. Stroke efficiency appears to depend on the development of optimum stroke mechanics for a particular set of physical characteristics.

F. RESPIRATION DURING SWIMMING

In most activities man simply breathes as needed. The coordination of inspiration and expiration with stroke mechanics is a necessity in prone swimming. Breathing in swimming is further complicated by the extra work required in inspiration (Karpovich, 1939).

Pulmonary ventilation and the number of strokes per minute are reasonably linear functions of swimming velocity (Pugh *et al.*, 1960), although considerable individual variation is found in the intercept and slope of the relationship. Tidal volumes are from 2 to 3 liters throughout a range of from 42 to 73 strokes per minute (Pugh *et al.*, 1960). Maximum pulmonary ventilations vary from an average of 109 liters/min (BTPS) for freestyle, breaststroke, and butterfly swimmers to 159 liters/min (BTPS) for backstroke swimmers. Backstrokers have a frequency of 64 breaths per minute with approximately two respirations per complete stroke cycle whereas other swimmers have a frequency of 38 breaths per minute with a maximum of one respiration per stroke cycle (Magel and Faulkner, 1967).

The number of liters of gas breathed for each liter of oxygen taken up (ventilation equivalent) were 26.2 for 8 front-crawl swimmers, 31.8 for 4 backstroke swimmers, and 30.1 for 6 runners.* All 18 subjects were of college age (18–22 years) and of intercollegiate caliber. Swimmers performing strokes other than backstroke display a relative hypoventilation of the alveoli (Rossier *et al.*, 1960). Pulmonary ventilations for a given oxygen uptake were routinely 30% less swimming front crawl than running or swimming backstroke (Magel and Faulkner, 1967). When ventilation is restricted, the oxygen uptake is maintained by a high oxygen extraction. Since the relationship between the energy cost of breathing and pulmonary ventilation is exponential rather than linear (Riley, 1954), alveolar hypoventilation reduces the energy cost of breathing at a given oxygen uptake.

G. Heart Rate during and after Swimming

Heart rates swimming have been recorded by direct leads (Irving, 1963). However, most of the heart rate data on swimming are based on heart rates palpated at the carotid or radial artery immediately after swimming (Faulkner and Dawson, 1966; Gavreesky, 1963) or from electrocardiograms after the swimmer leaves the water. A definitive study of heart rates during swims with variations in stroke, distance, and velocity has not been made. The availability of telemetry systems which are adaptable to underwater transmission should soon rectify this lack.

The heart rate taken for 15 sec immediately after swimming 50 m at various speeds is a reasonably linear function of velocity in the front crawl, back

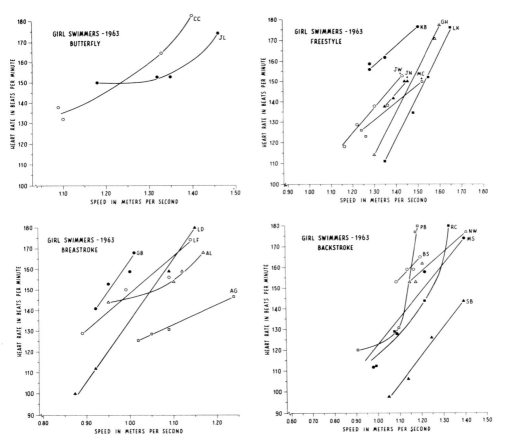

Fig. 4. Velocity–heart rate relationship in the four competitive strokes (from Faulkner and Dawson, 1966).

crawl, and breaststroke (Fig. 4). The relationship is curvilinear in the butter-fly stroke. Skilled swimmers swim at a given velocity with a lower heart rate than unskilled swimmers.

In a maximum effort of comparable time duration, swimmers appear to have maximum heart rates about 10 beats lower than runners.* Clarification of this difference will have to await studies in which the heart rates of comparable samples of swimmers and runners are telemetered during training and competition.

Oxygen transported per unit time from the lungs to the tissues depends on the interaction of oxygen utilization, oxygen capacity, and blood flow. Swimmers have a high oxygen utilization, a high oxygen capacity, and the potential to supply a high blood flow (Åstrand et al., 1963). Controlled longitudinal studies are necessary to clearly delineate the effects of swimming training on the cardiovascular and respiratory systems.

H. THERMAL EXCHANGE

Man maintains thermal balance in air throughout a moderately wide range of environmental temperatures by minimal physiological adjustments (Belding, 1949), whereas immersed in water a water temperature of 33°C is necessary to maintain a normal level of body temperature (Spealman, 1949). Heat production and/or body insulation must be increased to maintain heat balance in water colder than 33°C. The lowest temperature at which thermal balance can be maintained without an increase in heat production (critical temperature) varies from 22°C for fat men to 32°C for thin men (Cannon, 1963). Sufficient heat cannot be produced to maintain thermal balance even at reduced core temperatures in water colder than 15° to 20°C. The rapid heat loss in water is of particular consequence to distance swimmers, divers, and survivors of disasters at sea, who may undergo long periods of immersion.

Two temperature gradients exist in the flow of heat between the deep tissues of the body and the environment (Burton, 1934): the gradient from the interior of the body to the surface, and the gradient from the surface to the surrounding environment. The flow of heat across the internal physiological gradient takes place by the transport of heat by blood flow and by the process of conduction across tissues (Burton, 1934).

The internal temperature gradient is commonly taken as rectal (T_r) minus skin temperature (T_s). In water, skin temperature and water temperature are assumed to be the same (Burton and Bazett, 1936). Heat is conducted so rapidly from the immersed human body that heat loss is primarily limited by tissue conductivity. Tissue conductivity (K) is determined under stable conditions of rectal and skin temperature from Eq. (5):

$$K = [H/(T_r - T_s)] \text{ kcal/m}^2/\text{hr}/°C \tag{5}$$

where

> H = heat production in kcal/m² minus 12% to compensate for heat loss
> in respiration (Pugh and Edholm, 1955)

At rest, tissue conductivity is 9–10 kcal/m²/hr/°C in 33°C water and 2.5 kcal/m²/hr/°C in 7°C water (Carlson *et al.*, 1958). Swimming at an energy expenditure of 10 to 15 kcal/min doubles the resting tissue conductivity (Pugh and Edholm, 1955). Pugh and Edholm attribute the increased conductance to the localization of the extra heat production in the periphery. Tissue insulation (Ki in °C/kcal/m²/hr) is the reciprocal of tissue conductivity. Exposure to cold is quickly followed by constriction of the peripheral vessels and an increased tissue insulation and exposure to heat by vasodilatation and a decreased tissue insulation. Maximum tissue insulation is related to the percentage of body weight that is fat (Fig. 5). In air, the tissue insulation of the

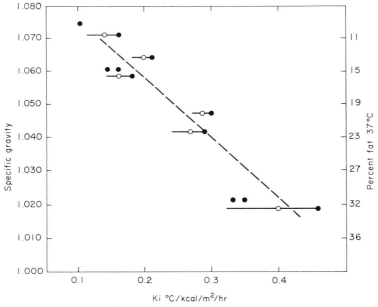

Fig. 5. Maximum values (solid circles) of body insulation found for various subjects in the water bath, average of several determinations (open circles). Lines denote the range between highest and lowest value (from Carlson *et al.*, 1958).

human head remains relatively constant between −21° and 32°C. The result is an increased heat loss from the head with decreasing temperature. Limited experiments on immersion indicate heat loss is greatly increased when the head and neck are immersed (Beckman, 1963).

The rapid loss of body heat in water compared to air results from the greater heat capacity of water and the greater heat conductivity of water. Since the specific heat of water is about 1 cal/cm³/°C compared to 0.000295 cal/cm³/°C for air, a given volume of water can take up approximately 3700 times more heat than a similar volume of air. The thermal conductivity is 53 kcal/m²/hr/cm/°C for water and 2 kcal/m²/hr/cm/°C for air. Therefore, heat is conducted 25 times as rapidly from the skin by water as by air. Man overheats at rest in water above 35.5°C and exercising strenuously in water above 30°C (Cooperative Underwater Swimmer Project, 1952). Competitive swimming except in water over 25°C presents the opposite thermal stress to that of running. Craig (1963a) has observed that swimmers can maintain 75% of maximum velocity for 4 min and 65% for 1 hr, compared to 68% and

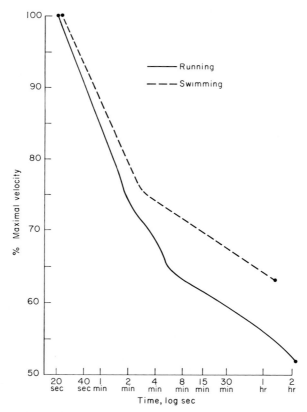

Fig. 6. Comparison of running and swimming velocity–duration curve based on the assumption that in each sport the maximal rates of energy expenditure are equal at the short distance (from Craig, 1965a).

subjectively the experience resembles alcoholic intoxication. Some impairment of skilled performance is encountered below 100 ft. An increased tolerance to nitrogen narcosis is developed through frequent deep diving (Miles, 1962). Even so, the United States Navy limits air diving to less than 300 ft. For deeper diving helium–oxygen mixtures are used.

B. OXYGEN PRESSURES

Chronic oxygen poisoning is not a serious hazard for divers breathing air since few deep dives are of sufficient duration for this condition to develop. A more common danger is acute oxygen poisoning, particularly for divers using closed-circuit oxygen-rebreathing apparatus in which extremely high partial pressures of oxygen may be encountered (Table VII). Acute oxygen

TABLE VII

A COMPARISON OF THE PARTIAL PRESSURE OF 100%
OXYGEN AND OXYGEN IN AIR (21%) AT SELECTED
PRESSURES

Equivalent depth in water (m)	Partial pressure of O_2 (mm Hg)	
	Air	100% O_2
0	160	760
10	320	1520
20	480	2280
30	640	3040
40	800	3800

poisoning culminates in a seizure of approximately 2 min duration similar to grand-mal epilepsy or electroshock therapy (Miles, 1962). The convulsions are sometimes preceded by symptoms of lip twitching, dizziness, nausea, choking sensation, dyspnea, and tremor. Symptoms disappear and the seizure is not repeated if the diver returns to air breathing. The danger for the self-contained diver is drowning due to the loss of his mouthpiece during a seizure in open water. Donald (1947) experimentally investigated over 2000 exposures to oxygen poisoning. Thirty-six men used breathing apparatus which gave 95% oxygen during exposures in a dry pressure chamber at 3.7 atm and in a wet pressure chamber at simulated depths of from 8 to 33 m. The exposure was terminated on the development of symptoms of oxygen poisoning or on the development of a seizure. Six percent suffered convulsions without any preceding symptoms. Extreme variation in tolerance was observed between individuals and in the same individual from day to day.

Symptoms occurred sooner (1) in the wet than in the dry chamber, (2) as oxygen pressure was increased, and (3) during work than during rest. Based on these data, a working dive on oxygen should not exceed 8 m (Table VII). For sport diving pure oxygen breathing equipment might well be abandoned altogether (Miles, 1962).

Based on the time–pressure relationship, two distinct mechanisms appear to be involved in oxygen poisoning (Miles, 1962). A high partial pressure of short duration produces acute effects on the central nervous system which are reversible. A smaller excess pressure over a considerable time period produces lung tissue damage which is not immediately reversible.

Oxygen is carried in both physical solution and combined with hemoglobin. The milliliters of oxygen dissolved in 100 ml of blood may be determined by: (O_2 dissolved) = ($a\ P_{O_2}/760$) × 100. The solubility constant a for oxygen in blood is 0.023 ml/ml of blood/atm of oxygen at a temperature of 38°C (Davenport, 1958). The amount of dissolved oxygen while breathing air is: (0.023 × 102/760) × 100 = 0.31 ml/100 ml; while breathing 100% oxygen at 760 mm Hg pressure (0.023 × 673/760) × 100 = 2.02 ml/100 ml; and while breathing 100% oxygen at 1520 mm Hg pressure (0.023 × 1520/760) × 100 = 4.34 ml/100 ml.

Breathing air, the oxygen tension of 102 mm Hg for hemoglobin assumes a 97.5% saturation. The hemoglobin becomes 100% saturated while breathing

TABLE VIII

ALVEOLAR, ARTERIAL, AND VENOUS OXYGEN TENSION, BREATHING AIR AND BREATHING 100% OXYGEN AT 760 MM HG PRESSURE

	Gas breathed		
	Air (760 mm Hg)	100% O_2 (760 mm Hg)	100% O_2 (1520 mm Hg)
O_2 tension air (mm Hg)	159	760	1520
O_2 tension alveoli (mm Hg)	102	673	1433
O_2 tension plasma (mm Hg)	102	673	1433
Hemoglobin saturation (%)	97.5	100	150
O_2 in solution (ml/100 ml blood)	0.31	2.02	4.34
O_2 hemoglobin (ml/100 ml blood)[a]	19.50	20.00	20.00
Total arterial oxygen (ml/100 ml blood)	19.81	22.01	24.34
Oxygen utilized (ml/100 ml blood)	5.00	5.00	5.00
Total venous oxygen (ml/100 ml blood)	14.81	17.01	19.34
Hemoglobin saturation (%)	75	85	95
O_2 tension venous (mm Hg)	40	60	90

[a]A hemoglobin of 15 gm/100 ml blood was assumed.

100% oxygen. Breathing pure oxygen at 760 mm Hg pressure; (1) increases the total oxygen carried in the blood by 11%; (2) "washes out" nitrogen quickly from the alveoli and gradually from the tissues and body cavities; and (3) impairs the transport of carbon dioxide from the tissues to the lungs because of a 50% increase in venous oxygen tension (for discussion, see Comroe and Dripps, 1950). At a pressure of 2 atm or a water depth of 10 m (Table VII), resting metabolism is almost supported by the oxygen dissolved in the plasma (Table VIII).

The physiological mechanism of oxygen poisoning has not been resolved. Physiological changes associated with exposure to high pressure oxygen include: (1) bradycardia; (2) a steady rise in tissue carbon dioxide; (3) stimulation of the respiratory center and an increased ventilation; (4) a 50% decrease in cerebral blood flow due to vasoconstriction; (5) an increased sensitivity of the respiratory center; (6) reflex stimulation of the respiratory center from pulmonary irritation; and (7) hypertrophy of the adrenal cortex (for discussion, see Miles, 1962).

C. Decompression Sickness

At sea level the nitrogen contained in the lungs, blood, and tissues is in equilibrium. At a partial pressure of 600 mm Hg, 1 ml of nitrogen dissolves in each 100 ml of blood and aqueous tissue, and 5 ml per 100 ml of fat (Miles, 1962). During descent, the partial pressure of nitrogen (and other gases) in the lungs increases and an increasing volume of nitrogen is dissolved in the blood and diffuses into the tissues until a new equilibrium is reached. During ascent, the excess quantities of gas which escape from the tissues and blood are expelled in expiration. However, bubbles may form in the tissues dependent on: (1) the depth and duration of the dive, and (2) the rapidity of ascent. The condition is termed "the bends" and decompression tables are available for safe ascents based on the interaction of depth and time (U.S. Navy Diving Manual, 1958).

D. Energy Expenditure in Diving

Energy expenditure in skin and SCUBA diving is limited by the restricted limb movements. Even the use of fins does not permit speed in excess of 60 m/min except for very brief periods of time. Oxygen uptakes of 1.3 to 1.9 liters/min have been reported for SCUBA divers swimming at a cruising speed of 18 to 24 m/min (Goff et al., 1957; Lanphier, 1954). Donald and Davidson (1954) recorded a maximum of 4.1 liters/min and a mean of 3.16 liters/min for a group of four finned underwater divers from the Royal Marine Commandos. The determinations were made during 10-min swims at 45 to 62 m/min. The maximum oxygen uptakes of the men were not available; however, it would appear that they were within 15 to 20% of maximum. The velocity, duration, and oxygen uptake achieved makes this a considerable physical feat even for Marine Commandos.

Seven to nine "booted" divers were studied during minimum and maximum movement at a depth of 7.6 m in tidal water (Donald and Davidson, 1954). Minimum movement required a mean oxygen uptake of from 0.83 to 1.61 liters/min, slightly less than the cost of walking at 2 mph in air. When the maximum distance possible was covered in 15 min, oxygen uptakes ranged from 1.41 to 2.35 liters/min with a mean of 1.96. Donald and Davidson (1954) observed that the powerful drive of the legs was not possible in submerged running because of the greatly reduced effective weight in water. The feet just touch the bottom lightly and fast propulsion is achieved by swimming movements of the arms and hands, often facing backwards. Although the uptakes were equivalent to the energy expenditure of walking at 4 mph in air, the divers were exhausted afterwards.

As the swimming velocity of finned swimmers was increased from 18 to 30 m/min the respiratory rate rose slightly from 14 to 17 breaths/min and the pulmonary ventilation increased from 20 liters/min to 36 liters/min. The ventilation equivalents were 15.4 liters of ventilation per liter of oxygen consumed at 18 m/min velocity and 18.8 at 30 m/min (Goff et al., 1956b).

E. Breath Holding

Underwater swimming is a popular recreational pursuit, a water safety skill, and the occupational task of the amas of Korea and Japan and the Torres Straits Islanders. Compared to an average human who can hold his breath for approximately one minute, trained sponge divers can hold their breath for 2–3 min (Irving, 1939). Generations of practice in breath-hold dives has not increased this capacity. The duration of breath holding is determined by the oxygen stores, the excess carbon dioxide, and neurogenic factors (Klocke and Rahn, 1959).

After a maximum inspiration, a 70-kg man has oxygen stores of 900 ml in the lungs, 1200 ml in the blood, and 250 ml in the tissue fluids for a total of 2350 ml. Three minutes of breath holding at a resting metabolism of 300 ml/min exhausts close to 50% of the oxygen stores which Irving (1939) cites as the maximum lack that man can tolerate. The increased performance capacity of the sponge divers is likely due to increased oxygen stores and an increased tolerance to both oxygen lack and excess carbon dioxide.

Hyperventilation increases voluntary breath holding to 5 or 6 min, and this procedure is commonly used prior to underwater swimming. The case histories of a number of fatal and near-fatal underwater accidents indicate an inherent danger in underwater swimming after hyperventilation (Craig, 1962;

Dumitru and Hamilton, 1964). The survivors reported that they had hyperventilated vigorously on the pool deck, attempted an underwater swim for distance, and lost consciousness with little or no warning.

Hyperventilation, breath holding, and exercise produce hypoxia under physiologically compromising circumstances. The hyperventilation may reduce alveolar P_{CO_2} from 40 to 15 mm Hg and increase alveolar P_{O_2} from 100 to 140 mm Hg (Davenport, 1958). The increased metabolism of swimming rapidly decreases the arterial P_{O_2} and increases the arterial P_{CO_2}. Under these circumstances it is possible to lose consciousness due to a decreased cerebral oxygen tension before the "breaking point" of breath holding is reached (Craig et al., 1962).

Teruoka (1932), Schaefer (1956), DuBois (1955), Hong and others (1963), and Lanphier and Rahn (1963) have observed that changes in ambient pressure during breath-holding dives produce unusual concentrations of oxygen (3.3%) and carbon dioxide (5%). The alveolar partial pressures increase during a breath-holding dive to 10 m, and CO_2 exchange may actually reverse and diffuse from the alveoli into the blood (Hong et al., 1963). The alveolar oxygen tension does not reach pre-dive levels of 120 mm Hg until 45 sec of mild work have transpired at 2 atm (Lanphier and Rahn, 1963). The danger of latent hypoxia occurs on ascent as the lung volume increases. All subjects had negligible oxygen uptakes during ascent, and oxygen may even be transferred from the blood to the alveoli (Lanphier and Rahn, 1963). On surfacing, oxygen tensions were as low as 24 mm Hg, and subjects displayed some confusion and loss of control.

Breathing 100% oxygen increases breath-holding time. The duration of breath holding varied from 3 to 8 min after normal breathing of 100% oxygen and from 6 to 14 min after hyperventilation of 100% oxygen. The range of the alveolar P_{CO_2} at the breaking point was 50 to 90 mm Hg after normal breathing and slightly less after hyperventilation. The correlation between breath-holding time and PA_{CO_2} was 0.89. With a constant oxygen consumption, the lung volume decreased linearly with breath-holding time (Klocke and Rahn, 1959). Three subjects maintained voluntary breath holding until the lung volume was reduced to the residual volume and no measurable amount of gas could be expired.

Impaired consciousness due to high P_{CO_2} tensions have been encountered in breath-holding dives preceded by oxygen breathing (Klocke and Rahn, 1959). A peak P_{CO_2} of 63 mm Hg was attained at 2 atm (Lanphier and Rahn, 1963). "CO_2 narcosis" could occur with greater exertion, deeper dives, more rapid descent, or higher P_{CO_2} prior to submergence. Hyperventilation decreases the possibility of CO_2 excess and increases the risk of hypoxia.

The amas of Korea and Japan collect food from the ocean floor at depths of 5 to 17 m, yet no cases of underwater blackout have been recorded in these groups (Hong *et al.*, 1963). Korean amas make an inhalation of approximately 85% of their vital capacity (in boat) just before submergence. Alveolar P_{CO_2} drops from 37 to 26 mm Hg and alveolar P_{O_2} increases from 102 to 120 mm Hg. This constitutes a relatively mild degree of hyperventilation compared to that possible on a pool deck.

The very limited heart rate data on humans during underwater swimming are rather unusual considering the extensive data telemetered from diving animals (Irving *et al.*, 1941). Scholander (1963) has observed bradycardia during submergence in every diving mammal studied. The extensive vasoconstriction which occurred concomitantly with the bradycardia maintained normal systolic and diastolic blood pressure (Irving *et al.*, 1941).

In man, most investigators have observed a slowing of the heart rate during breath-hold diving (Craig, 1963b; Harding *et al.*, 1965; Irving, 1939). In trained underwater swimmers a marked and persistent bradycardia is usually observed on submergence with the heart rate slowing to less than 50 beats/min. Even the elevated exercise heart rate of surface swimming was slowed from 115 to 36 beats/min during the first 12 sec of underwater swimming (Irving, 1963). The slowing of the heart rate during breath-hold diving has been demonstrated by children as well as adults and by both poor and competent swimmers. Wolf (1964) and Wolf and Groover (1965) have attributed the bradycardia of breath-hold diving to an "oxygen conservation reflex." Rather than a single reflex, it appears that diving bradycardia in man may be attributable to the interaction of a number of known physiological mechanisms. Craig (1963b) has observed that a slowing of the heart rate results from maneuvers that increase the venous return at the beginning of the breath hold and an increased heart rate from those maneuvers that decrease the venous return. Water temperature, intrathoracic pressure, body position, and degree of immersion may all play a role (Craig, 1963b). Down to 27 m, diving depth was not a factor. The mechanism suggested implies an important role for the carotid sinus.

III. Summary

Man is making increasing use of aquatic environments in recreational, commercial, military, and scientific programs. Water is a hazardous medium for man because of the lack of a respirable gas, the high pressure gradient, the rapid heat exchange, and man's reduced work efficiency in water. Over 5000 persons lose their lives annually in the United States in water accidents according to the Metropolitan Life Insurance Company Statistical Bulletin (1966), and Griffin (1966) estimates that an additional 7000 near-drownings occur.

In spite of the hazards, man is making significant progress in his adaptation to an aquatic environment. Competitive swimmers are swimming faster, marathon swimmers are swimming farther, and divers have increased the depth and the duration of their dives. Ambient pressure chambers anchored at depth have enabled man to live for over a month at a depth of 60 m (Medical Tribune, 1966).

Each advance requires a carefully planned interaction of man's physiological capacities, modern science and technology, and the demands of the aquatic task. Unfortunately, most training programs, work tasks, and exposure periods for swimmers and divers are still derived more empirically than scientifically. Largely because of the military and commercial implications the published data are more extensive and better organized in underwater swimming and diving than in competitive or marathon swimming.

Cross-sectional studies have indicated swimmers and/or divers are significantly different from control populations in body build, pulmonary function, cardiovascular function, and aerobic capacity. Swimmers and divers also appear to have performance capabilities different from other highly trained groups. The efficiency of highly trained swimmers and divers while performing tasks in and under the water is of particular significance. Controlled longitudinal investigations before, during, and after extensive training programs in swimming and diving are vitally needed to assess the interaction of hereditary self-selection and environmental adaptability. A scientific approach to aquatics is gradually evolving yet many challenging problems still limit man's performance capacity in the water and his use of the sea.

Acknowledgment

Grateful acknowledgment is given to Albert B. Craig, Josef Smith, and Hugh G. Welch for their critical reading of the manuscript. Most of the unpublished data from the University of Michigan were collected in collaboration with John R. Magel.

REFERENCES

Agostoni, E., Gurtner, G., Torri, G., and Rahn, H. (1966). *J. Appl. Physiol.* **21**, 251.
Alley, L. E. (1952). *Res. Quart.* **23**, 253.
Andersen, K. L. (1960). *Acta Chir. Scand.* Suppl. 253, 169.
Åstrand, P. O., and Saltin, B. (1961). *J. Appl. Physiol.* **16**, 977.
Åstrand, P. O., Eriksson, B. O., Nylander, I., Engstrom, L., Karlberg, P., Saltin, B., and Thoren, C. (1963). *Acta Paediat.* Suppl. 147, 75 pp.
Balke, B. (1963). *Proc. 1st Can. Fitness Seminar, Saskatchewan*, p. 5.
Beckman, E. L. (1963). *Proc. 2nd Underwater Physiol. Symp.* (C. J. Lambertsen and L. J. Greenbaum, eds.) Pub. 1181, p. 247. Natl. Acad. Sci.—Nat. Res. Council, Washington, D.C.
Belding, H. S. (1949). *In* "Physiology of Heat Regulation and the Science of Clothing" (L. H. Newburgh, ed.), p. 351. Saunders, Philadelphia, Pennsylvania.
Bloomfield, J., and Sigerseth, P. (1965). *J. Sports Med. Phys. Fitness* **5**, 76.
Burton, A. C. (1934). *J. Nutr.* **7**, 497.

Burton, A. C., and Bazett, H. C. (1936). *Am. J. Physiol.* **117**, 36.

Cannon, P. (1963). *J. Roy. Naval Med. Serv.* **49**, 88.

Carey, C. R., Schaefer, K. E., and Alvis, H. J. (1956). *J. Appl. Physiol.* **8**, 519.

Carlson, L. D., Hsieh, A. C. L., Fullerton, F., and Elsner, R. (1958). *J. Aviation Med.* **29**, 145.

Comroe, J. H., and Dripps, R. D. (1950). "The Physiological Basis for Oxygen Therapy." Thomas, Springfield, Illinois.

Conference for National Cooperation in Aquatics. (1962). "The New Science of Skin and SCUBA Diving." New York.

Cooperative Underwater Swimmer Project. (1952). National Research Council Committee on Amphibious Operations. Rept. NRC:CAO:0033.

Counsilman, J. E. (1955). *Res. Quart.* **26**, 127.

Cousteau, J. Y. (1966). "World Without Sun." Harper, New York.

Craig, A. B. (1962). *J. Sports Med. Phys. Fitness* **2**, 23.

Craig, A. B. (1963a). *J. Sports Med. Phys. Fitness* **3**, 14.

Craig, A. B. (1963b). *J. Appl. Physiol.* **18**, 854.

Craig, A. B., Halstead, L. S., Schmidt, G. H., and Schnier, B. R. (1962). *J. Appl. Physiol.* **17**, 225.

Cureton, T. K. (1930). *Res. Quart.* **1**, 87.

Cureton, T. K. (1940). *Res. Quart.* **9**, 68.

Cureton, T. K. (1951). "Physical Fitness of Champion Athletes." Univ. of Illinois Press, Urbana, Illinois.

Davenport, H. W. (1958). "The A.B.C. of Acid-Base Chemistry." Univ. of Chicago Press, Chicago, Illinois.

Deutsch, F., and Kauf, E. (1927). "Heart and Athletes." Mosby, St. Louis, Missouri.

Donald, K. W. (1947). *Brit. Med. I.* **I**, 172.

Donald, K. W., and Davidson, W. M. (1954). *J. Appl. Physiol.* **7**, 31.

DuBois, A. B. (1955). *Proc. 1st Underwater Physiol. Symp.* (L. G. Goff, ed.) Pub. 377, p. 90. Natl. Acad. Sci.—Natl. Res. Council, Washington, D.C.

Duffner, G. J., and Lanphier, E. H. (1960). *In* "Science and Medicine of Exercise and Sports" (W. R. Johnson, ed.), p. 348. Harper, New York.

Dumitru, A. P., and Hamilton, F. A. (1964). *Am. Acad. Gen. Practice* **29**, 123.

Faulkner, J. A. (1966). *Res. Quart.* **37**, 41.

Faulkner, J. A., and Dawson, R. (1966). *Res. Quart.* **37**, 282.

Gavreesky, W. (1963). *J. Sports Med. Phys. Fitness* **3**, 6.

Glasser, E. M. (1950). *Nature* **166**, 1068.

Goff, L. G. (1955). *Proc. 1st. Underwater Physiol. Symp.*, Pub. 377, p. 153. Natl. Acad. Sci.—Natl. Res. Council, Washington, D.C.

Goff, L. G., Brubach, H. F., Specht, H., and Smith, N. (1956a). *J. Appl. Physiol.* **9**, 59.

Goff, L. G., Frassetto, R., and Specht, H. (1956b). *J. Appl. Physiol.* **9**, 219.

Goff, L. G., Brubach, H. F., and Specht, H. (1957). *J. Appl. Physiol.* **10**, 197.

Griffin, G. E. (1966). *Military Med.* **131**, 12.

Harding, P. E., Roman, D., and Whelan, R. F. (1965). *J. Physiol. (London)* **181**, 401.

Herrington, L. P. (1949). *In* "Physiology of Heat Regulation and the Science of Clothing" (L. H. Newburgh, ed.), p. 262. Saunders, Philadelphia, Pennsylvania.

Hong, S. K., Rahn, H., Kang, D. H., Song, S. H., and Kang, B. S. (1963). *J. Appl. Physiol.* **18**, 457.

Horton, B. T., and Gabrielson, M. A. (1940). *Res. Quart.* **11**, 119.

Irving, L. (1939). *Physiol. Rev.* **19**, 112.

Irving, L. (1963). *J. Appl. Physiol.* **18**, 489.

Irving, L., Scholander, P. F., and Grinnell, S. W. (1941). *J. Cellular Comp. Physiol.* **17**, 145.

Kang, B. S., Song, S. H., Suh, C. S., and Hong, S. K. (1963). *J. Appl. Physiol.* **18**, 488.

Karpovich, P. V. (1933). *Res. Quart.* **4**, 21.

Karpovich, P. V. (1939). *Res. Quart.* **10**, 3.

Karpovich, P. V., and LeMaistre, H. (1940). *Res. Quart.* **11**, 40.

Karpovich, P. V., and Millman, N. (1944). *Am. J. Physiol.* **142**, 140.

Karpovich, P. V., and Pestrecov, K. (1939). *Inter. Z. Angew. Physiol.* **10**, 504.

Karpovich, P. V., Adrian, M. J., and Singh, M. (1966). *Federation Proc.* **25**, 334.

Keatinge, W. R. (1961). *Quart. J. Exptl. Physiol.* **46**, 69.

Keatinge, W. R., and Evans, M. (1961). *Quart. J. Exptl. Physiol.* **66**, 83.

Keys, A., and Brožek, J. (1953). *Physiol. Rev.* **33**, 245.

Klocke, F. J., and Rahn, H. (1959). *J. Appl. Physiol.* **14**, 689.

Kory, R. C., Callahan, R., Boren, H. G., and Syner, J. C. (1961). *Am. J. Med.* **30**, 243.

Lambertsen, D. J., and Greenbaum, L. J., eds. (1963). *Proc. 2nd Underwater Physiol. Symp.* Pub. 1181., p. 296. Natl. Acad. Sci.—Natl. Res. Council, Washington, D.C.

Lanphier, E. H. (1954). *Federation Proc.* **13**, 84.

Lanphier, E. H., and Rahn, H. (1963). *J. Appl. Physiol.* **18**, 471.

Magel, J. R., and Faulkner, J. A. (1967). *J. Appl. Physiol.* **22**, 929.

Malhotra, M. S., and Wright, H. C. (1960). *J. Physiol. (London)* **151**, 32.

Margaria, R. (1963). *J. Sports Med. Phys. Fitness* **3**, 145.

Medical Tribune. (1966). Full Fathom 34—Aquanauts Live for 43 Days. pp. 14–16, March 12–13.

Metropolitan Life Insurance Company Statistical Bulletin. (1966). Vol. 47, p. 1.

Miles, S. (1957). *J. Physiol. (London)* **137**, 85.

Miles, S. (1962). "Underwater Medicine." Lippincott, Philadelphia, Pennsylvania.

Molnar, G. W. (1946). *J. Am. Med. Assoc.* **131**, 1046.

Montoye, H. J., Epstein, F. H., and Kjelsberg, M. O. (1965). *Am. J. Clin. Nutr.* **16**, 417.

Mosterd, W. L., and Jongbloed, J. (1964). *Intern. Z. Angew. Physiol.* **20**, 288.

Newman, F., Smalley, B. F., and Thomson, M. L. (1961). *J. Physiol. (London)* **156**, 9P.

Olsen, C. R., Fanestile, D. D., and Scholander, P. F. (1962). *J. Appl. Physiol.* **17**, 938.

Passmore, R., and Durnin, J. V. G. A. (1955). *Physiol. Rev.* **35**, 810.

Pugh, L. G. C., and Edholm, O. G. (1955). *Lancet* **II**, 761.

Pugh, L. G. C., Edholm, O. G., Fox, R. H., Wolff, H. S., Hervey, G. R., Hammond, W. H., Tanner, J. M., and Whitehouse, R. N. (1960). *Clin. Sci.* **19**, 257.

Riley, R. L. (1954). *Ann. Internal Med.* [N.S.] **41**, 172.

Robinson, S. (1961). *In* "Medical Physiology" (P. Bard, ed.), p. 494. Mosby, St. Louis, Missouri.

Rossier, P. H., Buhlmann, A. A., and Wiesinger, K. (1960). "Respiration and Physiologic Principles and their Clinical Applications" (P. C. Luchsinger and K. M. Moser, eds.) Mosby, St. Louis, Missouri.

Rowell, L. B., Taylor, H. L., and Wang, Y. (1964). *J. Appl. Physiol.* **19**, 919.

Schaefer, K. E. (1956). *J. Appl. Physiol.* **8**, 524.

Scholander, P. F. (1962). *Harvey Lectures* **57**, 93.

Scholander, P. F. (1963). *Sci. Am.* **209**, 92.

Scholander, P. F., Hammel, H. T., LeMessurier, H., Hemmingsen, E., and Garey, W. (1962). *J. Appl. Physiol.* **17**, 184.

Song, S. H., Kang, D. H., Kang, B. S., and Hong, S. K. (1963). *J. Appl. Physiol.* **18**, 466.

Spealman, C. R. (1949). *In* "Physiology of Heat Regulation and the Science of Clothing" (L. H. Newburgh, ed.), p. 323. Saunders, Philadelphia, Pennsylvania.

Swegan, D. B., and Thompson, H. L. (1959). *Scholastic Coach* **28**, 22.
Teruoka, G. (1932). *Intern. Z. Angew. Physiol.* **5**, 239.
Tuttle, W. W., and Corleaux, J. F. (1935). *Res. Quart.* **6**, 24.
Tuttle, W. W., and Templin, J. L. (1942). *J. Lab. Clin. Med.* **28**, 271.
U.S. Navy Diving Manual. (1958). U.S. Govt. Printing Office, Washington, D.C.
Van Huss, W. D., and Cureton, T. K. (1955). *Res. Quart.* **26**, 205.
Wells, G. (1932). *Res. Quart.* **3**, 108.
Wolf, S. (1964). *Trans. Am. Climatol. (Clin.) Assoc.* **76**, 192.
Wolf, S., and Groover, M. E. (1965). *Federation Proc.* **24**, 204.

AUTHOR INDEX

Numbers in italics indicate the pages on which the complete references are cited.

447

Moses, C., 391, *392*
Mossfeldt, F., 126, *128, 229, 236*
Mosso, U., 38, *41*
Mosterd, W. L., 423, 424, *445*
Motley, E. P., 316, *319*
Motley, H. L., 252, *265*
Mottram, V. H., 160, *171*
Muido, L., *217*
Müller, 271, *321*
Müller, E. A., 36, *41,* 302, 304, 305, *321*
Müller, F., 248, *265*
Munro, A., 190, *196*
Murawski, B. J., 146, *150*
Musshoff, K., 118, 119, 120, *128*
Myhre, L. G., 260, *264*
Myllyla, G., 143, 144, *150*

N

Nagle, F. J., 204, 209, *217,* 257, 259, *263*
Naimark, A., 146, *150*
Nalbach, H., 214, *216*
Napier, J. A., 287, *321*
Nedbal, J., 132, *150*
Neil, E., 114, *128*
Neilson, C. H., 140, *150*
Nelms, J. D., 192, 193, *195, 196*
Nelson, D. O., 169, *171*
Nelson, R. A., 169, *170*
Nett, T., 399, 401, 410, *414*
Nevai, J., 234, *237*
Newburgh, L. H., 176, 177, *196*
Newman, F., 418, 419, *445*
Newton, J. L., 187, *196,* 257, 259, *264,* 316, *320*
Nielsen, B., 188, *196*
Nielsen, H. E., 257, *264*
Nielsen, M., 61, 70, 74, *77,* 111, *127,* 188, *196,* 213, *216*
Nikkilä, E., 229, *237*
Nilsson, N. J., 94, *128*
Noell, W., 245, 255, *265*
Nordan, H. C., 273, 277, *321*
Northrup, D. W., 141, *151*
Norton, E. F., 242, *265*
Nutt, M. E., 133, *148*
Nylander, I., 415, 417, 418, 419, 424, 425, 430, *443*

O

Obeg, S. A., 315, *320*
Öbrink, K. J., 139, *149*
Oda, T., 254, *265*
Ogston, D., 144, 145, *150*
Ohlson, M., 228, *237*
Oldham, P., 225, *237*
Olesen, K. H., 365, *386*
Olsen, C. R., *445*
Olson, H., 228, 233, *237*
Opitz, E., 245, 246, 248, 250, *264, 265*
Oqaua, S., 260, *263*
Orsini, D., 298, *321*
Osborn, S., 328, *356*
Otis, A. B., 48, *78,* 242, 244, 251, *265*
Ott, I., 185, *196*
Owen, J. R., 260, 261, *265*
Owen, S. G., 72, *77*

P

Pace, N., 379, *386*
Painter, R., 222, *238*
Palmer, M. A., 284, *321*
Parchwitz, E., 143, 144, *151*
Pare, A., 325, *357*
Parin, V. V., 202, *217*
Parish, H. H., Jr., 136, *148*
Parizkova, J., 389, *392*
Parker, H. V., 365, *386*
Parks, J., 222, *237*
Parlin, W., 223, *236*
Pascale, L. R., 389, *392*
Passmore, R., 146, *150,* 287, 298, *321,* 424, *445*
Paul, O., 208, *217*
Pauling, L., 279, *321*
Payne, R. B., *217*
Pearcy, M., 190, *196*
Pearl, D., 177, *194*
Pearl, R., 287, *321*
Pearlman, D., 225, *238*
Peltonen, T., 230, *236*
Percival, L., 169, *171*
Perrault, C., 326, *357*
Persson, B., 230, *237*
Pertuzon, E., 303, *319*
Pestel, C. V., 245, *264*

Subject Index

A

A-band, 9–11
Abdominal injury, 352
Acceleration sprinting, 407
Acclimatization, 342
  altitude, 247–249, 253–254, 258–259, 261, 336–338
  cold, 192–193
  heat, 189, 191, 315, 336–337
Acetylcholine, 14–15, 84
Actin, 12
Actin filaments, 16, 83
Action potential, 13, 16, 21
Actomyosin, 12, 14
Acute exercise, 388
Adenosine-triphosphate, 11–12, 38–40
Adiabatic calorimetry, 269–274
Adrenal cortex, 86, 145–146, 439
Adrenaline, *see* Catecholamines
Aerobic power, 61, 295, 302, 397, 399, 401–407, 410–413, *see also* Physical work capacity
Aerobic work capacity, 59–61, 312, *see also* Physical work capacity
Aging, 232, 391–392
Albumin, 136–137
Albuminuria, 131, 134–136, 339
Alcohol, 211
Aldosterone, 86
All-or-nothing principle, 83
Altitude
  acid-base balance, 251, 262
  athletic competition at, 256, 342
  blood flow at, 245, 250, 252, 255, 263

blood pressures, 246–247, 255
blood properties, 252–255, 263
cardiovascular dynamics at, 245–247, 252, 263
characteristics of life at, 240–242
gas tensions at, 242–245, 257
heart rate, 246
hypoxia of, 241–245, 247–250, 252–253, 255, 263
lung diffusion, 251–252, 263
and man, 240–242
muscular strength at, 257
oxygen
  consumption at, 248–249
  requirements, 247, 256
  transport at, 243–244, 253, 263
physical work capacity at, 255–259
pulmonary ventilation at, 249–252, 262
respiratory physiology at, 242–243
stroke volume, 246
tolerance, 251
training for, 260–263
working capacity, effect on, 60
Alveolar-arterial O_2 gradient, 70–71, 249, 252
Alveolar ventilation, 61
American College of Sports Medicine, 328
American Medical Association, 338
Amphetamines, 202–203, 206–209
Anaerobic work, 62–63, 397, 399, 405–407, 410–413
  capacity, 256, 300
Analytical dairy, 287
Androgens, 148

463

H

H^+ ion concentration, 71–72
Haldane gas analyzer, 280
Handball, 312
Harvard step test, 331–332
Head injury, 352
Heart, 82–89, 105–106, 117–121
  hormone effects, 84
  membrane potential, 83
  nervous mechanisms, 83–84, 106
  parasympathetic nerve, 84
  sympathetic nerve, 84
Heart patients, 308
Heart rate, 61, 85, 92, 94–97, 109, 122–125, 290, 295, 302–304, 312, 315, 331–332, 334, 401–403, 408–409, 417–419, 429–430, 439, 442
  age effects, 96–97
  physical conditioning effects, 97, 115, 292
  telemetered, 286, 290
  various activities, during, 112–113
Heart size, 118–121, 123, 400, 417
Heat balance equation, 175
Heat exchange, 175–185, 268, 314, 430–435
Heat exhaustion, 342
Heat stress, 174–193
Heat stroke, 342, 352–353
Hematocrit, 90, 252, 254
Hematuria, 135–136
Hemoconcentration, 253–255
Hemoglobin, 123, 253, 263, 418, 438
Hemoglobin concentration
  maximum aerobic power, effect on, 57–59, 61
Hemoglobinuria, 137–138
Hernia, 339
Hollow sprints, 407–408
Homeostasis, 397
  heat and cold exposure, 175–187
Homeotherm, 173–175
Horsepower, 299
Hydronephrosis, 136
Hydrostatic forces, 100
Hydrotherapy, 355
Hyman Cardiopulmonary Index, 332
Hypertension, 225–226
Hyperthermia, 177, 181
Hyper ventilation, 61, 262, 440–441
Hypoglycemic reaction, 340
Hypothermia, 177, 181

I

I-band, 9–11
Infectious disease, 351
Insulin, 229, 340
Interval sprinting, 407
Interval training, 401–402, 407–409
Intestines, 140–141
Intraintestinal pressures, 140–141
Isometric contraction, 16–19, 21–22, 27–28, 30–38, 40, 107–110, 299, 354
Isotonic contraction, 16–19, 22, 30–31, 34–38, 40, 354

J

Job classification, 290, 303
Joint injury, 353

K

Kidney function, 130–139
  exercise effects, 131–139
Kidney physiology, 131–134
Kilocalorie cost of work, 297, 302
Knee injury, 350
Kofranyi–Michaelis respirometer, 271, 275, 286

L

Lactic acid, 40, 56, 57, 61, 63–64, 397
Lean body mass, 332, 361, 364, 369, 371, 378, 380–384, 389–390, 416–417
Legal liability and sports injury, 335
Lipid metabolism disorders, 228–229
Longevity, 233–234
Lung capacities, 46–47
Lung diffusion, 61, 68–71
Lung ventilation, 43–47, 50, 55–56, 59–60, 67–70, 72, 291, 295, 419, 421, 428